For Cameron
and my four babies

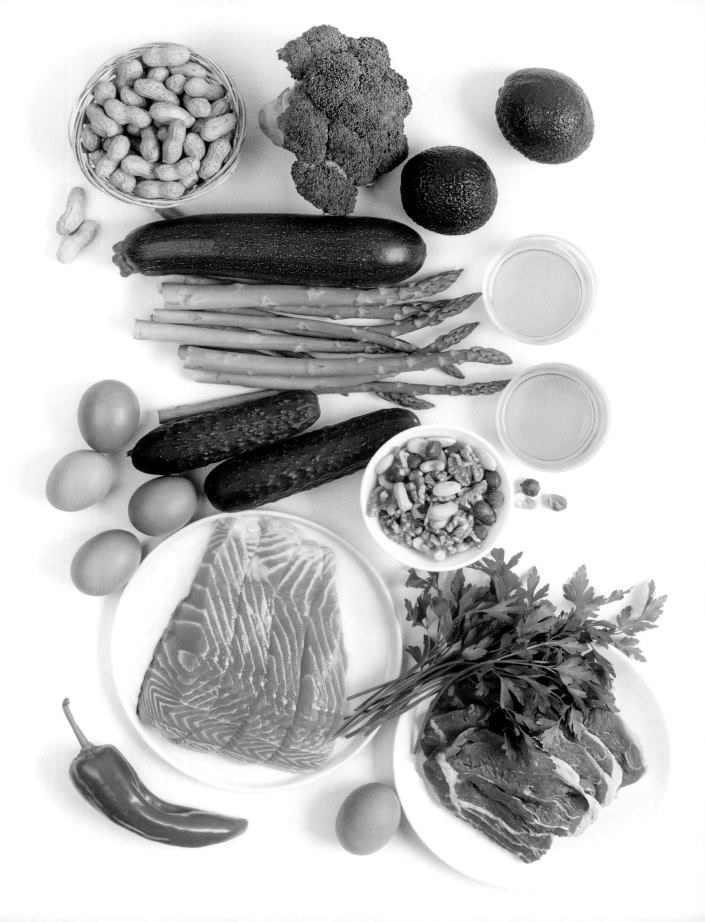

CONTENTS

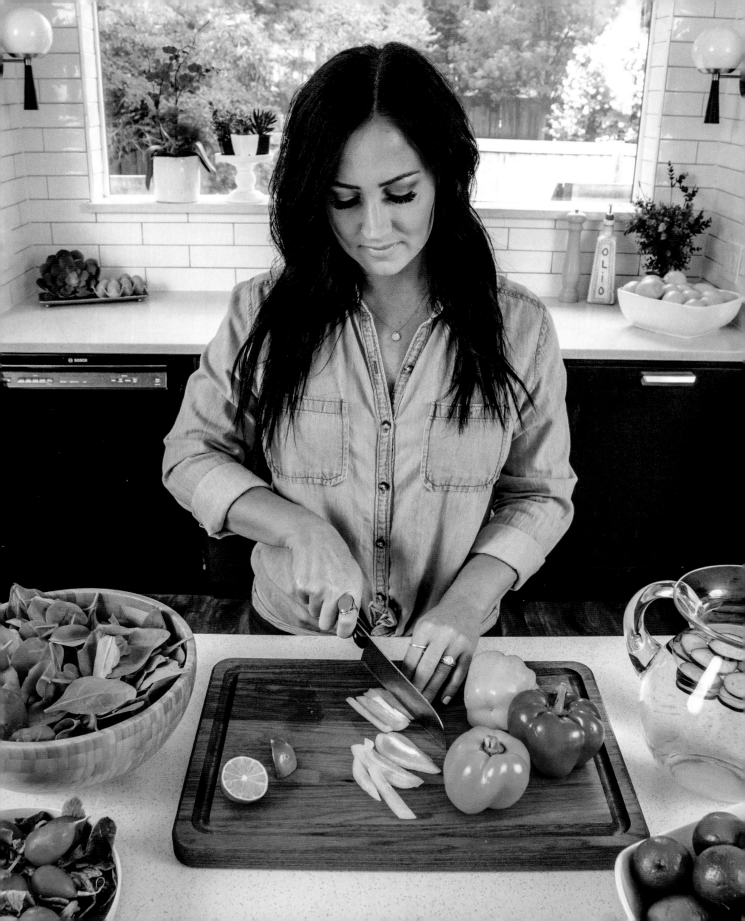

PREFACE

Oh hey! I'm Julie. I am a busy mom of four, the creator of the popular keto Instagram @ketomadesimple, and a total foodie at heart. I've struggled with my weight my entire life. I know how it feels to be chubby, to be uncomfortable in my own skin, and to simply feel like crap. Do you feel that way, too? If so, you're not alone. I'm here to show you how you can have your own keto success story while enjoying foods that'll heal you from the inside out.

So, what the heck is keto? How do I start? Do I have to like cauliflower now? These were just a few of the hundreds of questions that I asked before I started my keto journey. I was overloaded with information, and it all became so overwhelming. I created my @ketomadesimple Instagram because I wanted to show people that keto doesn't have to be complicated. You don't need any fancy or bizarre ingredients. You don't need pricey supplements or equipment. You just need good food options and a strong desire for change.

My hope for this book is to teach you a thing or two about keto, but more importantly to show you the best way to make it a sustainable way of living for you. Keto is not one-size-fits-all. Everybody is different, and everyone requires a unique approach. I'll take you through the ins and outs and then let you decide how to keto your way!

MY STORY

I am not one of those people who always envisioned myself writing a cookbook. In fact, I learned to cook by watching the Food Network! When my oldest child (who is now sixteen) was a baby, I had him on a very strict eating regimen. One of those daily feedings was at 4:00 p.m., which meant that we sat and watched Rachael Ray explain how to properly cut onions, mince garlic, and cook from the soul. This was my culinary school. My point in sharing this with you is not to rat myself out for the lack of training, but simply to tell you that if I can make these recipes, anyone can.

I've struggled with my weight for years. Between 2014 and 2016, my problems escalated. I was a single mom with three small children, working a job that I hated but needed, and battling hormonal issues that I didn't even know existed. It was almost as if I woke up one day and realized that I had packed on a bunch of weight without noticing. It was a gradual weight gain that had crept up on me, and I weighed the most I've ever weighed. In the midst of all this, I began feeling very anxious and depressed, two emotions I was not used to feeling. I was put on antidepressants and anti-anxiety meds, but I knew deep down that there was a much larger issue.

Long story short, I was diagnosed with polycystic ovary syndrome, or PCOS. If you're not familiar with this condition, it's basically a giant hormonal nightmare. To name just a few of the symptoms, PCOS causes acne, depression, and—yep, you guessed it—weight gain. I was relieved to have found out what was going on with my body, but I had no idea how to combat it. I did what any normal human being would do: I Googled it. And when I learned about what leads to PCOS, all things pointed to keto as the solution.

I began doing all the research I possibly could about the ketogenic diet, and within a few days, I jumped right in. I'll be honest with you, I didn't really know what I was doing, and I certainly didn't understand why I was doing it. All I knew was that I was loving eating all the foods that I had been taught to avoid my whole life, like bacon, rib-eye steak, and heavy cream. My keto journey began in February 2017, and I don't see it ending anytime soon. I have lost over 60 pounds, but more importantly, I have gained my life back. Food no longer controls me. I am in control. I tell my body what we are doing! I have fallen completely in love with this way of eating and with myself again. There's no better feeling in the entire world.

Although I do not have any formal culinary training, I *do* have the determination to make keto a sustainable way of living. In other words, I wanna love what I'm eating, so I'd better freaking figure out a way to make that happen! I have spent countless hours in the kitchen working to create keto recipes that you will love, and that will nourish your mind, body, and soul. Most of these dishes should be familiar to you; the only real difference is a slight shift in ingredients. Trust me, your body will thank you. The beautiful thing about keto is that you can keto-fy just about anything by making a couple of simple adjustments.

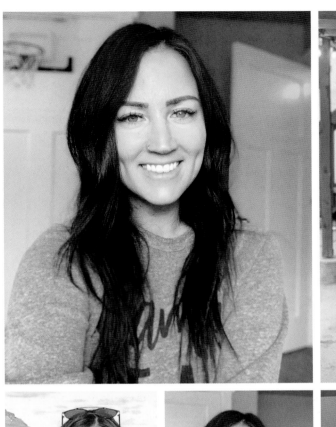
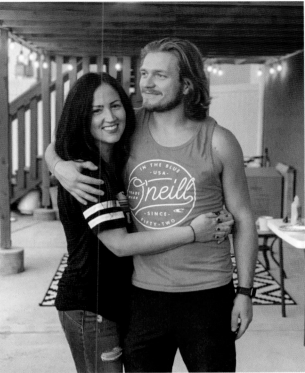
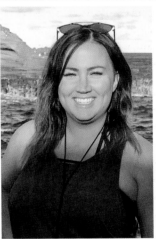
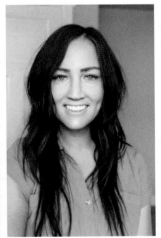
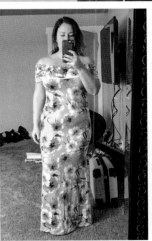
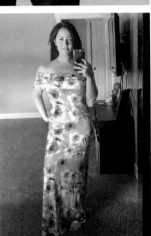

I hope you use this book as a lifeline throughout your journey. Whether you are doing keto for weight loss, to reduce inflammation, or to combat diabetes, autoimmune disease, or some other health issue, my goal is to provide you with the tools you need to be successful.

XOXO,

Julie *Julie Smith*

WHAT IS KETO?

The ketogenic diet is a high-fat, moderate-protein, low-carbohydrate diet that forces the body to burn fats rather than carbohydrates. After you eat a meal high in carbohydrates, your body produces insulin to deal with that glucose. Glucose is what your body will choose as its main energy source. When glucose is present, your body will resist burning fat. By removing carbohydrates and replacing them with fats, you force your body to burn fat for fuel. This is called ketosis. Once your body fully makes the switch to using fats for fuel rather than glucose, you are what's known as "fat adapted." Congrats! In ketosis, you are a fat-burning machine!

Not all fats are created equal. Keto is fat-focused, so you want to make sure that you are fueling your body with high-quality healthy fats. Healthy fats include saturated fats, monounsaturated fats, polyunsaturated fats, and naturally occurring trans fats. Stick with unprocessed oils like coconut oil, extra-virgin olive oil, and avocado oil, which are great sources of saturated and unsaturated fats. You want to avoid processed vegetable oils like soybean oil and canola oil, as they have negative effects on metabolism, inflammation and stress levels, and weight regulation. Low-fat dairy products should also be avoided. In other words, focus on fats that naturally occur in meats and dairy; cook with coconut oil, olive oil, and avocado oil; and eat those avocados!

DIFFERENT KETO STYLES

Keto is not one-size-fits-all. You need to figure out the best way to approach a ketogenic diet to fit your needs, goals, and lifestyle. These are some common terms that may help guide you on how you'd like to keto. There is no right or wrong way!

- **Standard Ketogenic Diet (SKD)**—The standard keto diet is the most common: low-carb, moderate-protein, high-fat. A typical rule is that your calories should consist of 70 percent fats, 25 percent proteins, and 5 percent carbs. Most people like to stay under 25 grams of net carbs a day, although some can go up to 50 grams and still stay in ketosis. The percentages vary from person to person. Your main source of carbs will be vegetables.
- **Lazy Keto**—Don't let the name "lazy keto" fool you; it isn't a negative thing at all. What it really means is that you eat freely, without tracking your macros. Most lazy keto-ers are mentally aware of what and how much they are eating and typically aim for no more than 20 grams of net carbs a day. I really love the lazy keto way because it's allowed me to be in tune with what my body needs. I don't aim to hit certain macros each day; I eat when I'm hungry, and I don't eat when I'm not. This has made it *very* sustainable for me and has significantly improved my relationship with food.

- **Dirty Keto**—The term "dirty keto" simply means that you're not picky about ingredient quality. You are constantly in a state of ketosis, but any food that'll get you into ketosis is fair game—fake sugars, processed meats and cheeses, diet sodas, etc. Plenty of people eat this way and see huge amounts of weight loss success. This is a great way to approach keto short term for weight loss. It is also great for people who have busy schedules and have no choice but to eat out frequently. Not to mention, you'll get the biggest bang for your buck because you're not concerned with organic, grass-fed everything. If you're doing keto for gut health, inflammation, or autoimmune diseases, I highly recommend *not* using this approach; in those cases, high-quality ingredients should be your focus.

- **Cyclical Keto**—The term "cyclical keto" refers to allowing yourself to go in and out of ketosis during the week. The standard format for this is five to six days of strict keto and one to two days of higher-carb eating. This approach is typically used by athletes who do high-intensity workouts multiple times a week. The goal is to switch from ketosis to refill muscle glycogen. This is also known as carb loading.

- **Targeted Ketogenic Diet (TKD)**—With the targeted keto approach, you follow the standard keto diet but add in carbs near your workouts. This approach is great for people who need extra carbs to provide fuel during a workout but don't want to do long-term carb loading, like cyclical keto.

- **High-Protein Keto**—The name is pretty self-explanatory. This approach is a spin-off of the standard keto diet, but with a slight shift in percentages. While carbs should still make up 5 percent of your calories and fats and proteins make up the rest, you place more emphasis on protein than fat. This approach is excellent for people with low iron or protein deficiencies or those looking to protect muscle mass. The downside is that so many people argue that too much protein will kick you out of ketosis. I happen to disagree, but hey, that's just me.

- **Carnivore Keto**—This way of eating is becoming very popular in the keto community. The diet consists of meats and animal fats, including dairy, and nothing else. Although it's a controversial way of eating, studies have shown that people who follow a carnivore diet have quicker weight loss, more mental clarity, and a healthier digestive system. It is also great for athletic performance. This way of eating takes out a lot of the complicated thought processes. Just eat meats and dairy—it's that simple.

If anyone cares to know, I'm a mix between lazy keto, dirty keto, and high-protein keto.

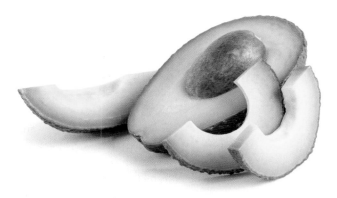

KETO LINGO

When I first became a part of the keto social media community, I saw a *lot* of unfamiliar abbreviations. Not gonna lie, I Googled most of these things the first time I encountered them. I hope this list saves you that step!

ACV—apple cider vinegar

BF—body fat

BG—blood glucose

BPC—bulletproof coffee (fatty coffee with butter and coconut oil; see page 34 for my recipe!)

CW—current weight

GW—goal weight

HWC—heavy whipping cream

IF—intermittent fasting

IIFYM—if it fits your macros

IR—insulin resistance

LCHF—low carb, high fat

NSV—non-scale victory

OMAD—one meal a day (this is an approach where you only eat one meal in your entire day)

SAD—standard American diet

SF—sugar-free

SKD—standard ketogenic diet

SW—starting weight

WOE—way of eating

KETO-FRIENDLY FOODS

I'm not here to tell you what you can and can't eat. That's not what this book is about. I want to show you what your options are so that you can decide for yourself how to make better choices.

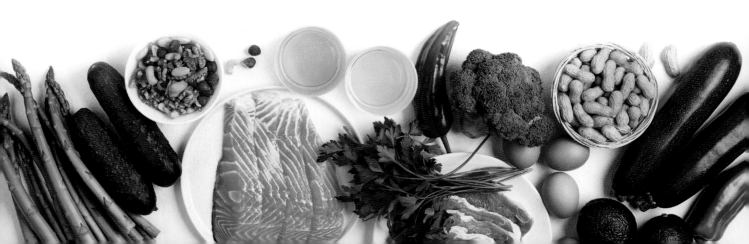

Vegetables

I have never eaten more vegetables in my life than I have on the ketogenic diet! Veggies truly are the healthy centerpiece of keto. This is where the majority of your daily carbs should come from. Some avid macro trackers don't even track their carbs from veggies because eating vegetables is an essential part of healing our bodies. Whether or not you want to track the carbs in veggies is up to you and your approach.

- Artichoke hearts
- Arugula
- Asparagus
- Bell peppers
- Bok choy
- Broccoli
- Brussels sprouts
- Cabbage
- Cauliflower
- Celery
- Chard
- Collard greens
- Cucumbers
- Eggplant
- Endive
- Fennel
- Garlic
- Green beans
- Jalapeño peppers
- Kale
- Kimchi
- Leafy greens
- Leeks
- Lettuce
- Mushrooms
- Okra
- Onions
- Pepperoncini
- Pickles
- Radicchio
- Radishes
- Romaine lettuce
- Sauerkraut
- Spinach
- Swiss chard
- Tomatoes
- Zucchini

Tip:

Fermented foods like kimchi and sauerkraut are some of the most powerful foods out there for improving gut health. They are loaded with cultures of beneficial bacteria that aid digestion, reduce inflammation, and strengthen your immune system.

Avoid:

- Corn
- Root vegetables such as beets, carrots, parsnips, and potatoes
- Sugar snap peas

Tip:

I do eat beets and carrots in small amounts because I've found that it works for me. Remember, keto isn't a set of hard-and-fast rules that apply to everyone; it's about experimenting to find what works best for you!

Fruits

With the exception of avocados, coconut, and olives, which I've listed under "Oils and Fats," fruits should be eaten in moderation, since they are naturally high in carbs. I like to refer to fruit as nature's candy. Opt for these fruits, which are lower in sugar than other types:

- Blackberries
- Blueberries
- Cranberries
- Lemons
- Limes
- Raspberries
- Rhubarb
- Strawberries

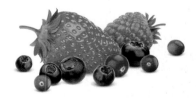

Proteins
Meat and Eggs

Whenever possible, choose organic, grass-fed/pasture-raised meats. If you can't, that's okay. You'll still be able to achieve ketosis with everything on this list. Opt for fatty cuts like rib-eye steak, pork shoulder, chicken thighs, and drumsticks with skin.

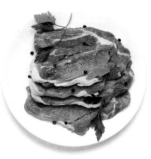

- Bacon (I recommend uncured center-cut)
- Beef
- Bison
- Bologna
- Chicken
- Cured meats
- Duck
- Eggs
- Ham
- Jerky
- Lamb
- Pork
- Pork rinds
- Rabbit
- Turkey
- Veal
- Venison

Fish and Seafood

Fish and seafood are a phenomenal way to get more potassium and vitamin B into your diet, along with keeping carbs low but nutrients high. Choose wild-caught fatty varieties whenever you can.

- Clams
- Cod
- Grouper
- Halibut
- Lobster
- Mackerel
- Muscles
- Oysters
- Salmon
- Sardines
- Scallops
- Shrimp
- Trout
- Tuna

Proteins to Avoid

- Beans and legumes
- Meat covered or mixed with breadcrumbs (but check out my keto breadcrumbs made from pork rinds on page 304!)
- Soy products such as tempeh and tofu

Dairy

While dairy is acceptable on keto, it's not always the best option for your body. In fact, it can be problematic for some people. Keep this in mind as you navigate your way through your journey. I always say that if you're looking for a way to trim down quickly, dairy should be the first thing to go. (See page 26 for more on handling stalls.) Use the full-fat versions of all dairy products.

- Butter
- Cheeses (hard, soft, and blue)
- Cottage cheese
- Cream cheese
- Half-and-half
- Heavy whipping cream
- Plain Greek yogurt
- Sour cream

Avoid:
- Cow's milk
- Low-fat/fat-free dairy products
- Yogurt sweetened with sugar

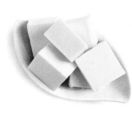

Oils and Fats

Healthy monounsaturated and saturated fats are an essential part of a ketogenic diet. They are what will fuel your body, keep you feeling fuller longer, and provide you with lots and lots of energy!

- Avocado oil
- Avocados
- Butter (preferably grass-fed)
- Cocoa butter
- Coconut
- Coconut butter
- Coconut oil
- Duck/Goose fat
- Ghee
- Lard
- Macadamia nut oil
- MCT oil
- Nut butters
- Nut oils
- Olive oil
- Olives
- Tallow

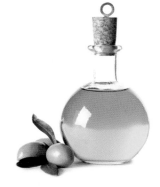

Avoid:

- Canola oil
- Corn oil
- Polyunsaturated fats marketed as "heart healthy," like margarine
- Safflower oil
- Sunflower oil
- Trans fats (except the ones naturally occurring in meat)
- Vegetable oil

Nuts and Seeds

It is so incredibly easy to overeat nuts and seeds (at least it is for me). Be mindful when eating them because the carbs can add up quickly!

- Almonds
- Brazil nuts
- Cashews*
- Chia seeds
- Flaxseeds
- Hazelnuts
- Hemp seeds
- Macadamia nuts
- Pecans
- Pine nuts
- Pistachios*
- Poppy seeds
- Sesame seeds
- Sunflower seeds
- Unsweetened coconut flakes
- Walnuts

Eat these nuts in moderation, as they are higher in carbs than most.

Flours and Other Baking Ingredients

- Almond flour
- Coconut flour
- Dark chocolate without soy lecithin
- Guar gum
- Oat fiber
- Psyllium husk powder
- Unsweetened cocoa powder
- Xanthan gum

Avoid:

- All grains, even "whole grains," barley, millet, quinoa, rice, wheat flour/wheat gluten

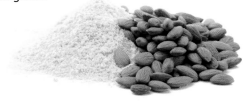

Condiments, Sauces, and Flavorings

- Balsamic vinegar
- BBQ sauce (sugar-free; I like AlternaSweets brand)
- Blue cheese dressing (see page 274 for my recipe)
- Bone broth, chicken and beef
- Caesar dressing
- Coconut aminos or gluten-free soy sauce (tamari)
- Dijon mustard
- Hot sauce (I like Frank's RedHot)
- Italian dressing (sugar-free)
- Ketchup (sugar-free; I like AlternaSweets brand)
- Maple syrup (I like ChocZero brand)
- Mayonnaise (made with avocado oil rather than unhealthy seed oils)
- Prepared yellow mustard
- Ranch dressing (look for the one with the least carbs, or make it yourself using the Ranch Seasoning Mix on page 310)
- Soy sauce (tamari is a gluten-free version)
- Spicy brown mustard
- Sriracha sauce
- Toasted sesame oil
- Vanilla extract
- Worcestershire sauce

Dried Herbs and Spices

- Garlic powder
- Garlic salt
- Ground cinnamon
- Ground cumin
- Ground nutmeg
- Italian seasoning
- Onion powder
- Paprika (regular and smoked)
- Parsley
- Red pepper flakes
- Turmeric powder

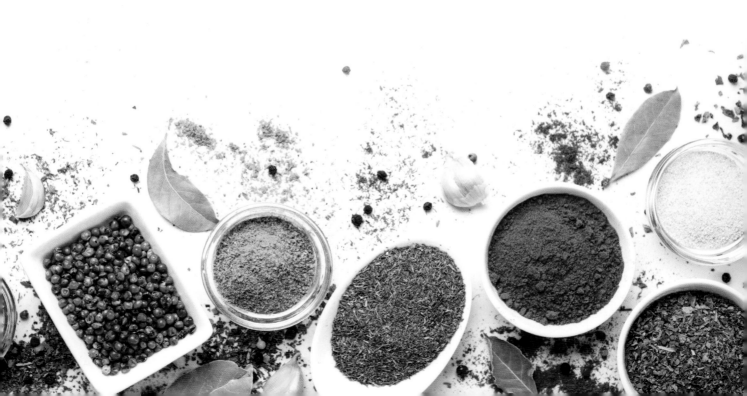

Sweeteners

My sweetener of choice is monk fruit. Monk fruit replaces sugar at a 1:1 ratio, so it's super easy to convert recipes that call for sugar into keto-friendly versions: if a recipe calls for ½ cup of sugar, simply use ½ cup of monk fruit sweetener instead. Be mindful when you are trying out a new keto sweetener and pay attention to how or if it affects your body. If one type doesn't agree with you, or you don't like the taste, another sweetener might be a better choice.

- **Erythritol** is a sugar alcohol that provides the least calories and net carbs. Erythritol doesn't affect blood sugar or insulin levels. Erythritol is very popular for baking. The downside is that it can leave a "cooling" effect in your mouth. Obviously, everyone has different taste buds, but this is the biggest complaint I've heard. Erythritol comes in granulated and confectioners'-style forms.

- **Monk fruit sweetener** comes from a small, round fruit grown in Asia. It is extracted by removing the seeds and skin, crushing the fruit, and collecting the juice. Sweeteners made with monk fruit don't impact blood sugar levels. Monk fruit has zero calories and has no evidence showing negative side effects. It comes in liquid, granulated, and powdered form.

- **Stevia** is a sugar substitute extracted from the leaves of the stevia plant. Stevia comes in liquid and granulated form. It is highly concentrated and is around 300 times sweeter than regular sugar. Stevia can help improve blood pressure, optimize blood sugar regulation, and decrease inflammation. It contains zero carbs, zero calories, and zero sugars. The downside is that because it is extremely concentrated, it can have be super potent and have a bitter aftertaste.

Brands I like:

- **Lakanto** is a monk fruit–based sweetener that measures 1:1 with sugar, so it makes it easy to convert recipes that call for sugar. This is my sweetener of choice!

- **Pyure** is a stevia/erythritol blend.
- **Swerve** is erythritol blended with other natural sweeteners. It also measures 1:1 to sugar, making converting recipes that call for sugar super easy.

Avoid:

- Artificial sweeteners (Equal, aspartame, acesulfame potassium, sucralose, saccharin, Sweet & Low, Splenda)

- Sugar (table sugar, high-fructose corn syrup, agave syrup, honey, maple syrup, fructose)

> Tip:
>
> *In this book, my main sweetener of choice is Lakanto Classic, which is a granulated-style sweetener. Feel free to use whichever keto-approved sweetener you like.*

Drinks

- Bone broth
- Coconut water
- Coffee
- Seltzer water
- Tea, especially green tea
- Unsweetened nut milks
- Water with lemon/lime juice

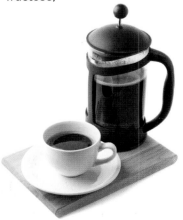

EAT THIS, NOT THAT

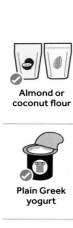 Almond or coconut flour — Regular flour

 Crushed pork rinds or almonds — Breadcrumbs

 Unsweetened almond or coconut milk — Milk

 Riced cauliflower or broccoli — Rice

Plain Greek yogurt — Flavored yogurt

Crispy Parmesan chips — Croutons

Unsweetened almond or coconut milk — Half-and-half

Dried spices — High-carb veggies

Low-carb tortillas or lettuce wraps — Tortillas

Zucchini fries — Fries

Fathead dough, chicken crust — Pizza crust

Spirits, low-carb beer, dry wine — High-carb alcohol

Shirataki noodles, zucchini noodles, spaghetti squash — Pasta

Bulletproof coffee — Latte

Cheese buns — Hamburger buns

Chia seed oatmeal with almond milk — Oatmeal

Mashed cauliflower — Mashed potatoes

Stevia, erythritol — Sugar

Rao's low-carb marinara sauce — Pasta sauce

Cream cheese & egg waffles — Waffles

Cauliflower hashbrowns — Hashbrowns

Low-carb, sugar-free ice cream — Ice cream

Chicken broth with spices — Soups

Almond flour pancakes — Pancakes

Pork rinds, parsnip chips — Potato chips

KETO-FRIENDLY SNACKS

If you're just starting out on keto, chances are you're looking for snack ideas. You're in the right place. I'm not a snacker anymore, and I'm willing to put money on it that you won't be, either, once you become fat-adapted; you'll stay fuller longer, and your meals should satisfy your hunger. But until you no longer feel the need to snack, these items should help hold you over! Most of these snacks are grab-and-go, with very little prep required.

Almonds	Bacon	Beef jerky	Bell peppers with ranch dressing	Blackberries	Blueberries
Celery with peanut butter	Cheese Crackers (page 82)	Fat bombs	Hard-boiled eggs	Macadamia nuts	Meatballs
Olives	Pecans	Pepperoni	Pickle, cheese, and lunch meat roll-ups	Pickles	Pork rinds
Raspberries	Sausage links	Strawberries	String cheese	Sunflower seeds	Walnuts

ALCOHOL ON KETO

I'm probably stating the obvious here when I say that alcohol is not the best thing for you. The more alcohol you drink, the more the weight loss will slow down, because your body will burn the alcohol before burning anything else. However, I understand the concept of real life, and let's be honest, people like to drink.

I personally do not drink alcohol. This is obviously a choice made by me, for me. However, if you enjoy a drink here and there, just be smart about it. Know what you're drinking, how much you're consuming, and what you are mixing it with. Here's a handy cheat sheet showing the best options.

ALCOHOL CHEAT SHEET	CARBS	CAL	ABV
VODKA			
Burnett's	0	96	40%
Smirnoff	0	97	40%
Absolut	0	100	40%
Svedka	0	103	40%
Grey Goose	0	103	40%
Stolichnaya	0	103	50%
Ciroc	0	103	40%
Skyy	0	105	40%
WHISKEY			
Crown Royal	0	96	40%
Jack Daniels	0	98	40%
Jim Beam	0	104	40%
Seagram's	0	104	40%
Dewar's	0	104	40%
Wild Turkey	0	104	50%
Chivas Regal	0	105	40%
Johnnie Walker	0	105	40%
TEQUILA			
Don Julio	0	96	40%
Tres Agaves	0	102	40%
El Jimador	0	102	40%
Patron	0	103	40%
1800 Tequila	0	103	40%
Milagro	0	103	50%
Cazadores	0	103	40%
Sauza	0	104	40%
RUM			
Malibu Island Spiced	0	72	30%
Captain Morgan Spiced	0.4g	86	35%
Bacardi Superior	0	96	40%
Myer's Original Dark	0	97	40%
Castillo	0	97	40%
Sailor Jerry	0	103	40%
The Kraken	0	105	40%
GIN			
Gordon's	0	96	40%
Seagram's	0	103	40%
Bombay	0	114	47%
Beefeater	0	115	47%
Tanqueray	0	116	47.3%
BRANDY			
Honey Bee	0	103	40%
Courvoisier	0	104	40%
McDowell's	0.1g	104	40%
Martell	0.4g	126	40%
Hennessy	1g	103	40%
Remy Martin	3g	103	40%

ALCOHOL CHEAT SHEET	CARBS	CAL	ABV
RED WINES			
Pinot Noir	3.4g	121	10.4%
Merlot	3.7g	122	10.6%
Cabernet	3.8g	122	10.3%
Syrah	3.8g	122	10.5%
Zinfandel	4.2g	129	11.1%
SKINNYGIRL WINES			
SkinnyGirl Prosecco	2g	100	12%
SkinnyGirl Pinot Grigio	4g	100	12%
SkinnyGirl Moscato	5g	100	12%
SkinnyGirl Chardonnay	5g	100	12%
SkinnyGirl Rose	5g	100	12%
SkinnyGirl Cabernet Sauvignon	5g	100	12%
WHITE WINES			
Sparkling White Wine	1.5g	96	12%
Brut Cava	2.5g	128	12%
Brut Champagne	2.8g	147	12%
Pinot Blanc	2.9g	119	12.5%
Pinot Grigio	3g	122	10.7%
Chardonnay	3.1g	123	13%
Albarino	3.5g	143	13%
Riesling	5.5g	128	9.5%
BEER			
Green Trailblazer	0.5g	119	4.7%
Budweiser Select 55	1.9g	55	2.4%
Miller 64	2.4g	64	2.8%
Rolling Rock Green Light	2.4g	83	3.7%
Michelob Ultra	2.6g	95	4.2%
Budweiser Select	3.1g	99	4.3%
Beck's Premier Light	3.2g	64	2.3%
Miller Lite	3.2g	96	4.2%
HARD SELTZER			
Truly Spiked	2g	100	5%
White Claw	4g	110	5%
Spiked Seltzer	5g	140	6%
Nauti Seltzer	5g	110	5%
ALCOHOL & MIXERS TO AVOID			
Peach Schnapps	9.8g	108	15%
Margarita Mix	10g	41	–
Curacao	10.5g	108	31%
Baileys Irish Cream	11.3g	147	17%

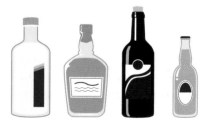

DINING OUT ON KETO

One of my favorite things to do is eat out at a restaurant that I've never tried before. All you foodies know exactly what I'm talking about! However, dining out can be a little tricky when you have food restrictions. My biggest piece of advice here is to plan ahead. Look up the menu beforehand and then go in with a game plan. I find it super easy to find keto-friendly options almost anywhere. Here are some tips for navigating restaurant menus:

- Bunless burgers are always a win. Avoid ketchup and BBQ sauce, though—those are filled with sugar. Stick with mayo and mustard.

- Meat dishes typically come with a side of fries or something similar. Swap that out for a side salad or some grilled veggies. You may end up paying a little extra, but that's your life now. Accept it.

- Use your best judgment when it comes to dressings and sauces. Vinaigrettes usually have sugar in them, so it's best to opt for oil and vinegar. Ranch and blue cheese are usually great choices, too. *Always* ask for dressings and sauces on the side so you can do a teeny taste test first.

- If the meal comes with complimentary rolls, bread, or chips and salsa, simply ask your server to not bring it to you. It's not weird, I promise. Plus, it cuts down on the restaurant's food costs and prevents food waste. This may not affect you, but the restaurant will appreciate you for it.

- Do not order anything that is described with words like "sweet," "glazed," "honey," "teriyaki," "maple," "candied," and "BBQ." Those dishes are loaded with sugars.

- Don't be afraid to ask the kitchen to modify your order. I like to tell my server that I'm gonna be a pain in the ass with my order. I find that when I admit that, servers are less likely to be annoyed with me. They usually giggle, too, which lightens the mood. Servers deal with food allergies all the time. Treat your keto diet the same way.

- When in doubt, look for simple, whole foods. The more complicated the dish, the more questionable the ingredients. Salads are always a fantastic option, as are simple meats and veggies.

MACROS

What are macros? This question stumped me for weeks when I first started keto. What the heck is a macro? I'll explain to you in the simplest way I know how. *Macro* is short for *macronutrient*. All foods and drinks consist of three macronutrients: fats, proteins, and carbohydrates. When figuring out your personal macros, you're essentially trying to calculate the percentages of protein, fat, and carbs that you should be eating.

How do you find your personal macros?

I recommend finding a macro calculator online (my favorite is on my website, www.
ketomadesimple.life). As mentioned earlier, the macros for a keto diet typically look like
this: fats make up 70 percent of your calories, proteins take up 25 percent of your calories,
and the remaining 5 percent of your calories come from carbohydrates.

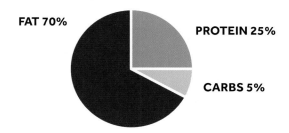

FAT 70% PROTEIN 25% CARBS 5%

Now, your personal macros may differ depending on your goals, weight, activity level, and
so on. So just make sure that you find *your* macros. Don't forget to recalculate them every
once in a while. If you are losing weight at a very fast pace, I recommend recalculating your
macros once a month. If you're a slow loser like I am, adjust your macros every couple of
months, or after every 10-pound weight loss.

Macro tracking versus intuitive eating

I cannot emphasize this enough: you have to find what works for you and your lifestyle.
If you are just starting out on keto, tracking your macros is probably a good idea, at
least until you are at a point where you are aware of what you're eating. By tracking your
macros, you are able to learn which foods are keto-friendly and how to manage your
portion sizes.

My personal approach is intuitive eating. This is the number-one question I'm asked
on Instagram: "How do you do keto without tracking?" My answer is simple: I eat when
I'm hungry and don't eat when I'm not. I make sure that when I do eat, my meals are full
of healthy fats, proteins, and non-starchy veggies. I do keep a mental note of my carbs
and always stay under 20 grams of net carbs a day. I do this thing where I give myself a
countdown. For example, if I eat breakfast with 6 grams of net carbs, I know that I have
14 grams left for the day. And the countdown begins. This is my way of tracking, and it
works for me. There may be days when I go over on my protein limit. And you know what?
That's okay! There are definitely days when I don't even come close to my daily calorie goal
because I'm just not that hungry. That's also okay! Some days, I am hungrier than others,
and it's incredibly freeing to know that I am able to recognize those hunger signs rather
than having a chart tell me I need to eat more. I never want to be a slave to tracking for
the rest of my life. Keto is how I eat now and probably what I'll do forever. I am very happy
to be at a point where I can recognize the foods that I need and what my body is lacking.
This takes practice, but if you're up for it, I find it to be the most freeing and healthy
relationship with food possible.

TESTING FOR KETONES

When first starting out on a ketogenic diet, you'll probably be dying to know if you're in ketosis. I get it! I've been there. There are a few ways of testing for ketones that are fairly inexpensive.

 Blood testing—Blood testing is the most accurate way to test your ketone levels. With most meters, you prick your finger and the meter gives you a digital reading of your current level. This method measures BHB (the predominant ketone) in the bloodstream. Most blood ketone readers also have the ability to measure blood glucose levels; the only difference is that you use a different type of test strip. The downside of a blood ketone meter is getting used to pricking your finger.

 Urine testing—Urine testing is the least expensive way to test your ketone levels. You simply pee on a strip, and it tells you your current ketone level by color; the darker in color the strip, the more ketones are present in your urine. However, this method is not as accurate as blood testing. All the liquids you drink can dilute your urine. As time goes on, you will no longer be peeing out ketones because your body will be using them as fuel. However, urine test strips are great if you are just starting out and are dying to know whether you're in ketosis.

Breath testing—Breath ketone meters measure the amount of acetone excreted in your breath. They are not as accurate as blood meters but supposedly are more reliable than urine test strips.

The good old-fashioned way—I think the best (and cheapest!) way to know whether you're in ketosis is to recognize your body's natural symptoms. Here are a few ways to detect that you're on the right track:

- **Bad breath**—This is probably the most common side effect. If you are in ketosis, your breath will be funky, at least in the beginning. You will produce a fruity smell in your breath and in your urine (acetone). Sounds fun, I know. But I promise, the outcome is worth the temporary funk!

- **Cloudy pee**—Yes, I know this is gross, but it is such a good indicator of ketone levels. If you're noticing that you have stinky/cloudy pee, congratulations! You're likely in ketosis. This, too, is likely to be a temporary side effect.

- **Reduced appetite**—When you've achieved ketosis, you will be less hungry. If you feel full and don't need to eat as often, you're probably in ketosis.

- **Increased focus and energy**—When you first start a ketogenic diet, you will likely feel lethargic and perhaps a little sick. This is your body's way of adjusting to your new eating style. Once you reach ketosis, you should feel a huge surge in energy and mental focus. This means that your body has started using ketones for fuel and no longer needs to yo-yo with glucose.

- **Digestive changes**—You may experience short-term digestive issues like constipation and diarrhea. These symptoms are very common when first starting out. Don't freak out—your levels should balance out soon! Just try to remember that digestive changes are a good sign of beginning ketosis.

INTERMITTENT FASTING (IF)

I'm sure you're familiar with fasting and its benefits, but let me explain how fasting goes hand in hand with a ketogenic diet. Do you *have* to fast while doing keto? No, but there are tremendous benefits. I did keto for about a year and a half *without* fasting. Why? Because I didn't like the thought of being hungry, but I also didn't understand how beneficial it could be for my body. I wish I would've started fasting sooner.

Intermittent fasting is an eating pattern where you cycle between eating and fasting. The most common form of IF is a 16:8 schedule, meaning that you eat during an eight-hour window and spend the remaining sixteen hours of the day fasting. Your body's fat-burning process peaks after you've been fasting for twelve to fourteen hours. For the first twelve hours, your body burns glycogen (a molecule that stores sugar), and after twelve hours, it starts to burn fat stores. This is the reasoning behind the popular 16:8 schedule, as it gives your body enough time to move into the fat-burning state. Intermittent fasting gives your body a break from constantly digesting foods. Instead of working on digestion, your body will repair itself and work on balancing your hormones. Fasting also has been proven to help you reach ketosis sooner. If you are struggling to get into ketosis, try fasting for sure. Research has also shown that IF preserves muscle mass while burning fat.

There are many ways to approach a fast, and I'll share my approach with you here. But first, I'd like to make it very clear that everyone is different. What works for me may not work the same way for you. Trial and error are a part of your life now. Don't be afraid of it. Use it as an opportunity to grow.

My fasting/eating window looks like this: I eat my meals between 8:00 a.m. and 4:00 p.m. This works for me because I've never been a late-night eater, and I *love* breakfast. So for me, this schedule is the best of both worlds. Obviously, you'll need to tailor fasting to your schedule. If you're not that into breakfast, for example, you might consider an eating window of noon to 8:00 p.m. instead.

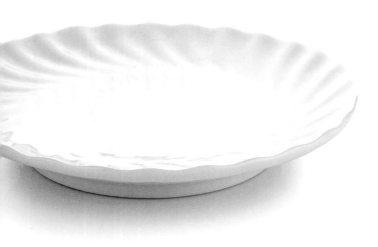

TIME- AND MONEY-SAVING TRICKS

- **Plan ahead!** Make a grocery list of items you need, and do not stray from your list! Not only will this help cut down on your grocery bill, but it will also keep you from making poor decisions in the moment.

- **Prep your fruits and veggies right away.** You are more prone to making good food choices when healthy items are easily accessible.

- **Bulk chop your veggies.** When I come home from the store with a big batch of onions, I chop them all, place them in a gallon-sized freezer bag, and put them in the freezer. Then I just pull them out when I'm ready to use them for cooking. This also works for broccoli, cauliflower, Brussels sprouts, bell peppers, and many other vegetables. Lettuce is another great item to bulk chop, but store it in the refrigerator; it does not freeze well.

- **Hard-boil your eggs!** Hard-boiled eggs are a great snack or on-the-go breakfast. I love making a huge batch.

- **Buy meat in bulk.** When I buy ground beef, it's usually on sale and needs to be cooked right away or frozen. Cook it! You can cook large batches of ground beef and store them in the freezer. I like to separate it by the pound and then just bring the meat out when I am ready to use it in a recipe. Simply add the seasonings you want when reheating. Same goes for chicken!

- **Portion out snacks such as nuts and berries.** Nuts and berries are very easy to overindulge in, not to mention costly, so measuring them out will prevent you from going overboard.

- **When making soups or casseroles, double the batch and freeze half.** You can freeze individual servings or family-sized portions for those days when you just don't feel like cooking.

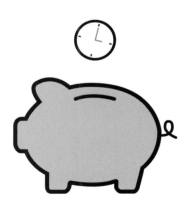

HANDLING STALLS

Let's face it, you're going to experience a weight loss stall every once in a while. That's just a part of life. Trust me, I know how frustrating stalls can be! While I'm not a doctor or a nutritionist, I have lived through stalls and figured out ways to beat them. Keep in mind that everyone is different, and you'll need to play around to figure out what works for you and how your body operates. But maybe these tips can help. Please don't get mad at me for some of these suggestions!

Dairy—You could be eating too much dairy. Gasp! I hate to even mention this because the idea of giving up dairy makes people so sad. Eating too much cheese and heavy cream can cause bloating and inflammatory issues. If you're not seeing a drop on the scale and you feel like dairy could be the culprit, try eliminating it for a week or two. I think you'll be surprised at the results!

Keto sweeteners—While most "keto-approved" sweeteners shouldn't spike blood sugar levels, there are always people who don't react well to them. Try eliminating them gradually. Don't add that erythritol to your coffee, skip keto desserts for a week, and stay away from sugar-free sauces for a while, and see how your body reacts! I think you'll find that your palate can do without sweetness, even in coffee.

Nuts—Nuts (and nut butters) are sneaky. It's so easy to overindulge because they are such convenient foods. However, those carbs can add up quickly if you're not careful. I'm not saying to eliminate them altogether; I'm just saying to be mindful.

Flours—Cut out almond flour and coconut flour. I bake with these ingredients frequently, and my body likes them. But again, we are all different. I've heard of people being kicked out of ketosis after consuming too much almond and coconut flour, so be careful here. It's easy to get carried away with these things because it feels like you're cheating, even when you're not. Take fathead pizza, for example. It's so yummy and keto-friendly that I sometimes think I can eat the whole thing, but we have to remind ourselves that not all keto-friendly foods are a free-for-all.

Greens—UP YOUR GREENS!!! I know that keto can be super enjoyable because you get to indulge in foods like bacon and sausage, but do not forget to eat those veggies! Greens are so important, and I'm certainly guilty of not eating enough of them. I've noticed that as soon as I up my veggie intake, I feel fantastic, and then I see some movement on the scale.

Calories—Again, I know it's easy to love the foods you're eating, but it's also easy to go over your calorie limit when you're eating high-fat. Some say calories don't matter, but let's be real; they do. I personally am not one for tracking my calorie intake. Why? Because I do not overeat. Portion control is my strong suit. You may be different, so just be aware of your calorie intake if you're not seeing much progress.

I'm hoping that these tricks can help you through your stalls, but I also want to make sure that you're focusing on how you feel and not on how much you weigh. Easier said than done, I know. But my theory with keto is, if you feel substantially better than you used to, then you're on the right track. Get yourself in the right head space. Rather than focusing on a number on the scale, try focusing on the steps you are taking to improve your health. If you stay consistent, the weight will fall off eventually. Stressing won't do you any favors, so hang in there and keep your head up!

KETO AND HAIR LOSS

I remember my early keto days, pulling out clumps of hair in the shower and thinking I was legitimately going bald. You're there, too? Okay, here's the scoop.

Hair loss is a totally normal symptom with any low-carb diet. But don't freak out! It's only temporary. Here are a few reasons why it could be happening:

- Calorie deficit
- Vitamin deficiencies
- Not enough protein
- Stress
- Lack of biotin

Here are some helpful tips to keep that hair of yours in place:

- Take a biotin supplement. These can be found over the counter. Start with a smaller dosage of 500 to 1,000 micrograms (MCG). You can also get biotin from foods such as eggs, salmon, avocados, cauliflower, spinach, and nuts, to name a few.
- Take a collagen supplement. Collagen not only helps with cellular repair but also is an excellent source of protein. There are several on the market, but my favorite is from Perfect Keto. It comes in a powder form to put in coffee, almond milk, or water. Or you can get it in pill form and skip the hassle of remembering to add it to your drinks. Collagen is also excellent for skin and nails.
- Eat foods that are high in zinc, such as grass-fed beef, lamb, chicken, cacao powder, and cashews.
- Coconut oil everything! Although coconut oil will not help stimulate hair growth, it can help prevent hair loss. Add it to veggies and meats, or eat it straight up like a weirdo (me).

Bottom line is, don't let the hair loss scare you from continuing your keto way of living. Once your metabolism adjusts to your new eating habits, the situation should improve.

KETO FLU

The keto flu can happen when your body switches from burning sugar to burning fat for energy. Going from a standard American diet to a low-carb diet lowers your insulin levels. This is the goal of a ketogenic diet. However, it will take your body some time to adjust to this huge change. Be patient and trust the process.

You may or may not get the keto flu. I was one of the lucky ones who didn't, but it happens to a lot of people when just starting out on keto. Around day three, you may start to feel irritable, feel sick to your stomach, and develop a killer headache. Congrats, you have the keto flu! Don't give up just yet. This phase is so temporary—a few days, maybe even a week. Once you get past it, you'll feel better than ever.

You can help prevent keto flu symptoms by supplementing with electrolytes. My favorite supplement is from Keto-Beam. It provides all essential electrolytes and trace minerals, such as magnesium, potassium, sodium, and calcium.

THE IMPORTANCE OF A SUPPORT SYSTEM

When I first started my keto journey in February 2017, I did it by myself. I'm not saying that I didn't have support from my family, because I absolutely did, 100 percent. But my family didn't really understand keto. They knew I was making a lifestyle change, and they supported me in all the ways they knew how, but I still felt pretty alone. I would make dinner for my family and then make a keto version of whatever they were eating for myself. It was hard, but it was mostly just a pain in my butt. I mean, my kids are *serious* carb people: mac 'n' cheese, pasta, cereal, beans, and bread. So. Much. Bread. It was hard for me to be around all those high-carb foods, but I wanted results more than I wanted a piece of bread as a temporary pleasure.

I found myself spending time on social media, searching for fellow keto people. I stumbled on a few who truly inspired me on a deep level. Some of those people didn't even know I existed, but I felt connected to them. They were my support system. Those Instagram accounts paved the way for me to figure out what I was doing and inspired me to continue. They were my most treasured online friends, and they had no idea!

It wasn't until July 2018, when my husband started keto, that I truly understood the significance of having a support system. I no longer have to make separate meals for

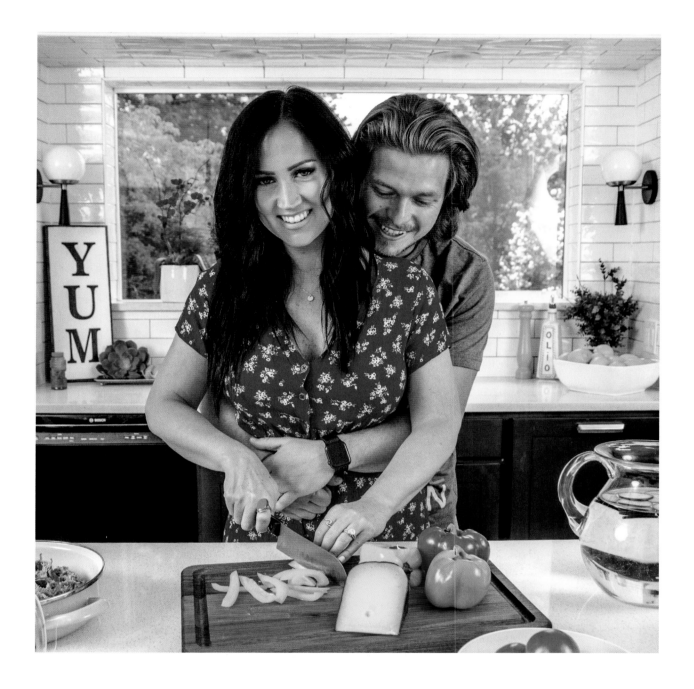

myself and my family. Our kids eat what I make and that's that! My husband and I can sit and talk keto for hours at a time. It's such a fun common ground for us.

My point in sharing this with you is that you *need* a support system. It is crucial for you to stick with your goals. If you do not have someone in real life who will do keto with you, look for strangers online! I can guarantee you that there are people out there who need you, too. There are a ton of online support systems across social media. Find a buddy, and your life will be so much more pleasant! Trust me, there's a support system out there somewhere for you.

MY FAVORITE KITCHEN TOOLS

I highly recommend grabbing some good-quality kitchen tools. Having reliable items to work with makes life in the kitchen so much easier!

In the recipes, I assume that you have the basics on hand, such as saucepans, skillets, baking pans and sheets, a blender, and a mixer. In addition to those essentials, the following tools are really handy to have:

Griddle—I love my griddle for making cream cheese pancakes! The banana-flavored "pan-crepes" on page 52 are out of this world.

High-powered blender—I love my Blendtec high-powered blender. It makes whipped cream, pancake batter, and smoothies (like my Strawberry Coconut Smoothie on page 202) so incredibly fast and easily. You don't have to have a high-powered blender to make any of the recipes in this book, but it definitely helps.

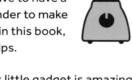

Milk frother—This little gadget is amazing for bulletproof coffee (see page 34 for my recipe). You can find one just about anywhere and for relatively cheap.

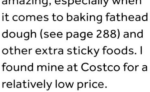

Silicone baking mats—These mats are amazing, especially when it comes to baking fathead dough (see page 288) and other extra sticky foods. I found mine at Costco for a relatively low price.

Silicone donut pan—I never owned a donut pan until I started keto. This is great for making sweet keto treats, like my Old-Fashioned Chocolate Donuts (page 226)!

Waffle iron—I never owned a waffle iron until I started keto, either. I found one for $20, and it is the perfect tool for weekend waffles! (See my Flourless Waffles recipe on page 48.)

HOW TO USE THIS BOOK

So how do you use this book? Short answer: apply it to *your* life.

Let me explain further. You are more prone to stick with a diet that fits perfectly into your lifestyle than with one that requires you to switch your entire life around to be something you're not. Don't set yourself up for failure. If you're not one for meal prepping, you don't have to meal prep. If you eat fast food a few times a week because you have a super busy schedule and convenience wins out, you can still do keto! Don't have the budget (or desire) to eat 100 percent grass-fed, organic everything? That's okay! This is the beauty of a ketogenic lifestyle: you can make it your own and still succeed.

I'm a firm believer in eating foods you love. I really feel like that's what keto is for me. I can't even tell you how many times I've said to myself, "I can't believe I get to eat this way and still lose weight." The trick is to adjust things according to your liking. Here are a few random thoughts that may help you figure out how to keto *your* way:

- **Thoughts on grass-fed and organic everything**—I live in a smallish town that doesn't offer many grocery options. It's either Walmart, Costco, or places that charge an arm and a leg for everything. Or I could drive twenty minutes, but who has the time for that? I don't. My go-tos are Walmart and Costco. We are a family of six with an already outrageous grocery budget. I don't buy grass-fed/organic all the time because it's one way to cut down on our grocery bill. For optimal health, grass-fed and organic are the best choices. However, it's just not feasible for me all the time. Guess what? I'm still alive. And I've lost over 60 pounds doing it my way. Do it your way!

- **Thoughts on ingredient substitutions**—This is a total personal preference. In my recipes, I recommend certain ingredients, but if you'd rather use something else (that's still keto-friendly), do it! Can't eat dairy? Plenty of my recipes offer a dairy-free option. (I've got coconut-free and nut-free options, too.) Hate cauliflower? No one is making you eat it! My goal with this book is to give you good base recipes so that you can alter them to your tastes and learn how to make keto a sustainable way of living for you.

- **Thoughts on tracking**—I have provided the macros for all of my recipes. Use them as guidelines, but I hope that at some point, you'll be able to eat without having to track. There is nothing more powerful than being in control of the foods you put in your mouth. This is what intuitive eating does for me, and I can talk all day about how amazing it is. The ability to eat freely and listen to my body rather than an app is the single reason why I have been able to sustain this lifestyle. It is so empowering!

Before you get cooking, I'd like to point out a few handy features in the recipes. At the top, I've placed icons to indicate which recipes are free of coconut, dairy, eggs, and/or nuts or can be modified to eliminate those ingredients. You'll also find the net carbs per serving of the recipe. At the bottom of each recipe page, I've included full nutritional information for each dish. Note that these totals do not include any optional ingredients or toppings.

Now it's time to head to the kitchen and make some delicious keto food! Please visit me on Instagram (@ketomadesimple) and tell me which recipes from this book are your favorites.

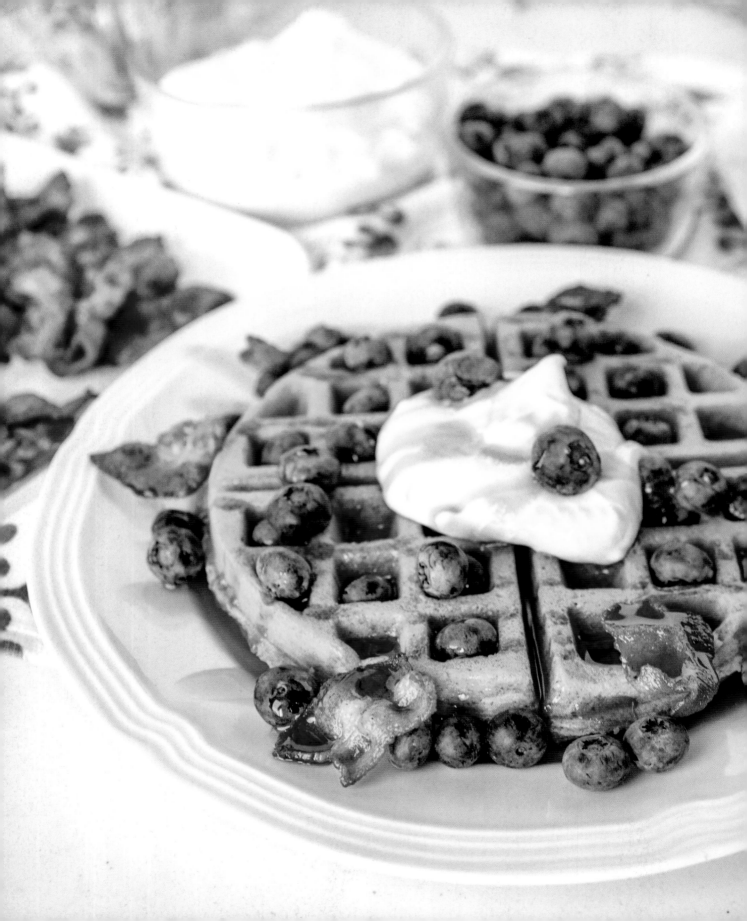

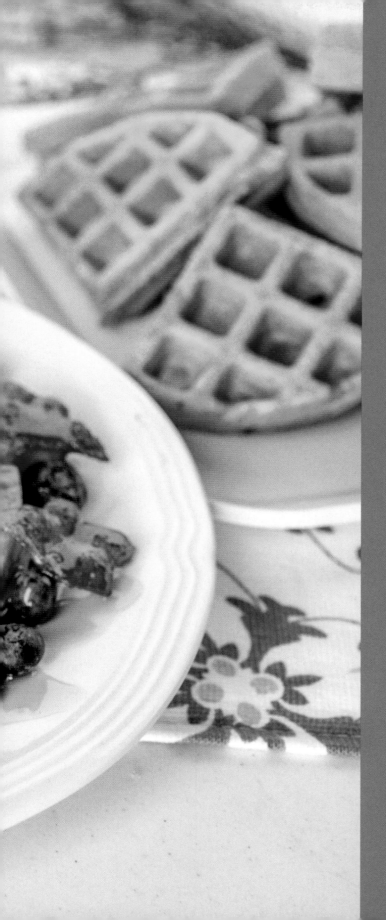

① GOOD MORNING

BULLETPROOF COFFEE

MAKES 1 serving   PREP TIME: 2 minutes   COOK TIME: —

Bulletproof coffee is a staple for most keto folks. It's a great way to add fats first thing in the morning. It'll boost your energy and keep you feeling full. There are a million ways to make bulletproof coffee, so don't be afraid to play around with this recipe!

INGREDIENTS

1 cup freshly brewed coffee

1 tablespoon unsalted butter or ghee

1 tablespoon coconut oil

Granulated sweetener, to taste (optional)

Ground cinnamon, for garnish

Special Equipment (optional):

Milk frother

Variation: Not a coffee drinker? Try this with warmed unsweetened almond or coconut milk instead of coffee!

DIRECTIONS

1. Pour the coffee into a mug and add the butter, coconut oil, and sweetener, if using. Use a milk frother (or a blender if you don't have a frother) to blend everything together.

2. Top the coffee with a sprinkle of cinnamon and enjoy!

Nutritional information

Calories: 224   Total Carbs: 0g
Fat: 26g   Fiber: 0g
Protein: 0g   Net Carbs: 0g

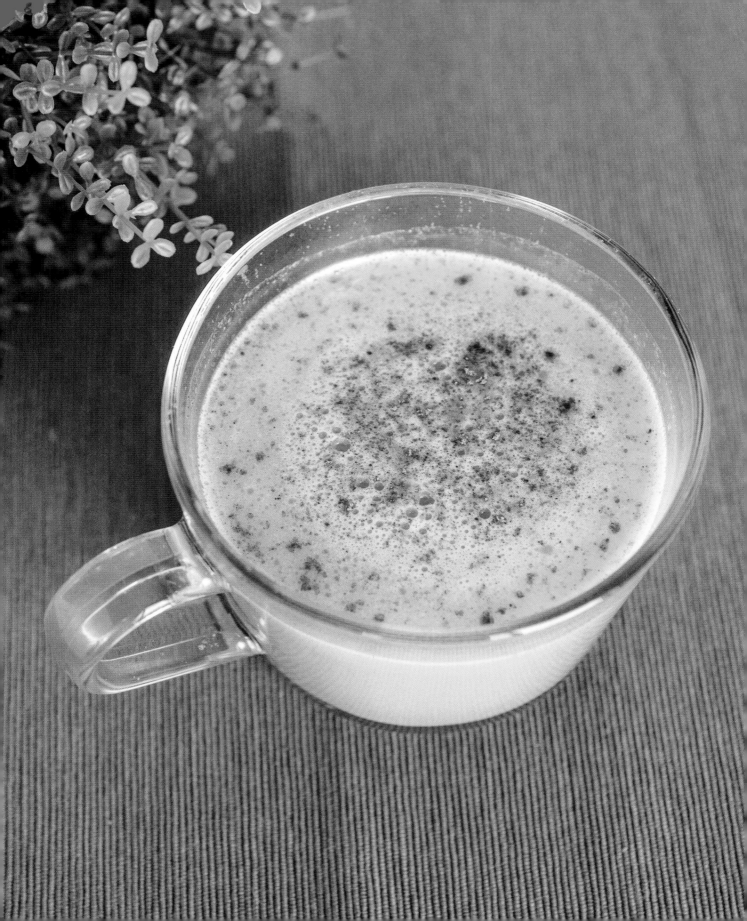

BANANA MUFFINS

MAKES 12 to 15 muffins (2 per serving)   PREP TIME: 10 minutes   COOK TIME: 45 minutes

This was one of the first keto baked goods that I attempted, and I was shocked when the recipe turned out as good as it did. I mean, I have decent baking skills, but something about the imitation banana flavoring in this recipe made me nervous. If there's one food I miss, it's bananas. These muffins do not disappoint! This batter can also be made into banana bread. Add some chocolate chips or nuts, and you have a delicious banana-flavored treat. We love our muffins topped with Cream Cheese Frosting (page 302).

INGREDIENTS

Cooking spray

¼ cup (½ stick) unsalted butter, softened

½ cup granulated sweetener

4 ounces cream cheese (½ cup), softened

1 teaspoon vanilla extract

4 large eggs

2 teaspoons banana extract

1¼ cups blanched almond flour

1 teaspoon baking powder

¼ teaspoon salt

¼ cup sour cream

DIRECTIONS

1. Preheat the oven to 300°F. Spray a standard-size 12-well muffin pan with cooking spray.

2. In a large bowl, cream the butter and sweetener with a hand mixer. Add the cream cheese and vanilla and mix well.

3. Add the eggs one at a time, making sure to mix well before adding the next egg.

4. Mix in the banana extract, then add the remaining ingredients and continue mixing until well combined.

5. Divide the batter evenly among the wells of the greased muffin pan, filling them about three-quarters full, and bake for 40 to 45 minutes, until a tester inserted into the center of a muffin comes out clean. Let cool in the pan for about 10 minutes before removing and eating.

6. Store leftover muffins in a resealable plastic bag in the refrigerator for up to 1 week.

Nutritional information (per serving)

Calories: 323	Total Carbs: 5g
Fat: 29g	Fiber: 2g
Protein: 9g	Net Carbs: 3g

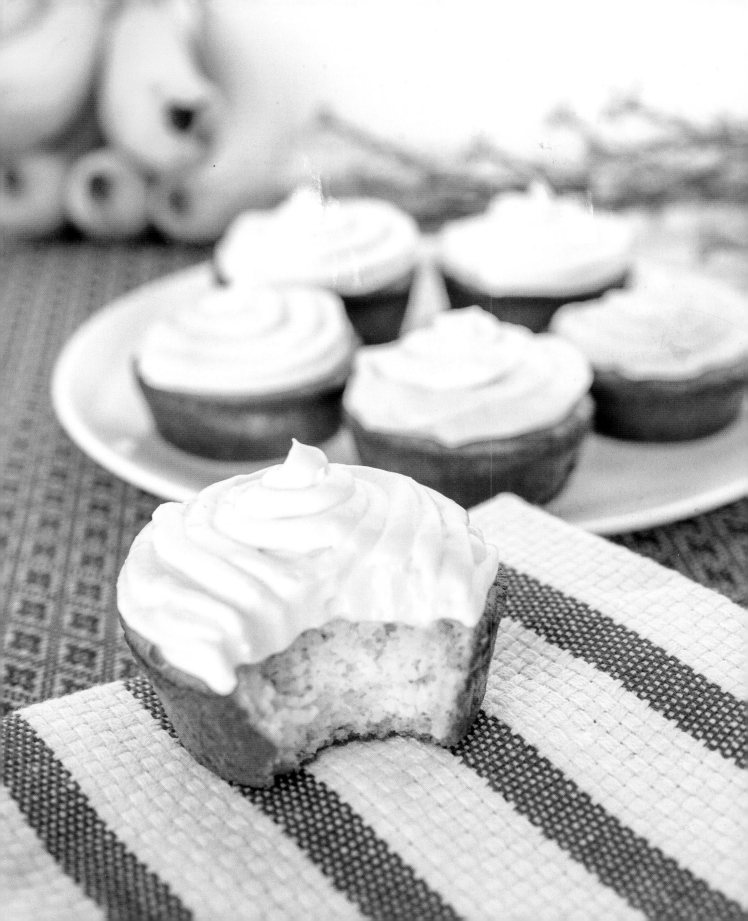

CYLIS'S CHIA PUDDING

MAKES 2 servings   PREP TIME: 5 minutes, plus 4 hours to chill   COOK TIME: —

Cylis is our youngest child and toughest critic when it comes to food. He knows what he wants and isn't afraid to tell us. He loves yogurt and frog-eye salad, so I tried to figure out a way to make a keto-friendly version of those two things, and that's how Cylis's Chia Pudding was born. I'll admit, I had never tried chia anything until I was in the process of writing this book. I was always afraid of chia seeds, and I didn't know where to buy them, and making a pudding out of them always sounded way too over my head to even attempt it. I was so wrong. This recipe could not be easier. I'm bummed that I waited so long to try chia pudding because we honestly can't get enough of it—especially Cylis, which speaks volumes about how delicious this pudding is! You can find chia seeds in the baking aisle at almost any grocery store.

INGREDIENTS

1 cup unsweetened almond milk or full-fat coconut milk

2 tablespoons heavy whipping cream or coconut cream

¼ cup chia seeds

1 tablespoon granulated sweetener

1 teaspoon banana extract

1 teaspoon coconut extract

Fresh raspberries, for garnish (optional)

DIRECTIONS

1. Place all the ingredients in a jar or mixing bowl. Shake the jar or whisk the ingredients so that the chia seeds get mixed in with the liquids.

2. Cover and refrigerate for at least 4 hours.

3. Garnish with raspberries, if desired.

4. Store leftovers in the refrigerator for up to 1 week.

Nutritional information (per serving)

Calories: 203	**Total Carbs:** 13g
Fat: 15g	**Fiber:** 10g
Protein: 5g	**Net Carbs:** 3g

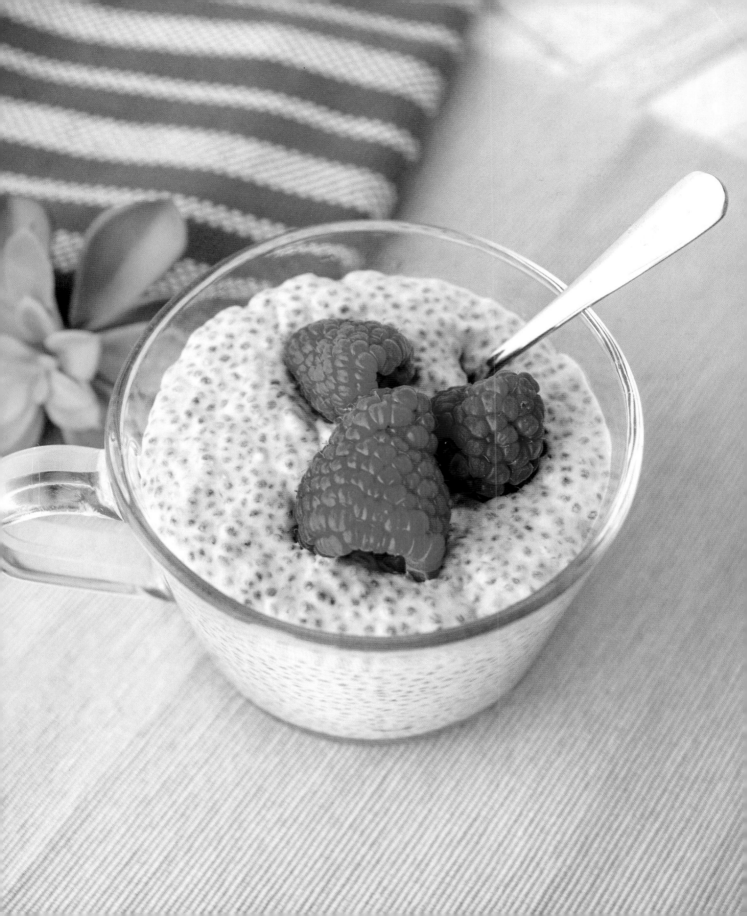

COUNTRY SAUSAGE GRAVY

MAKES 4 servings   PREP TIME: 2 minutes   COOK TIME: 15 minutes

Cameron's all-time favorite meal is biscuits and sausage gravy—hands down. When he started keto, I knew I had to come up with a low-carb version that he approved of. It took some tweaking, but I think I nailed it! This gravy is so rich, so hearty, and so easy to make. Cameron approves. Serve it over my Sour Cream and Cheddar Biscuits (page 128) for an authentic biscuits and gravy experience.

INGREDIENTS

1 teaspoon unsalted butter or ghee

1 pound bulk (ground) pork sausage, mild or hot

¼ teaspoon red pepper flakes

Salt and ground black pepper (optional)

½ teaspoon xanthan gum

1 cup heavy whipping cream

DIRECTIONS

1. Melt the butter in a large skillet over medium-high heat. Add the sausage and red pepper flakes and cook until the sausage is browned, about 10 minutes. Season with salt and pepper, if desired.

2. Sprinkle the xanthan gum over the cooked sausage and stir. Reduce the heat to low. Add the heavy cream and continue stirring until the gravy begins to thicken, about 5 minutes. Remove from the heat and serve.

3. Store leftovers in the refrigerator for up to 5 days. Reheat in the microwave or on the stovetop.

Nutritional information (per serving)

Calories: 595   Total Carbs: 2g
Fat: 55g   Fiber: 0g
Protein: 21g   Net Carbs: 2g

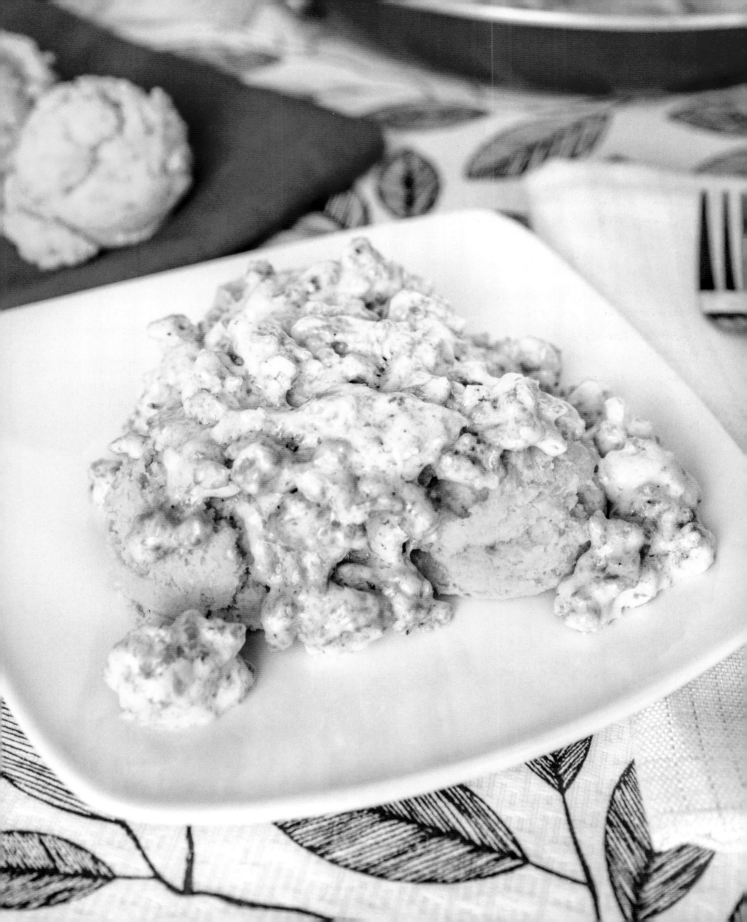

DUTCH BABY

MAKES 4 servings   **PREP TIME:** 8 minutes   **COOK TIME:** 20 minutes

When I used to scour the internet for keto-friendly recipes, I would immediately exit out of any recipe that seemed too hard or time-consuming. I prefer the laziest way of cooking possible. Ladies and gentlemen, this is it. Pop a few ingredients in a blender, bake, and voilà! You have a simple, delicious, and crowd-pleasing breakfast! We love ours topped with butter and sugar-free syrup.

INGREDIENTS

½ cup (1 stick) plus 3 tablespoons unsalted butter, softened, divided

6 large eggs

1 cup heavy whipping cream

1 cup blanched almond flour

1 tablespoon vanilla extract

2 teaspoons granulated sweetener

Pinch of salt

DIRECTIONS

1. Preheat the oven to 425°F.

2. Place 3 tablespoons of the butter in a 9 by 13-inch or similar-sized glass or ceramic baking dish. Place the dish in the oven while it's preheating so that the butter melts and coats the bottom of the dish. Keep an eye on it; you don't want the butter to burn.

3. While the oven is heating, place the remaining ingredients in a blender. Blend on high speed until everything is incorporated and there are no lumps.

4. Once the oven has reached temperature, slowly pour the egg mixture into the baking dish. Pouring very slowly makes the final product super fluffy!

5. Bake for 20 minutes or until the top is golden brown.

6. Store leftovers in the refrigerator for up to 5 days. Reheat in the microwave or in a toaster oven.

Nutritional information (per serving)

Calories: 764	Total Carbs: 7g
Fat: 74g	Fiber: 3g
Protein: 17g	Net Carbs: 4g

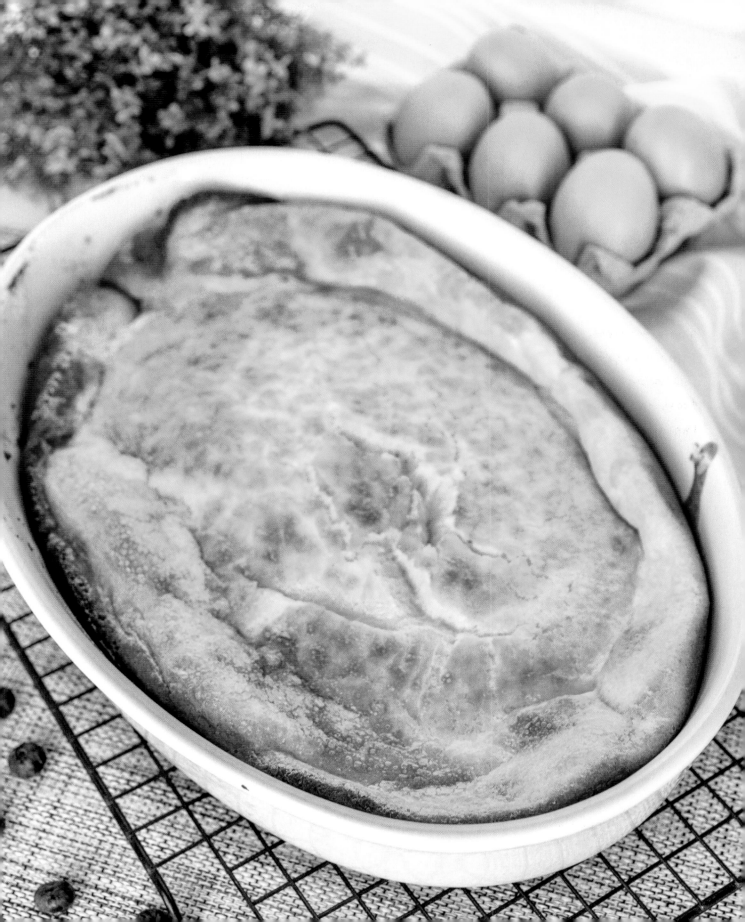

ORANGE ROLLS

MAKES 6 servings   PREP TIME: 30 minutes   COOK TIME: 25 minutes

While I was writing this book, I woke up in the middle of the night one night with the biggest lightbulb moment. I knew I had to make orange rolls! First thing in the morning, I ran downstairs and immediately got to work. I nailed it on my first try, and these bad boys were born. I think this is my favorite recipe in the entire book. It's a bit more labor-intensive than most of my recipes, but it is so, so worth every minute. I hope you love these rolls as much as I do!

INGREDIENTS

FOR THE DOUGH:

12 ounces mozzarella cheese, shredded (about 3 cups)

4 ounces cream cheese (½ cup)

1½ cups blanched almond flour

2 large eggs

1 tablespoon baking powder

1 teaspoon orange extract

FOR THE FILLING:

½ cup granulated sweetener

½ cup (1 stick) unsalted butter, softened

2 tablespoons grated orange zest, plus extra for garnish if desired

FOR THE ICING:

½ cup powdered sweetener

5 tablespoons heavy whipping cream

2 tablespoons water

1½ tablespoons unsalted butter, softened

½ teaspoon lemon extract

½ teaspoon orange extract

Nutritional information (per serving)

Calories: 627	Total Carbs: 8g
Fat: 57g	Fiber: 3g
Protein: 26g	Net Carbs: 5g

DIRECTIONS

1. Make the dough: Place the mozzarella and cream cheese in a large microwave-safe bowl. No need to stir at this point. Microwave for 1 minute. Take it out and stir with a fork, then microwave for another minute. At this point, you want the cheeses to be fully melted and smooth. Microwave for another 30 seconds, if necessary.

2. Add the almond flour, eggs, baking powder, and orange extract to the bowl with the melted cheeses and combine the ingredients with your hands. If the dough gets sticky, simply wet your hands and continue working it until it is well combined.

3. Place the dough in the refrigerator for 10 minutes to chill.

4. Preheat the oven to 425°F. Grease a 9-inch square glass baking dish.

5. While the dough is chilling, make the filling: Place the granulated sweetener, butter, and orange zest in a medium-sized bowl and mix until well combined.

6. Take the dough out of the fridge and place it on a sheet of parchment paper. Place another sheet of parchment on top of the dough and use a rolling pin to roll out the dough between the two sheets until it is about ¼ inch thick. Form the dough into a rectangle. Remove the top layer of parchment paper and discard.

7. Spread the filling evenly across the dough. Then, starting at one short end, roll the dough all the way to the other end so that it forms a large log.

8. Cut the log into 1½-inch slices and place the rolls in the greased baking dish, spacing them an inch apart to allow them space to expand.

9. Bake for 22 to 25 minutes, until golden brown.

10. Meanwhile, make the icing: In a medium-sized bowl, whisk the powdered sweetener, heavy cream, water, butter, and extracts until well combined and smooth.

11. Remove the rolls from the oven, pour the icing on top, and serve warm! Garnish with orange zest, if desired.

12. Store leftovers in the refrigerator for up to 1 week.

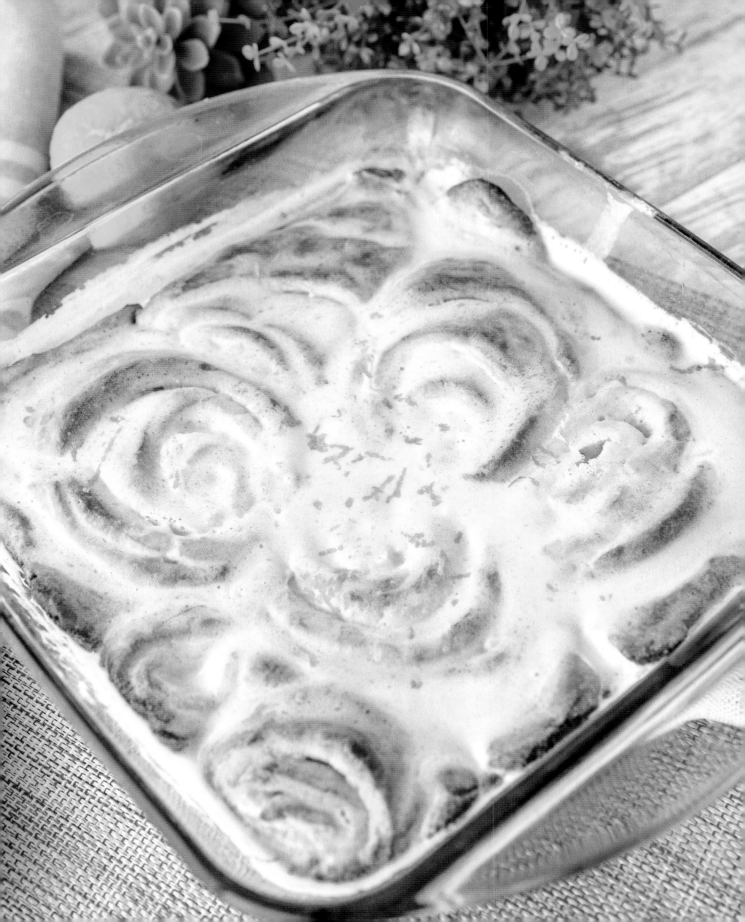

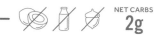

BAE (BACON AND EGGS)

MAKES 1 large serving   **PREP TIME:** 2 minutes   **COOK TIME:** 10 minutes

I know what you're thinking; this is just a recipe for bacon and eggs—what could be so special about it? Well, let me tell you... it's all in the method. Cooking eggs in bacon grease makes them incredibly fluffy and flavorful. Give this recipe a try! It will be your new favorite way to make bacon and eggs.

INGREDIENTS

4 slices bacon

4 large eggs

Salt and ground black pepper

DIRECTIONS

1. Cut the bacon into very thin, bite-sized pieces. (I use kitchen scissors for this task.)

2. Heat a medium-sized skillet over high heat. When hot, place the bacon pieces in the pan. Cook until browned and crispy, or to your desired doneness. Remove all but 3 tablespoons of the bacon grease from the pan.

3. Crack the eggs directly into the pan with the bacon. Stir with a spatula, scrambling the eggs with the bacon pieces, until the eggs are fluffy and cooked all the way through. Season with salt and pepper and serve immediately.

Nutritional information (per serving)

Calories: 472	Total Carbs: 2g
Fat: 32g	Fiber: 0g
Protein: 36g	Net Carbs: 2g

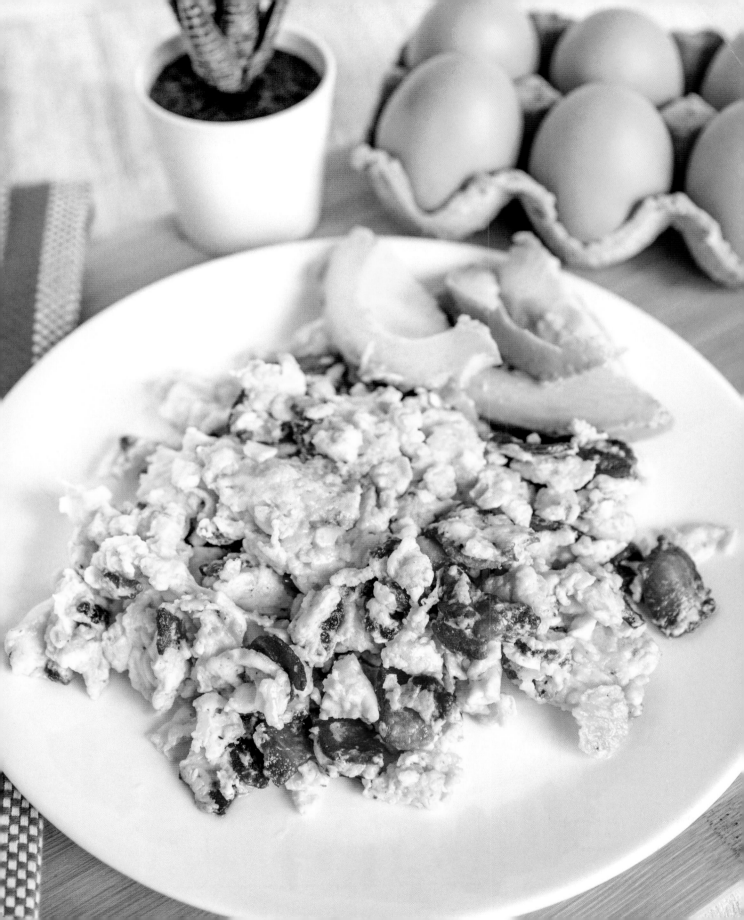

FLOURLESS WAFFLES

MAKES about 5 waffles (1 per serving)   PREP TIME: 4 minutes   COOK TIME: 15 minutes

I've experimented with a ton of keto waffle recipes in search of the perfect one. These are by far the densest, most filling waffles I've ever made—so filling that you could feed them to your kids for breakfast and not even need to make them dinner later! Win!

INGREDIENTS

8 large eggs

1 cup smooth unsweetened almond butter (see Tip)

1 tablespoon granulated sweetener

1 teaspoon baking powder

1 teaspoon vanilla extract

Cooking spray

FOR SERVING (OPTIONAL):

Sugar-free maple syrup, store-bought or homemade (page 269)

Next-Level Whipped Cream (page 268)

Fresh blueberries or other berries of choice

Chopped cooked bacon

Special Equipment:
Waffle maker

DIRECTIONS

1. Preheat a waffle maker.

2. Place all the ingredients in a blender and blend until smooth.

3. Once the waffle maker is hot, spray it with cooking spray. Pour the recommended amount of batter into each section of the waffle maker and cook according to the manufacturer's instructions. Repeat until all the batter has been used. My waffle maker gives me roughly five 5-inch waffles.

4. Serve topped with sugar-free maple syrup, whipped cream, berries, and/or chopped cooked bacon, if desired.

5. Store leftovers in the refrigerator for up to 1 week. Reheat in a toaster oven.

Tip: For almond butter, I love to use the grind-your-own machine at the grocery store. That way, I know I'm getting only almonds.

Nutritional information (per serving)

Calories: 390	**Total Carbs:** 8g
Fat: 33g	**Fiber:** 5g
Protein: 21g	**Net Carbs:** 3g

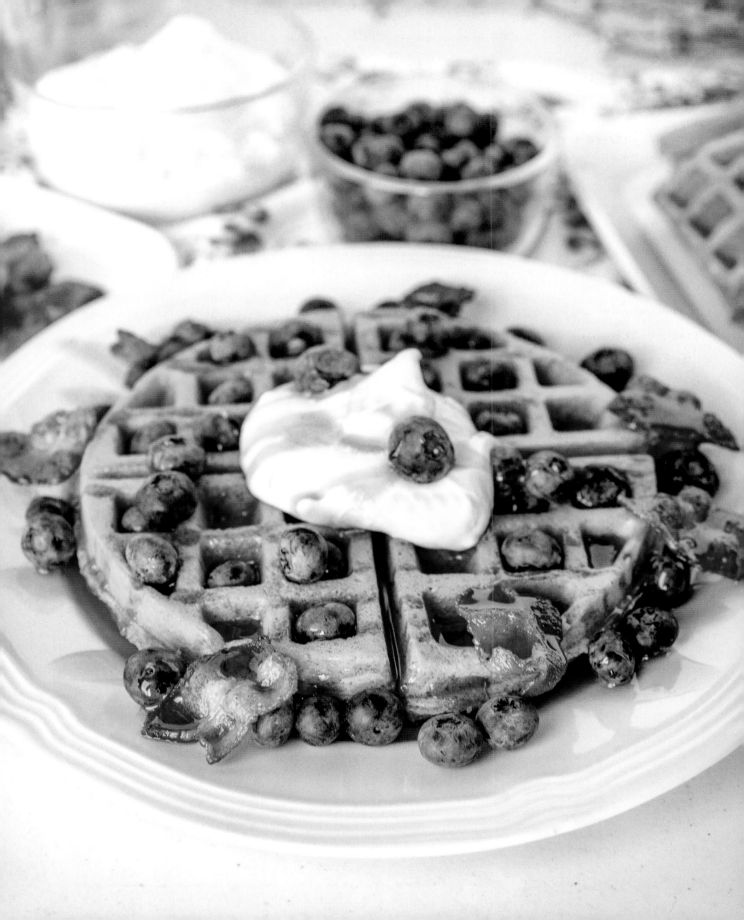

MILA'S PIZZA EGGS

MAKES 1 serving   PREP TIME: 2 minutes   COOK TIME: 15 minutes

I named these eggs after my daughter, Mila, because she asks for them literally every morning. They are her favorite food ever, and that makes me happy because they are so easy to make and always turn out delicious.

INGREDIENTS

2 tablespoons low-sugar tomato sauce

3 large eggs

1 ounce mozzarella cheese, shredded (about ¼ cup)

6 slices pepperoni

1½ tablespoons grated Parmesan cheese

¼ teaspoon Italian seasoning

Salt and ground black pepper

1 tablespoon unsalted butter or ghee, cut into small chunks and softened

DIRECTIONS

1. Preheat the oven to 400°F.

2. Place the tomato sauce in a small glass or ceramic baking dish. I use a 3-inch square baking dish, but any small baking dish will work; you could also use a large ramekin.

3. Crack the eggs on top of the tomato sauce. Sprinkle the mozzarella cheese over the eggs, then scatter the pepperoni on top.

4. Sprinkle with the Parmesan cheese and Italian seasoning and season with salt and pepper. Top with the chunks of butter—this doesn't need to look fancy.

5. Bake for 12 to 15 minutes, until the whites are set and the yolks are cooked to your liking. Enjoy!

Nutritional information

Calories: 509	Total Carbs: 4g
Fat: 40g	Fiber: 1g
Protein: 34g	Net Carbs: 3g

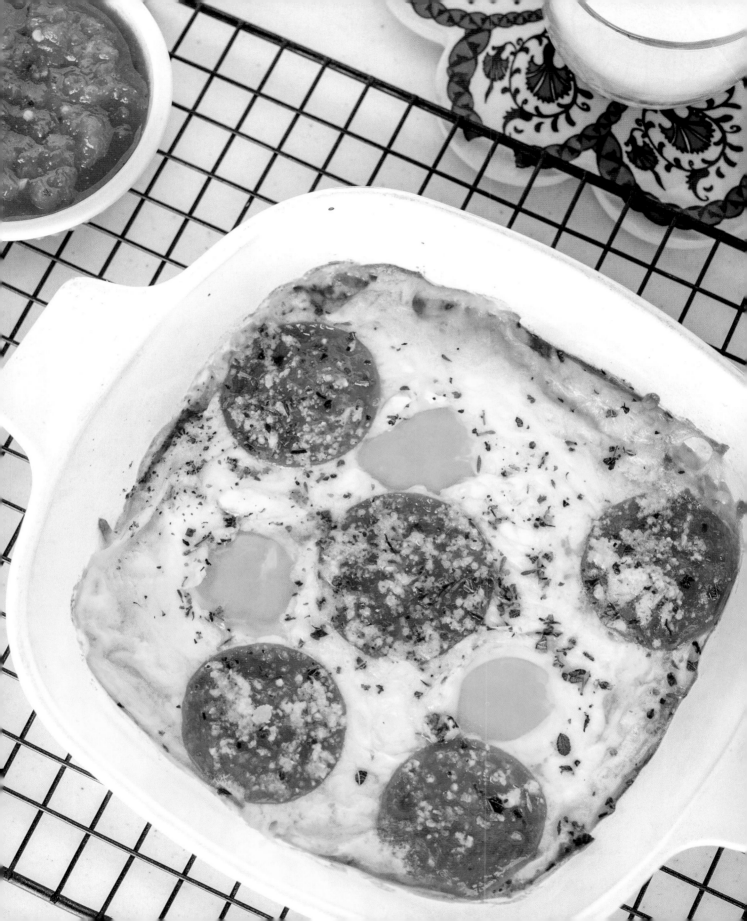

BANANA CREAM CHEESE PAN-CREPES

MAKES 24 pancakes (3 per serving)   PREP TIME: 10 minutes   COOK TIME: 15 to 30 minutes (depending on size of griddle)

One of the questions I'm asked most frequently is "what food do you miss that you can't eat on keto?" My answer is always bananas. There's just something about them that I crave. When given the chance, I'll add banana extract to anything! These thin banana-flavored pancakes have been a huge hit with my Instagram followers. The egg to cream cheese ratio is 1:1 (one egg per ounce of cream cheese), so if you don't want to make a large batch, you can follow that guideline to scale down the recipe. If you're not a banana fan (weirdo), you could substitute vanilla, lemon, or maple extract for the banana.

INGREDIENTS

1 (8-ounce) package cream cheese, softened

8 large eggs

1 tablespoon banana extract

1 teaspoon ground cinnamon

1 teaspoon baking powder

Cooking spray

Sugar-free maple syrup, store-bought or homemade (page 269), for serving

Butter, for serving

DIRECTIONS

1. Preheat a griddle or a large nonstick skillet over medium-high heat (about 350°F if using an electric griddle).

2. Place all the ingredients in a blender and blend until well combined, then let the batter rest for 5 minutes.

3. Spray the hot griddle with cooking spray. Pour ¼ cup of the batter onto the griddle for each pancake. (My griddle comfortably fits 8 pancakes.) Cook until the bottoms of the pancakes are golden brown, about 3 minutes. Flip the pancakes and cook the other side until golden brown, about 2 minutes. Repeat with the remaining batter.

4. Serve the pancakes with sugar-free maple syrup and butter.

5. Store leftovers in a resealable plastic bag in the fridge for up to 5 days, or freeze for up to 1 month. When you're ready for them, simply pop them into the microwave or toaster oven for a quick breakfast!

Nutritional information (per serving)

Calories: 484	Total Carbs: 4g
Fat: 38g	Fiber: 0g
Protein: 21g	Net Carbs: 4g

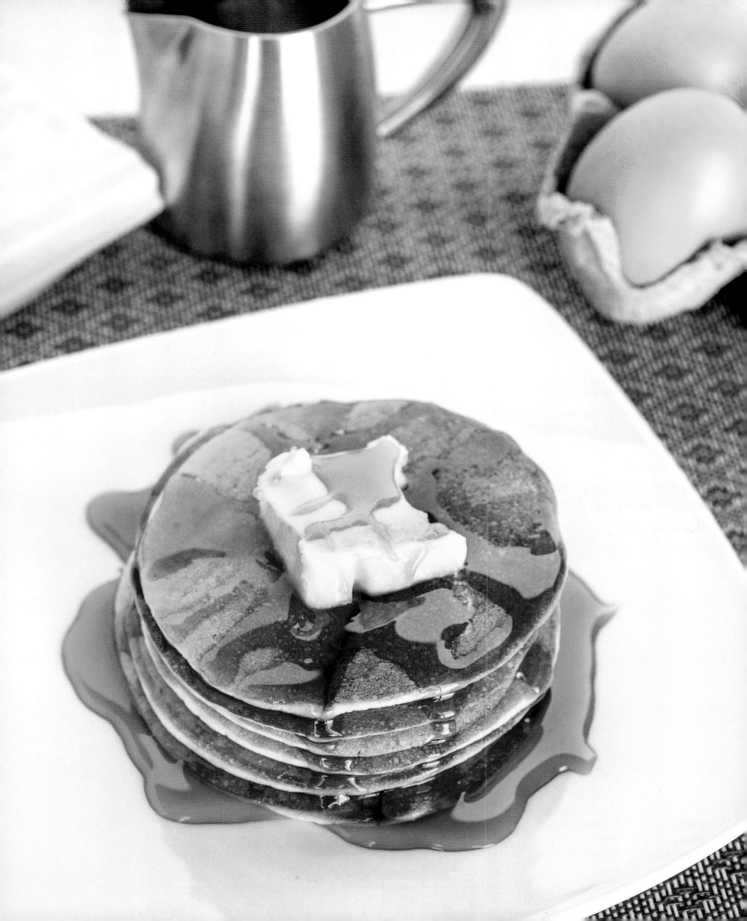

NET CARBS
1g

BACON AND MOZZARELLA FRITTATA MUFFINS

MAKES 12 muffins (2 per serving)   **PREP TIME: 15 minutes**   **COOK TIME: 25 minutes**

The ratio here is one egg per muffin. If you want a smaller batch, cut this recipe in half and you'll get six muffins. This recipe is so incredibly versatile, too. Add whatever meats or veggies to the basic ingredients, and you have a pretty damn good breakfast. These muffins are also great for taking with you on the go!

INGREDIENTS

Cooking spray

12 large eggs

Splash of heavy whipping cream (omit for dairy-free)

6 slices bacon, cooked and crumbled

4 ounces shredded mozzarella cheese (about 1 cup) (omit for dairy-free)

Salt and ground black pepper

DIRECTIONS

1. Preheat the oven to 350°F. Spray a standard-size 12-well muffin pan with cooking spray.

2. Crack the eggs into a large bowl and add a splash of heavy cream. Whisk until the yolks are mixed in with the whites.

3. Add the bacon and cheese. Sprinkle with salt and pepper and mix well.

4. Fill each well of the greased muffin pan about three-quarters full. Bake for 25 minutes or until golden. Serve immediately.

5. Store leftovers in a resealable plastic bag in the refrigerator for up to 5 days. Reheat in the microwave.

Nutritional information (per serving)

Calories: 213   **Total Carbs:** 1g

Fat: 15g   **Fiber:** 0g

Protein: 16g   **Net Carbs:** 1g

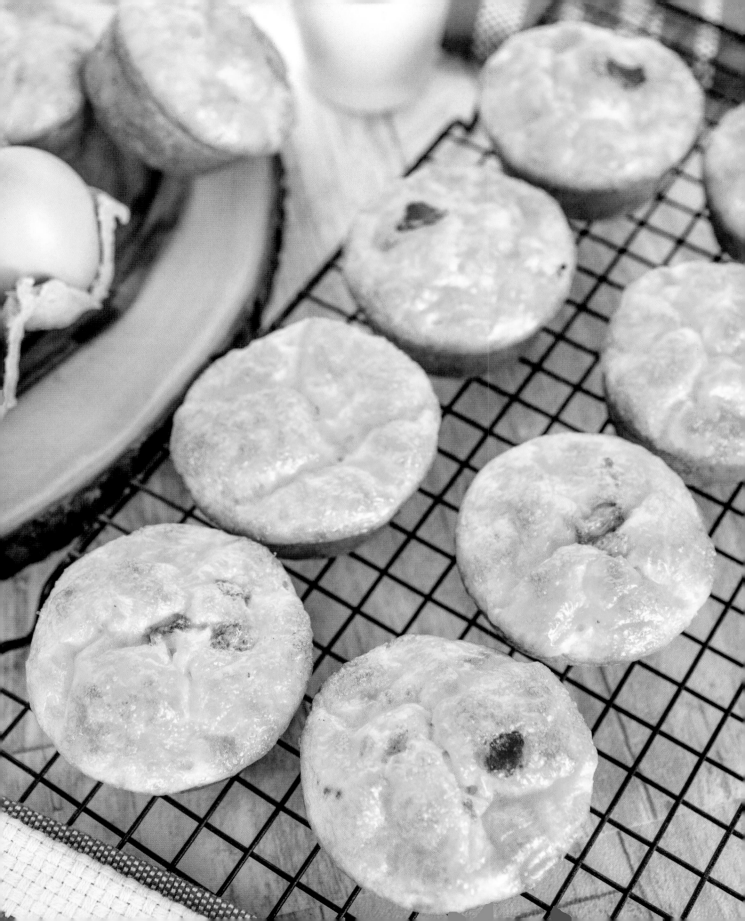

BUTTERY BAKED EGGS

MAKES 1 serving   **PREP TIME:** 2 minutes   **COOK TIME:** 15 minutes

This recipe is awesome because you can vary it in so many ways. Throw in some cheese, salsa, sliced jalapeños, prosciutto, and/or your favorite veggies—endless possibilities here!

INGREDIENTS

3 large eggs

2 slices bacon, cooked, or ½ cup cooked and crumbled breakfast sausage

1 tablespoon unsalted butter or ghee, cut into small chunks and softened

Salt and ground black pepper

DIRECTIONS

1. Preheat the oven to 350°F.

2. Crack the eggs into a small casserole dish. (I use a 3-inch square baking dish, but any small baking dish will work; you could also use a large ramekin.)

3. Tear the bacon into small pieces and sprinkle on top of the eggs. If you're using sausage, just crumble it on top of the eggs.

4. Scatter the chunks of butter on top of the eggs. Season with salt and pepper.

5. Bake for 10 to 15 minutes, until the eggs are cooked to your liking. At around the 10-minute mark, you'll have runny yolks; cooking the eggs for an additional 5 minutes will give you hard yolks.

6. Serve immediately!

Nutritional information

Calories: 416	**Total Carbs:** 2g
Fat: 33g	**Fiber:** 0g
Protein: 24g	**Net Carbs:** 2g

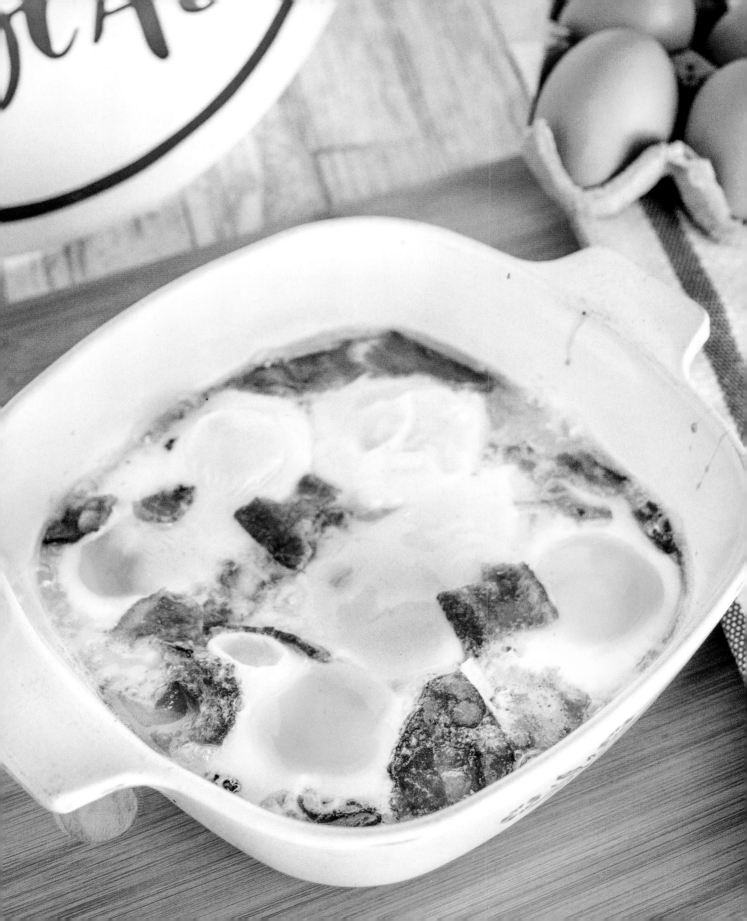

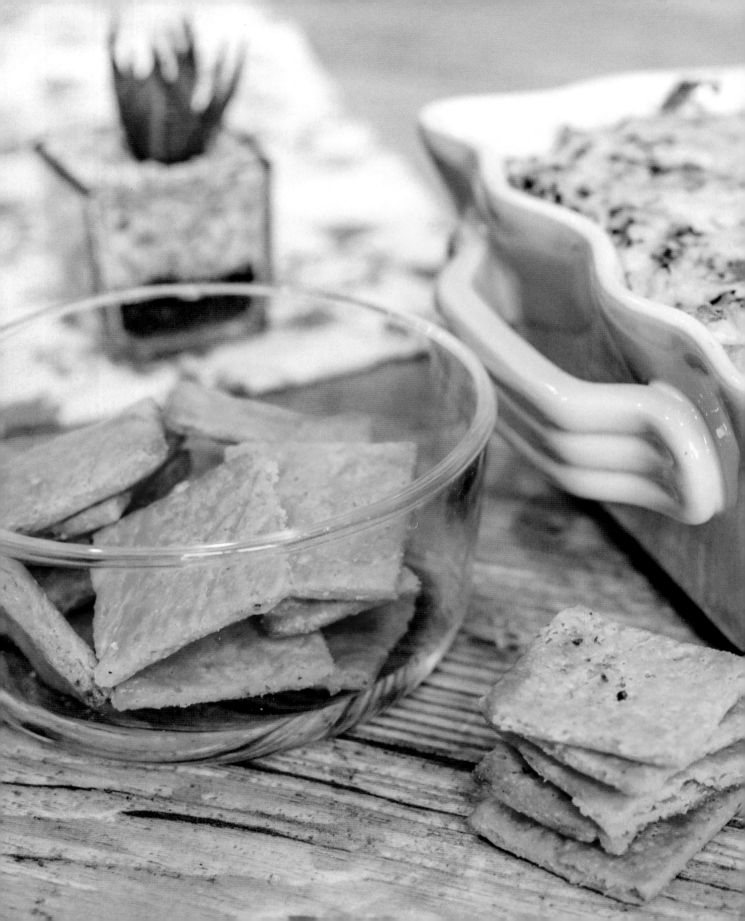

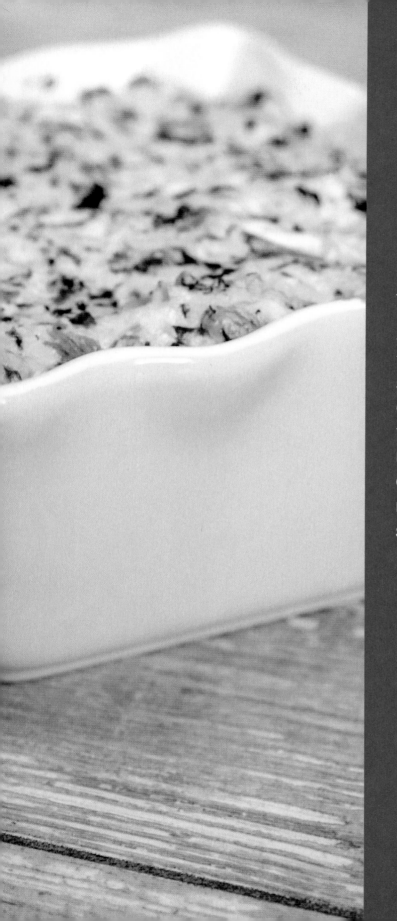

(2) MUNCHIES

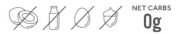

PEPPERONI CHIPS

MAKES 24 chips (12 per serving)   PREP TIME: 2 minutes   COOK TIME: 8 minutes

My favorite keto snack is pepperoni. It's cheap, easy to grab on the go, and pretty dang close to zero-carb. But have you ever tried pepperoni baked? Pepperoni chips are a whole new level of yummy. They are a fantastic replacement for regular chips and are perfect for all your favorite dips! Just make sure to keep a close eye on them while baking. They can go from absolutely perfect to burned to a crisp in 0.2 seconds. Try pairing them with Smoked Gouda Fondue (page 66) or dipping them in Blue Cheese Dressing (page 274)!

INGREDIENTS

24 slices pepperoni

DIRECTIONS

1. Preheat the oven to 400°F. Line a rimmed baking sheet with aluminum foil.

2. Spread the pepperoni on the foil in a single layer. Bake for 6 to 8 minutes, until crispy.

3. Serve on their own or with your favorite dip.

4. Store leftovers in the refrigerator for up to 1 week.

Nutritional information (per serving)

Calories: 105   Total Carbs: 0g
Fat: 10g   Fiber: 0g
Protein: 5g   Net Carbs: 0g

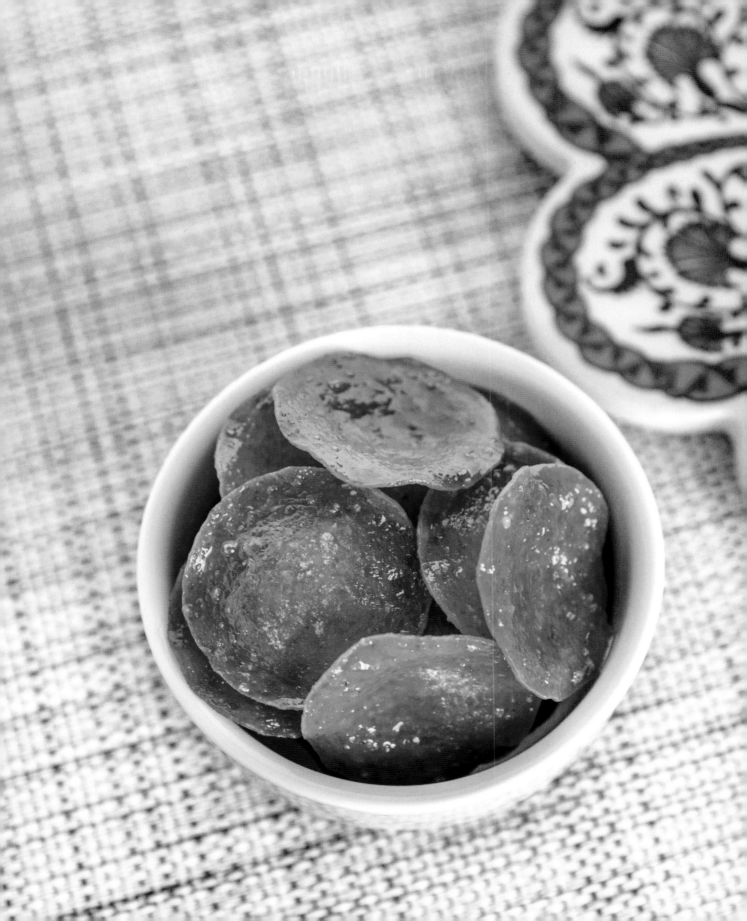

TUNA AVOCADO TACOS

MAKES 6 tacos (2 per serving)   PREP TIME: 2 minutes (not including time to make tuna salad)   COOK TIME: —

This dish was inspired by a fellow Instagrammer, Maggie Sterling (@lowcarbllama). When I first saw it, I thought to myself, "Wow, I'm so dumb for not thinking of that." Then I posted it to my Instagram feed (@ketomadesimple), and almost every commenter said the very same thing: such a genius idea that needs to be shared with the keto world! Feel free to jazz up these tacos however you like. Any type of tuna mixture or sliced cheese will get the job done.

INGREDIENTS

½ batch Tuna Avocado Salad (page 78)

6 slices provolone cheese (about 5 ounces)

Everything bagel seasoning, for garnish (optional)

DIRECTIONS

Place 2 tablespoons of tuna salad in each cheese slice and eat it like a taco! Sprinkle some everything bagel seasoning on the salad, if desired.

Nutritional information (per serving)

Calories: 652	Total Carbs: 6g
Fat: 44g	Fiber: 3g
Protein: 55g	Net Carbs: 3g

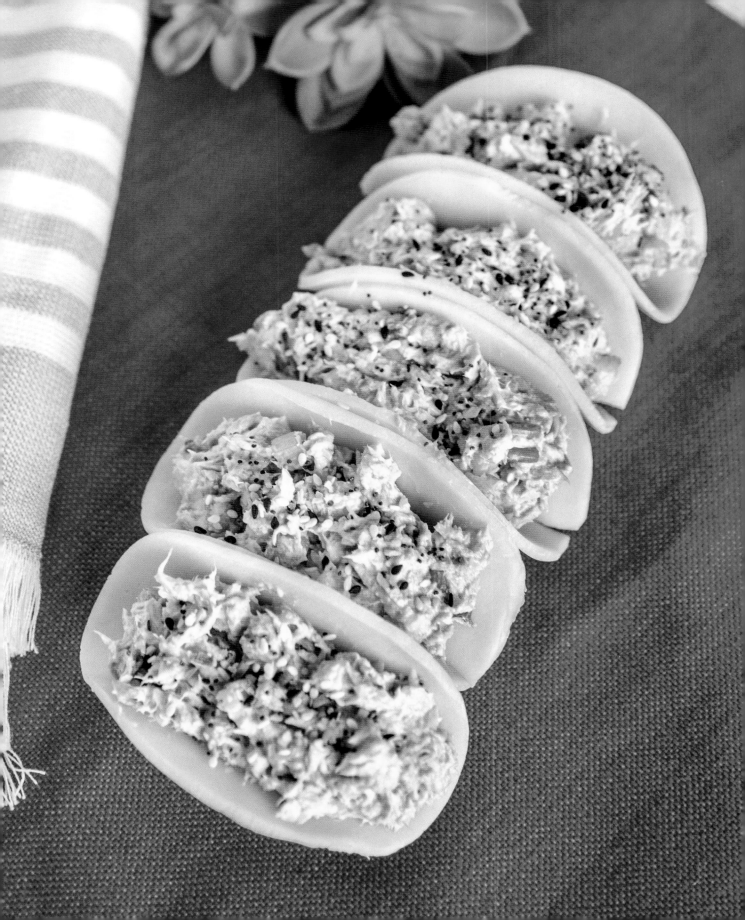

SWEDISH MEATBALLS

MAKES 24 meatballs (4 per serving)   PREP TIME: 15 minutes   COOK TIME: 20 minutes

Meatballs are a great keto dish—plenty of fat, tons of flavor, and awesome for meal prep! The sauce in this recipe is creamy, tangy, and perfect for the meatballs.

INGREDIENTS

FOR THE MEATBALLS:

1 pound bulk (ground) Italian sausage

1 pound ground beef

1 large egg

½ teaspoon salt

¼ teaspoon ground black pepper

¼ teaspoon ground nutmeg

2 tablespoons extra-virgin olive oil or unsalted butter, for the pan

FOR THE SAUCE:

1½ cups beef bone broth

½ cup sour cream

2 ounces cream cheese (¼ cup)

2 teaspoons prepared yellow mustard

1 tablespoon Worcestershire sauce

½ teaspoon onion powder

Chopped fresh parsley, for garnish

DIRECTIONS

1. Make the meatballs: Place the sausage, ground beef, egg, salt, pepper, and nutmeg in a large bowl and mix thoroughly with your hands to combine. Be careful not to overmix; you don't want the meatballs to be tough.

2. Form the meat mixture into twenty-four 1½-inch balls, rolling each portion between the palms of your hands to get a nice round shape.

3. Heat the oil in a large skillet over medium-high heat. Once hot, add the meatballs. Do not crowd the pan; you want to give the meatballs some room to brown. Try to keep about 1 inch of space between them. Cook them in batches if necessary.

4. Cook the meatballs for 6 to 9 minutes, turning them frequently, until browned on all sides. They do not need to be fully cooked at this point; you will add them back to the pan with the sauce to finish cooking. Remove the meatballs from the pan and set aside.

5. Make the sauce: In the same skillet, whisk together the sauce ingredients until well combined. Bring to a boil.

6. When the sauce is boiling, return the meatballs to the pan. Simmer for 10 to 12 minutes, uncovered, until the meatballs are cooked all the way through.

7. Garnish with parsley and serve.

8. Store leftovers in the refrigerator for up to 5 days or freeze for up to 1 month. Reheat in a skillet or in the microwave.

Nutritional information (per serving)

Calories: 527	Total Carbs: 2g
Fat: 42g	Fiber: 0g
Protein: 32g	Net Carbs: 2g

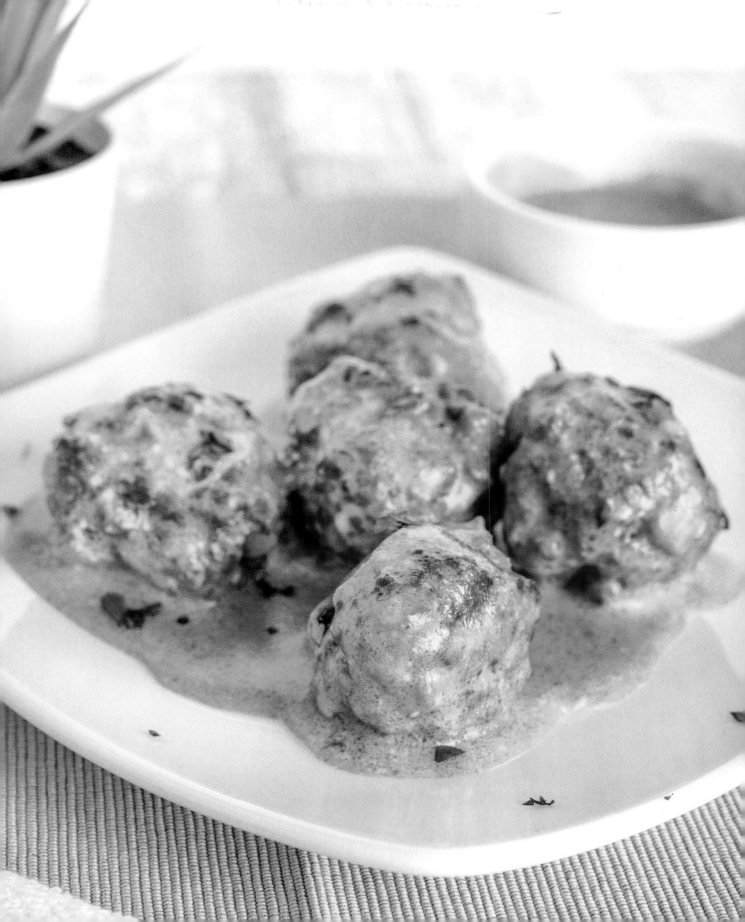

SMOKED GOUDA FONDUE

MAKES 8 servings (¼ cup per serving)   **PREP TIME: 3 minutes**   **COOK TIME: 15 minutes**

Do you have a fondue pot? Yeah, me neither. The good news is that you don't need one for this recipe. Simply place the fondue over low heat on the stovetop to keep it gooey and melty. Serve it with chicken, kielbasa, bell peppers, or bacon chips. Also, don't be afraid to substitute different cheeses if there's something you like better. The possibilities are endless here!

INGREDIENTS

¾ cup chicken bone broth

2 teaspoons lemon juice

½ teaspoon xanthan gum

8 ounces smoked Gouda cheese, shredded (about 2 cups)

6 ounces Gruyère cheese, shredded (about 1½ cups)

DIRECTIONS

1. In a medium-sized saucepan, whisk together the broth, lemon juice, and xanthan gum and bring to a boil over high heat.

2. After the broth mixture reaches a boil, reduce the heat to low. Slowly add the cheeses, ½ cup at a time, stirring until completely melted before adding more cheese.

3. Serve the fondue with your favorite meats or veggies for dipping.

4. Store leftovers in the refrigerator for up to 1 week. Reheat in a saucepan over low heat.

Nutritional information (per serving)

Calories: 186	Total Carbs: 1g
Fat: 14g	Fiber: 1g
Protein: 13g	Net Carbs: 0g

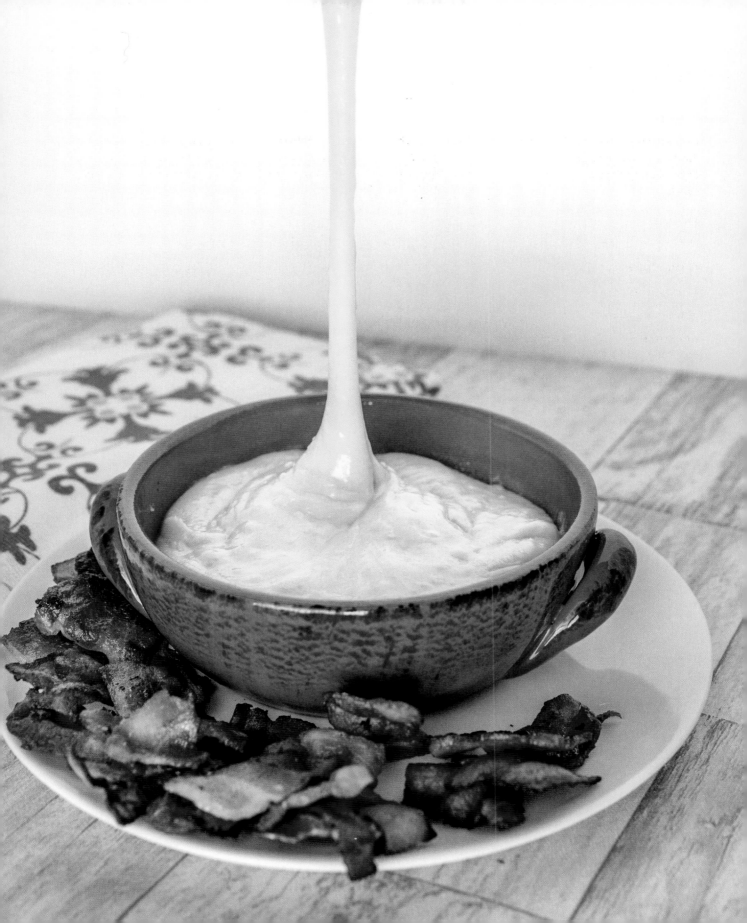

GAVIN'S GUAC

MAKES 8 servings (about 2 cups)   **PREP TIME: 5 minutes**   **COOK TIME:** —

I grew up in San Diego, where avocados grow freely in people's backyards. I've used this same recipe since I was in high school; it's just that good! The drizzle of olive oil adds an incredibly rich and buttery texture. I named this beautiful guacamole after our oldest son because he is the avocado king and begs for guac every chance he gets.

INGREDIENTS

4 to 5 medium-sized ripe avocados

2 cloves garlic, minced

¼ cup diced red onions

¼ cup diced tomatoes

Juice of ½ lime

¼ to ½ teaspoon salt

2 tablespoons chopped fresh cilantro

Drizzle of extra-virgin olive oil

DIRECTIONS

1. Cut the avocados in half lengthwise. Remove the pits and discard. Scoop the flesh of the avocados into a large mixing bowl. Mash with a fork.

2. Gently fold in the rest of the ingredients. I say "gently" because you don't want to crush the tomatoes. (And I think it looks pretty when there are a few large chunks of avocado in the guac.)

3. Serve or store leftovers in the refrigerator for up to 3 days. When storing, place plastic wrap directly on top of the guac and gently press down so that there is no air. This will keep your guac from browning.

Nutritional information (per serving)

Calories: 133	Total Carbs: 7g
Fat: 12g	Fiber: 5g
Protein: 2g	Net Carbs: 2g

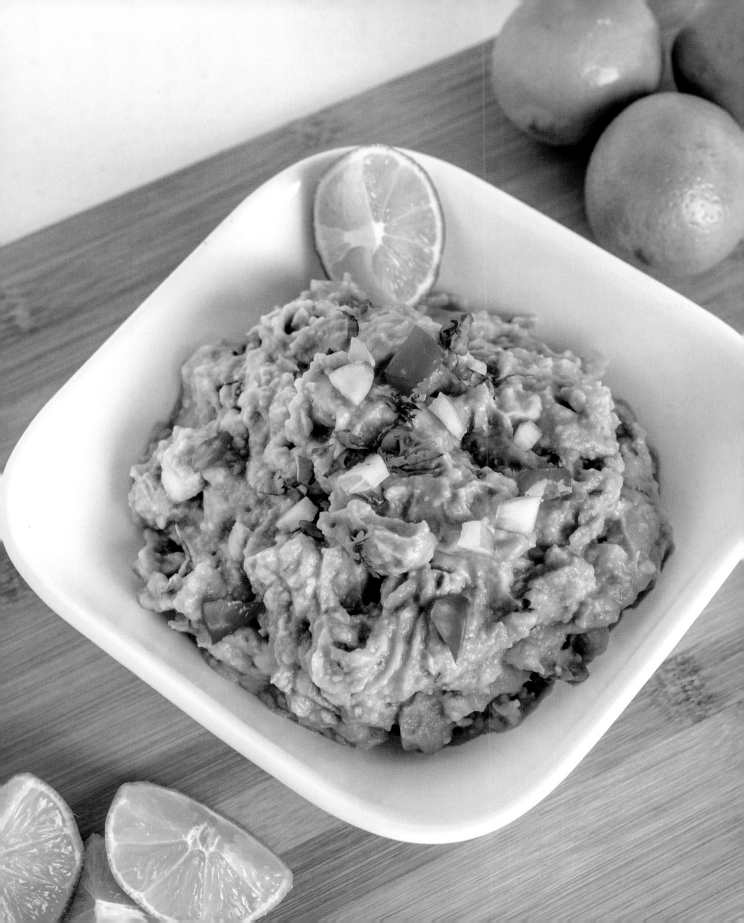

BEST 90-SECOND BREAD EVER

MAKES 1 serving   PREP TIME: 5 minutes   COOK TIME: 1½ minutes

In my early keto days, I tried every single 90-second bread recipe I could find. None of them even came close to curbing my bread cravings. They were all dry, chalky, and disappointing. I almost gave up and surrendered to the fact that I would never make a good bread substitute. Then I created this bad boy! I really think I nailed it with this one. It's buttery and breadlike and makes the perfect bun for any sandwich. It's been a huge hit with my social media followers, and I know you'll love it, too! This recipe is so versatile; feel free to get creative with how you use it. Two words: grilled cheese!

INGREDIENTS

Cooking spray

3 tablespoons blanched almond flour

1 large egg

½ teaspoon baking powder

3½ tablespoons unsalted butter, softened, divided

½ teaspoon granulated sweetener

1 teaspoon sour cream

1 tablespoon shredded mozzarella cheese

DIRECTIONS

1. Spray an 8-ounce ramekin or similar-sized shallow microwave-safe bowl with cooking spray. Set the ramekin aside.

2. Place the almond flour, egg, baking powder, 1½ tablespoons of the butter, the sweetener, sour cream, and cheese in a small mixing bowl. Mix well until the flour is evenly incorporated. The batter will be very thick and chunky because of the cheese.

3. Place the batter in the prepared ramekin and use the back of a spoon to smooth the top. Microwave on high for 90 seconds, or until the bread is fluffy and spongy.

4. Remove the ramekin from the microwave and flip it over to release the bread. When the bread is cool enough to handle, cut it in half.

5. To toast the bread, melt the remaining 2 tablespoons of butter in a skillet over medium-high heat. Put each half of the bread in the pan and cook until perfectly toasted, about 2 minutes. Flip and toast the other sides for 1 minute. Enjoy!

Nutritional information

Calories: 403   Total Carbs: 5g
Fat: 38g   Fiber: 2g
Protein: 14g   Net Carbs: 3g

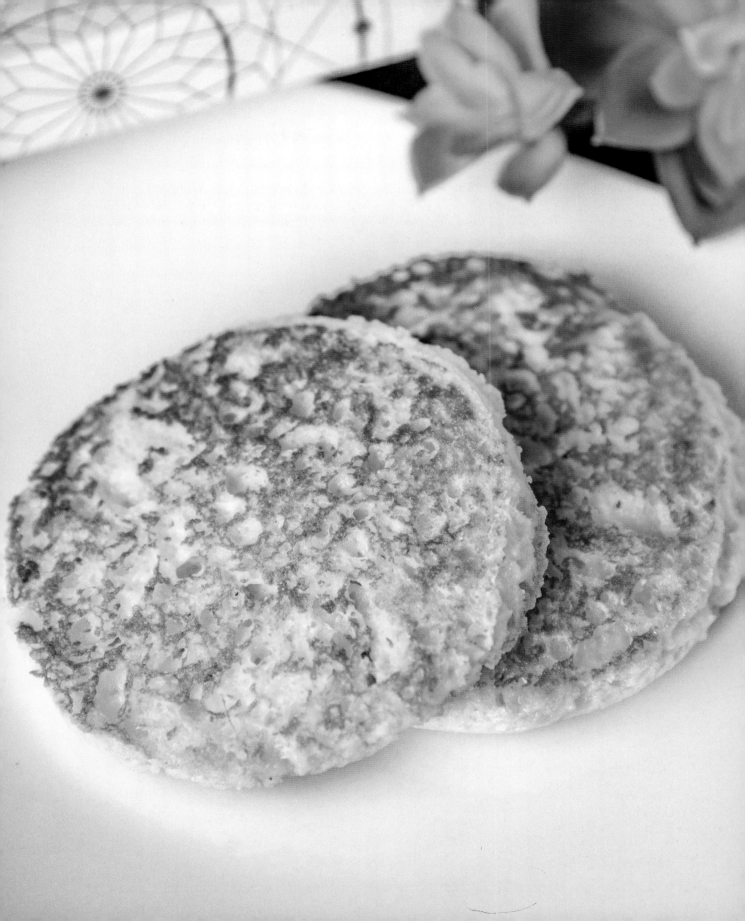

JALAPEÑO CHEESE CRISPS

MAKES 8 crisps (4 per serving)   PREP TIME: 2 minutes   COOK TIME: 5 to 10 minutes

In my early keto days, I struggled to find a quick but satisfying snack that took minimal effort. Then I started making these babies. This quickly turned into a phase where I ate these crisps every day for lunch. Plus, the jalapeños will set your mouth on fire, making you drink more water! These crisps are perfect for dipping in sour cream or ranch dressing.

INGREDIENTS

3 ounces cheddar cheese, shredded (about ¾ cup)

8 jalapeño pepper slices

DIRECTIONS

1. Preheat a large nonstick skillet or griddle over medium-high heat (about 350°F if using an electric griddle).

2. Using your fingers, grab about a tablespoon of the cheese and place in the skillet. Put a slice of jalapeño on top of the cheese, then cover with another tablespoon of cheese. Repeat, making a total of 4 piles.

3. Cook for 2 minutes, or until the cheese is stiff enough to flip. Flip the cheese over and cook until melted and starting to crisp, about 2 minutes.

4. Repeat, making another 4 crisps with the remaining cheese and jalapeño slices. Serve immediately.

Nutritional information (per serving)

Calories: 128	**Total Carbs:** 2g
Fat: 10g	**Fiber:** 0g
Protein: 8g	**Net Carbs:** 2g

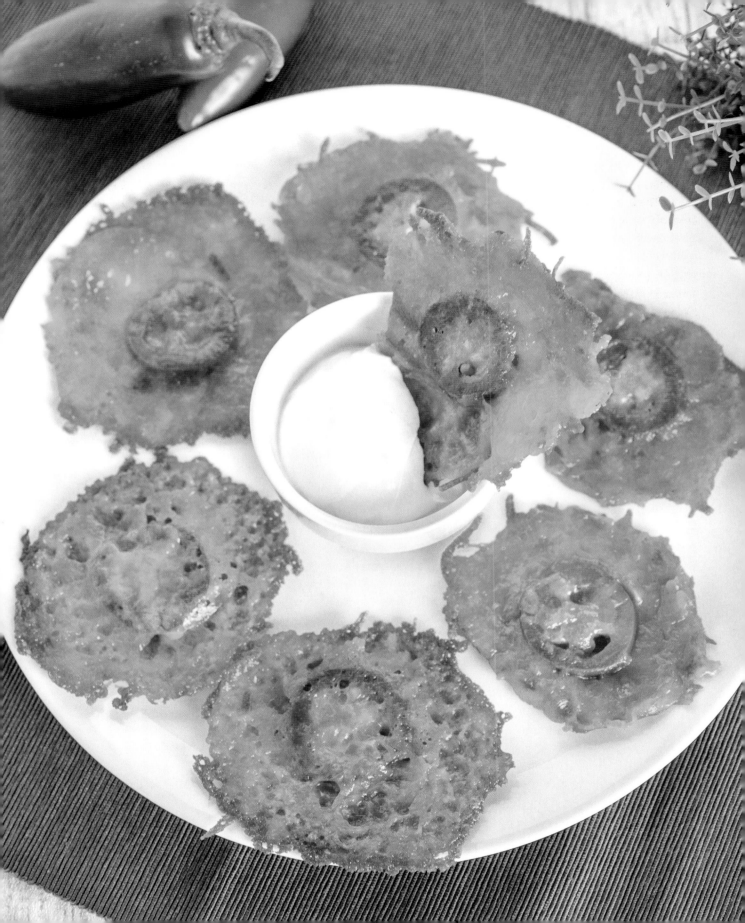

BACON CHEESE DIP

MAKES 5 servings (½ cup per serving)   **PREP TIME:** 5 minutes (not including time to cook bacon)   **COOK TIME:** —

You cannot go wrong with this dip—bacon, cheese, and more cheese! This stuff is a total crowd-pleaser, so plan on making it for your next party. You may even want to double the recipe. It's that good. I like to serve it with Cheese Crackers (page 82).

INGREDIENTS

1 (8-ounce) package cream cheese, softened

1 cup mayonnaise

8 ounces cheddar cheese, shredded (about 2 cups)

½ cup chopped green onions

¾ cup cooked and crumbled bacon (about 6 slices)

½ teaspoon garlic powder

DIRECTIONS

1. Place all the ingredients in a large bowl. Stir until everything is well combined.

2. Store leftovers in the refrigerator for up to 6 days. Reheat in the microwave or eat it cold!

Nutritional information (per serving)

Calories: 724	Total Carbs: 4g
Fat: 68g	Fiber: 0g
Protein: 22g	Net Carbs: 4g

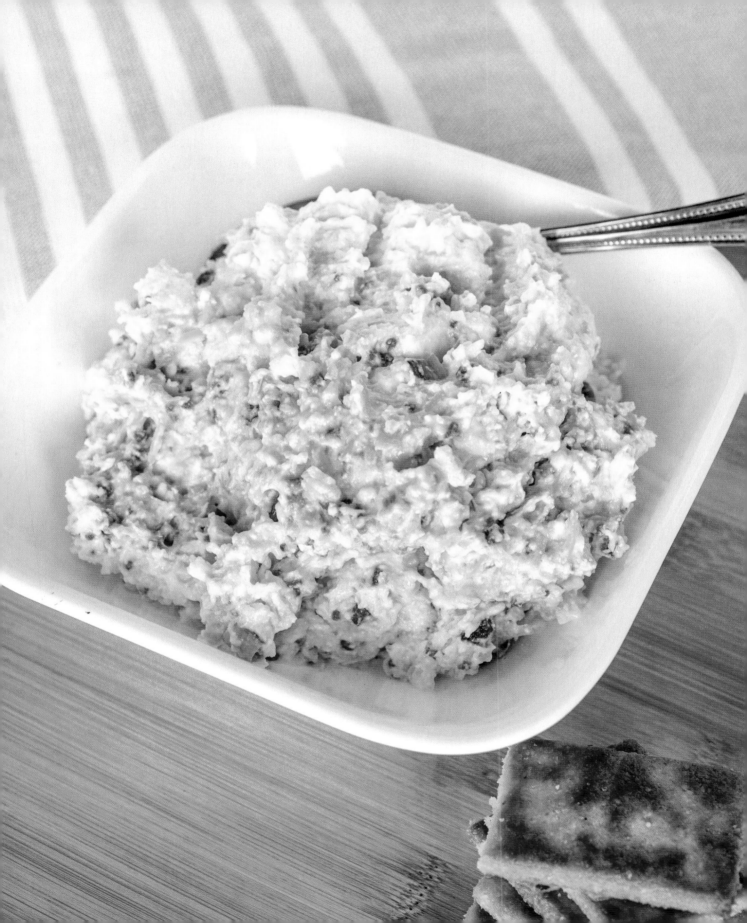

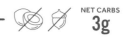

SPINACH ARTICHOKE DIP

MAKES 6 servings (½ cup per serving)   **PREP TIME: 8 minutes**   **COOK TIME: 25 minutes**

When I think of game-day food, spinach artichoke dip is the first thing that comes to my mind. It's the perfect dish to serve a crowd. Every time I make it, it's always the dish that everyone is gathered around, dipping away! Serve with Cheese Crackers (page 82).

INGREDIENTS

1 (10-ounce) bag frozen spinach

2 cups shredded Parmesan cheese (about 8 ounces)

1 (14-ounce) can quartered artichoke hearts

⅔ cup sour cream

⅓ cup mayonnaise

1 (8-ounce) package cream cheese, softened

¼ cup (½ stick) unsalted butter, softened

½ teaspoon garlic powder

DIRECTIONS

1. Preheat the oven to 375°F.

2. Thaw the spinach in the microwave according to the package instructions (usually 4 to 6 minutes on high).

3. Meanwhile, place the Parmesan cheese and artichoke hearts in a large bowl. The artichokes should be in small chunks, so you may need to chop them smaller than they come in the can.

4. When the spinach is done, remove it from the microwave and empty it into a clean dish towel. Squeeze out the excess liquid and then add the spinach to the artichoke mixture. Set aside.

5. In a small bowl, mix together the remaining ingredients until well incorporated.

6. Add the sour cream mixture to the spinach and artichoke mixture and stir to combine. Transfer to an 8-inch square or similar-sized baking dish. (The pan shown in the photo is 6 by 10 inches, but that size is really hard to find.)

7. Bake for 25 minutes, or until the top is golden brown and the cheese is melted.

8. Store leftovers in the refrigerator for up to 5 days. Reheat in the microwave or oven.

Nutritional information (per serving)

Calories: 470   Total Carbs: 7g
Fat: 42g   Fiber: 4g
Protein: 17g   Net Carbs: 3g

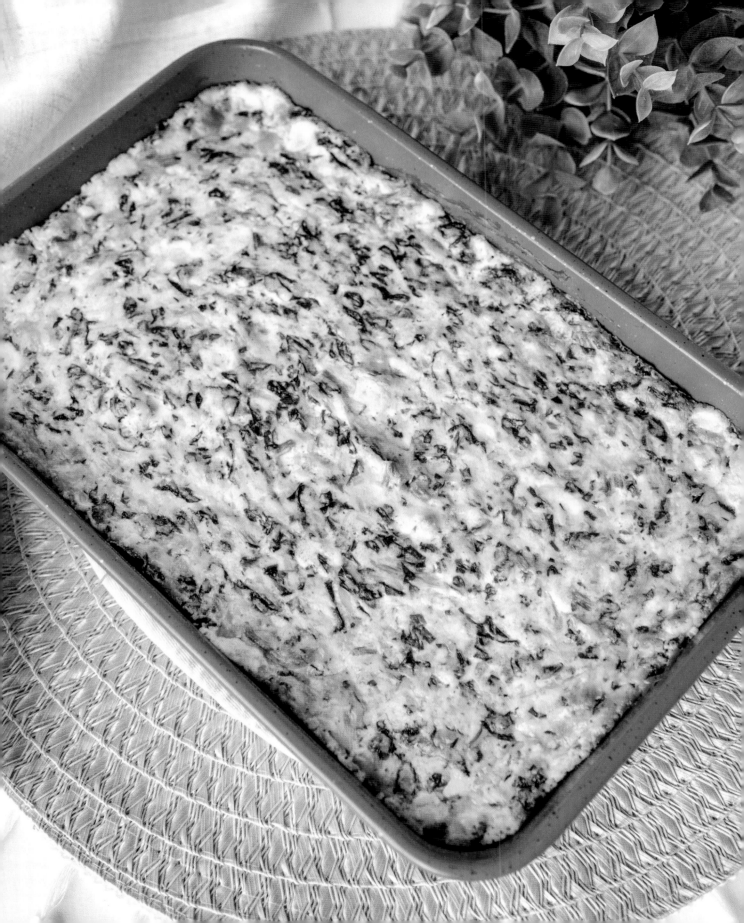

TUNA AVOCADO SALAD

NET CARBS
1g

MAKES 2 servings   **PREP TIME:** 5 minutes   **COOK TIME:** —

Canned tuna is one of those foods that we always keep in our pantry. It's such a quick and easy thing to have on hand when you don't feel like making anything extravagant. Adding avocado and celery really makes this dish fresh! Serve the salad alone, in cheese or lettuce wraps, or even as a dip for bell peppers when you're in the mood for some crunch.

INGREDIENTS

2 (5-ounce) cans tuna packed in water, drained

3 tablespoons mayonnaise

1 teaspoon prepared yellow mustard

1 stalk celery, chopped

1 green onion, chopped

¼ teaspoon garlic powder

¼ teaspoon onion powder

½ medium avocado, diced

DIRECTIONS

1. Place the tuna, mayonnaise, mustard, celery, green onion, garlic powder, and onion powder in a medium-sized bowl. Stir until everything is well combined.

2. Add the avocado and gently stir. Serve immediately or store leftovers in the refrigerator for up to 2 days.

Nutritional information (per serving)

Calories: 357	Total Carbs: 4g
Fat: 22g	Fiber: 3g
Protein: 34g	Net Carbs: 1g

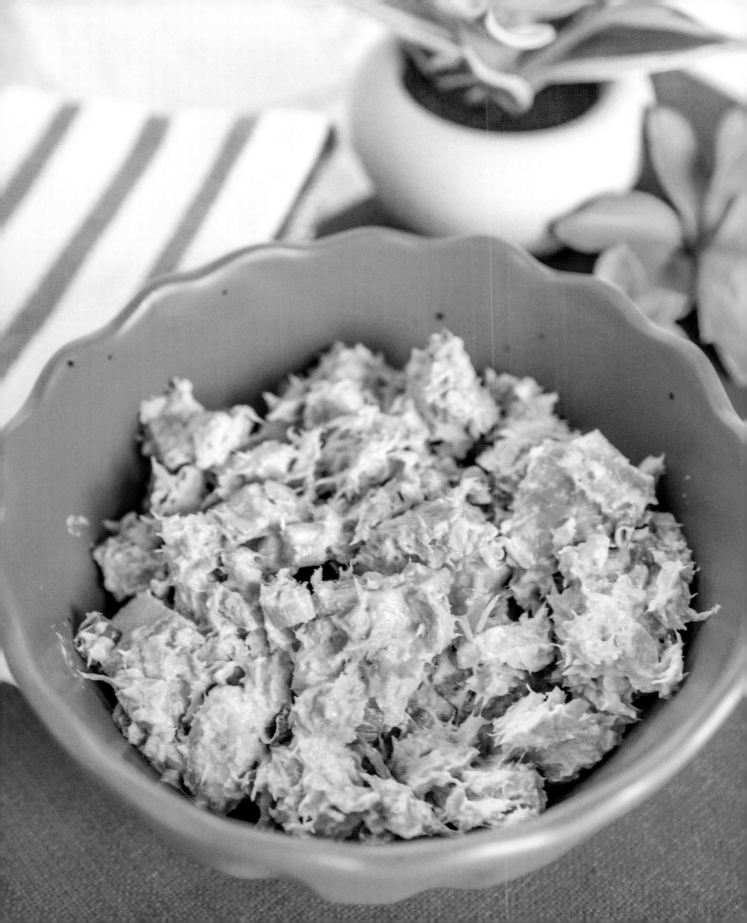

SAUSAGE-STUFFED MUSHROOMS

NET CARBS
3g

MAKES 14 mushrooms (2 per serving)   PREP TIME: 12 minutes   COOK TIME: 30 minutes

I've always been a huge mushroom fan. I got oddly excited recently when one of my boys decided that he was obsessed with mushrooms. He's the only other person in our family who will eat them, so this has become one of our favorite snacks to enjoy together. These are perfect for parties as well, even for the non-keto people in your life.

INGREDIENTS

2 tablespoons extra-virgin olive oil, for the pan

1 pound bulk (ground) breakfast sausage

¼ cup diced yellow onions

2 cloves garlic, minced

6 ounces cream cheese (¾ cup)

2 ounces Parmesan cheese, grated or shredded (about ½ cup)

¼ teaspoon red pepper flakes

Salt and ground black pepper

14 baby portobello mushrooms

2 tablespoons Savory Breadcrumbs (page 304)

Fresh flat-leaf parsley, for garnish (optional)

DIRECTIONS

1. Preheat the oven to 400°F.

2. Set a medium-sized skillet over medium-high heat. Coat the pan with the olive oil. Add the sausage, onions, and garlic and cook until the sausage is browned, about 10 minutes.

3. Add the cream cheese, Parmesan cheese, and red pepper flakes to the sausage and onion mixture. Cook until the cheeses are melted and everything is well incorporated, about 5 minutes. Sprinkle with salt and pepper. Set aside.

4. Remove the stem from each mushroom and wipe the entire mushroom with a damp paper towel. (This is the best way to clean mushrooms so the texture isn't compromised.)

5. Place the mushrooms cavity side up in an 8-inch square glass baking dish. Fill each mushroom with a spoonful of the stuffing. Top with the breadcrumbs.

6. Bake for 15 minutes, or until the tops are golden brown. Garnish with parsley, if desired, and serve!

7. Store leftovers in the refrigerator for up to 1 week. Reheat in the microwave or oven.

Nutritional information (per serving)

Calories: 383	Total Carbs: 3g
Fat: 32g	Fiber: 0g
Protein: 18g	Net Carbs: 3g

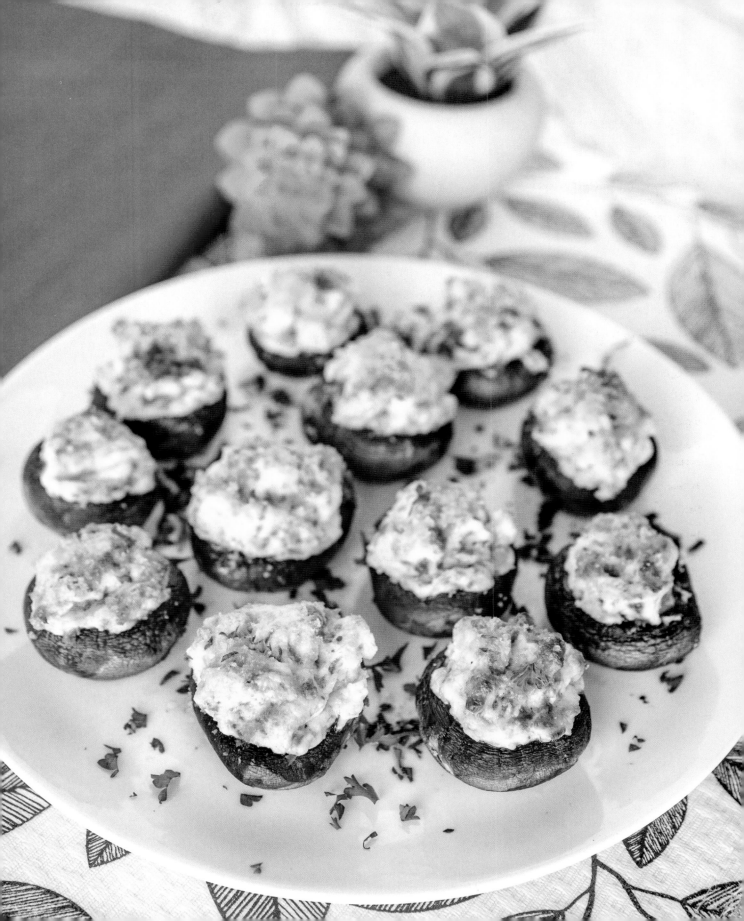

CHEESE CRACKERS

MAKES about 36 crackers (6 per serving)   PREP TIME: 15 minutes   COOK TIME: 15 minutes

These crackers make the perfect snack! Think flatbread meets Cheez-Its. The cheddar cheese gives these crackers the best flavor. You can make them as crispy or as breadlike as you want. The instructions below give you crunchy crackers. Want them to be more like flatbread bites? Roll the dough out thicker, and bake it for a little less time. Even non-keto eaters tend to love these.

INGREDIENTS

6 ounces cheddar cheese, shredded (about 1½ cups)

2 ounces Parmesan cheese, shredded (about ½ cup)

2 ounces cream cheese (¼ cup), softened

1 cup blanched almond flour

1 large egg

1 teaspoon garlic powder

½ teaspoon Italian seasoning

½ teaspoon salt

DIRECTIONS

1. Preheat the oven to 425°F. Line a baking sheet with parchment paper.

2. Place the cheddar cheese, Parmesan cheese, and cream cheese in a large microwave-safe bowl; there is no need to stir yet. Microwave on high for 1 minute. Stir the cheeses with a fork, then microwave for another 30 seconds. Remove from the microwave and stir until well combined. The mixture should be very soft and gooey at this point. If it isn't, microwave it for another 15 seconds. Repeat as necessary until the mixture is very soft and gooey.

3. Add the almond flour and mix with your hands. The dough will be hot, so you may need to let it cool for a minute before mixing. Squeeze the dough until the flour mixes in completely. It may take a couple minutes to get it to fully incorporate.

4. Add the egg, garlic powder, Italian seasoning, and salt. Mix until the egg and seasonings are fully incorporated. If the dough starts sticking to your hands, wet your hands slightly and then continue to work the dough.

5. Once the dough is mixed, place the dough on the lined baking sheet. Take another piece of parchment paper and place it on top of the dough. Using a rolling pin or your hands, flatten the dough evenly until it reaches the thickness of a cracker (about ⅛ inch thick).

6. Remove the top piece of parchment paper and use a pizza cutter to cut the dough into 1½-inch-wide strips. Then make horizontal cuts, forming small squares. Pull the squares apart slightly.

7. Bake for 7 minutes. Flip the squares over and bake for another 5 to 7 minutes, depending on the desired crunch. (The longer they bake, the crunchier they will be.) Eat them hot or let them cool on the baking sheet before enjoying.

8. Store leftovers in the refrigerator for up to 1 week.

Nutritional information (per serving)
Calories: 269   Total Carbs: 5g
Fat: 22g   Fiber: 2g
Protein: 15g   Net Carbs: 3g

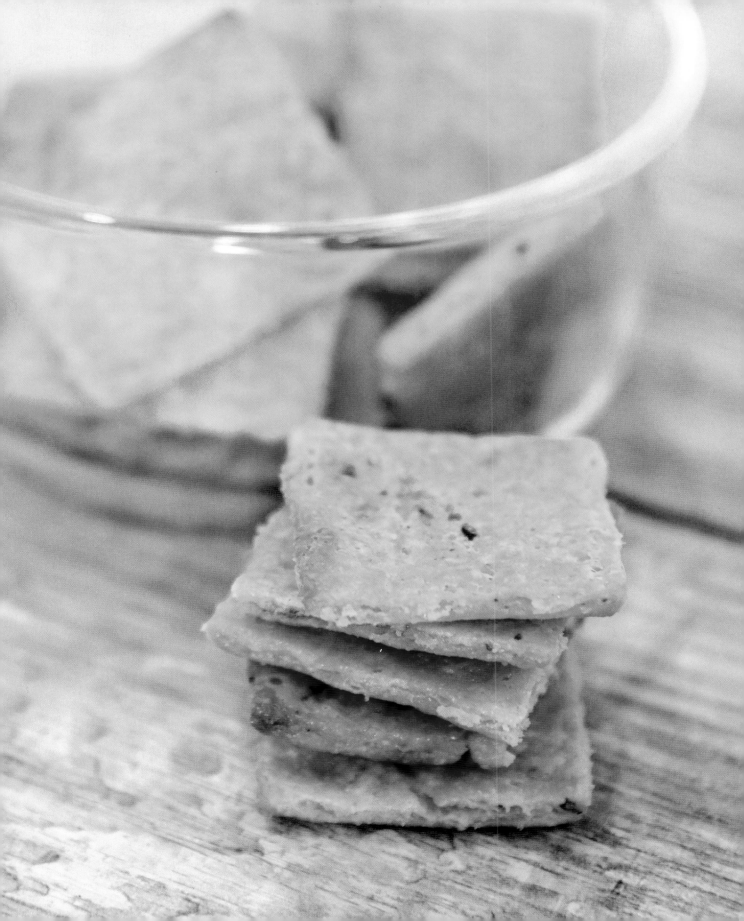

THE BEST DAMN DEVILED EGGS

MAKES 12 deviled eggs (4 per serving)   PREP TIME: 10 minutes (not including time to hard-boil eggs)   COOK TIME: —

I don't know about you, but we cannot keep deviled eggs in our house for more than 30 minutes. If I leave these on the counter, the kids turn into vultures. The eggs can be made a million different ways. Here's my favorite version—the sweetener counteracts the heat from the hot sauce and adds such a nice touch. I hope you love them, too!

NET CARBS
1g

INGREDIENTS

6 large hard-boiled eggs

2 tablespoons mayonnaise

1 tablespoon granulated sweetener (optional)

1 teaspoon prepared yellow mustard

1 teaspoon Worcestershire sauce

1 teaspoon hot sauce (optional)

Salt and ground black pepper

Paprika, for garnish

DIRECTIONS

1. Slice the eggs in half lengthwise. Empty the yolks into a small mixing bowl. Set the whites aside.

2. Add the mayonnaise, sweetener (if using), mustard, Worcestershire, and hot sauce (if using) to the bowl with the yolks. Sprinkle with salt and pepper. Mix well with a fork until the ingredients are well incorporated.

3. Place the yolk mixture in a small resealable plastic bag, then cut off a small portion of one corner of the bag. Pipe some of the yolk mixture into each egg white so that the cavity is completely filled.

4. Garnish the deviled eggs with paprika and serve!

5. Store leftovers in the refrigerator for up to 5 days.

Nutritional information (per serving)

Calories: 208	Total Carbs: 1g
Fat: 16g	Fiber: 0g
Protein: 13g	Net Carbs: 1g

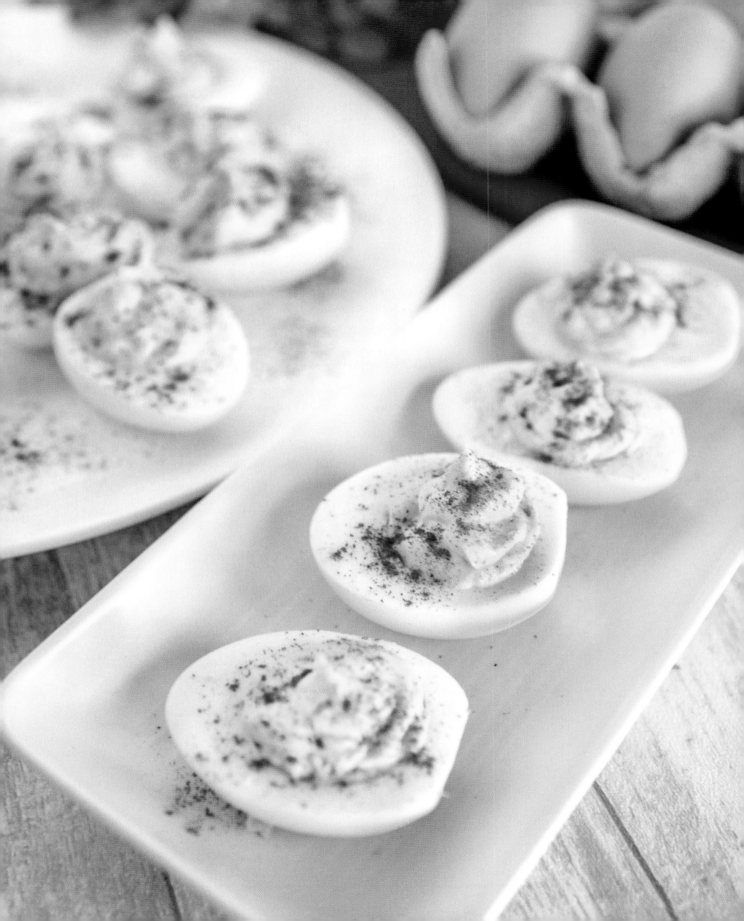

BBQ JALAPEÑO POPPERS

MAKES 20 poppers (4 per serving)   PREP TIME: 30 minutes   COOK TIME: 50 minutes

Jalapeño poppers have always been a favorite of mine, even in my pre-keto days. There are a million different recipes out there, and I'm convinced that they are all delicious. However, this one uses BBQ sauce, and you just can't get better than that!

INGREDIENTS

10 large jalapeño peppers

1 (8-ounce) package cream cheese, softened

4 ounces cheddar cheese, shredded (about 1 cup)

1 tablespoon garlic powder

1 tablespoon onion powder

4 to 5 slices bacon, cut in half crosswise

¾ cup sugar-free BBQ sauce

DIRECTIONS

1. Preheat the oven to 300°F. Line a rimmed baking sheet with aluminum foil for easy cleanup.

2. While wearing gloves (trust me on this!), cut the jalapeños in half lengthwise. Scoop out the seeds and veins. (That's where all the heat is, so if you don't like heat, make sure to get them all out!)

3. In a mixing bowl, mix together the cheeses, garlic powder, and onion powder until everything is well incorporated.

4. Place a spoonful of the cheese mixture in each hollowed-out jalapeño half. Depending on the size of your jalapeños, you'll use 1 to 2 tablespoons of the cheese mixture per pepper half.

5. Wrap a half-slice of bacon around each filled jalapeño and secure with a toothpick. Place on the lined baking sheet.

6. Bake for 45 minutes, or until the tops are golden brown.

7. Remove the baking sheet from the oven and turn the oven to the broil setting.

8. While the oven is heating, brush the jalapeños with the BBQ sauce. Broil for 5 minutes, or until the bacon is cooked to your desired doneness, then serve.

9. Store leftovers in the refrigerator for up to 1 week. Reheat in the oven to keep the bacon crispy.

Nutritional information (per serving)

Calories: 317	Total Carbs: 9g
Fat: 25g	Fiber: 1g
Protein: 12g	Net Carbs: 8g

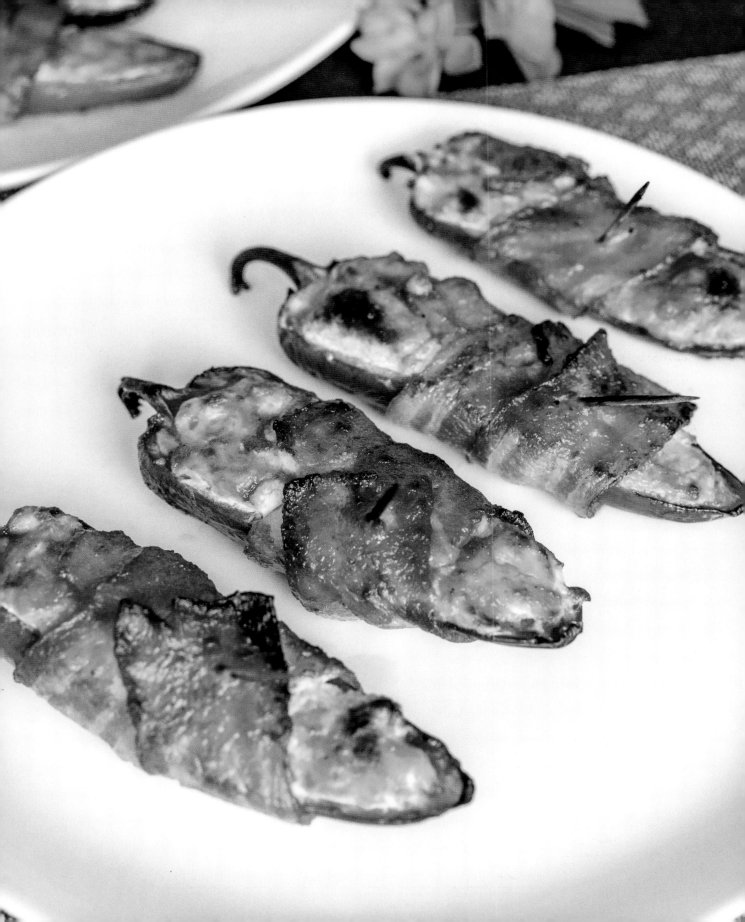

OVEN-BAKED CHEESY TUNA BITES

MAKES 20 mini muffins or 10 standard-size muffins (2 mini/1 standard muffin per serving) PREP TIME: 15 minutes   COOK TIME: 15 minutes

This combination sounds incredibly weird, but my kids love these things! They are perfect for making in advance and then grabbing on the go. Or pack them in lunches. They are good hot or cold, so they make a super-versatile snack. I always use a mini muffin pan for this recipe because we like them bite-sized, but you can use a regular-size muffin pan if you prefer.

INGREDIENTS

Cooking spray

2 (5-ounce) cans tuna packed in water

4 large eggs

1 ounce cheddar cheese, shredded (about ¼ cup), plus more for topping if desired

2 tablespoons grated Parmesan cheese

2 tablespoons heavy whipping cream

¼ teaspoon garlic powder

¼ teaspoon onion powder

Pinch of salt

Pinch of ground black pepper

Special Equipment (optional):
Mini muffin pan

DIRECTIONS

1. Preheat the oven to 350°F. Spray 20 wells of a mini muffin pan or 10 wells of a standard-size muffin pan with cooking spray. (If your mini muffin pan has fewer than 20 wells, you'll need to bake the muffins in batches.)

2. Open the cans of tuna, then drain and discard all the liquid; make sure to get out as much liquid as possible.

3. Place all the ingredients in a large bowl. Using a fork, stir until everything is well incorporated.

4. Spoon the tuna mixture into the greased wells of the muffin pan, filling them three-quarters full. If desired, top each muffin with a small amount of shredded cheddar.

5. Bake for 15 to 20 minutes, or until the eggs are fully cooked and the bites are firm, with a muffin-like texture. (Regular-sized muffins will take closer to 20 minutes, and mini muffins will take closer to 15 minutes.) Serve hot or cold!

6. Store leftovers in the refrigerator for up to 5 days. If desired, reheat in the oven.

Nutritional information (per serving)

Calories: 84	Total Carbs: 0g
Fat: 5g	Fiber: 0g
Protein: 10g	Net Carbs: 0g

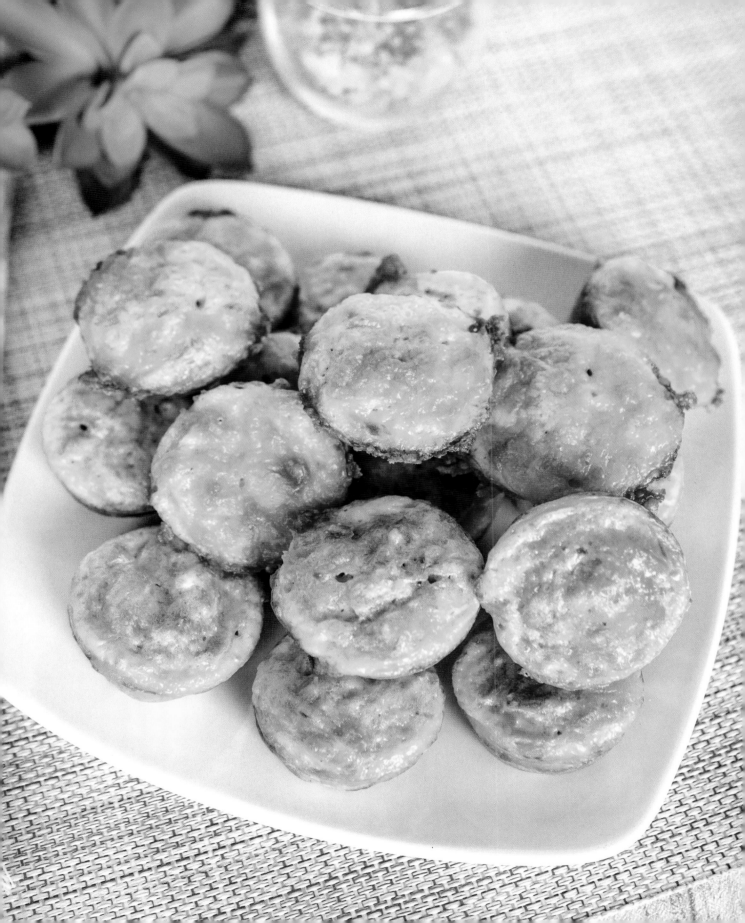

PORK BELLY STRIPS

MAKES 2 servings   PREP TIME: 5 minutes   COOK TIME: 28 minutes

I had seen pork belly at Costco, but I'd never bought it because it intimidated me. I mean, obviously it's very similar to bacon, but I always feared that I wouldn't cook it correctly. I don't know why I waited so long! Pork belly is honestly my favorite cut of meat, and here's why: it's super fatty and incredibly easy to make, and you can eat it for breakfast, lunch, or dinner. It also helps that the flavor is out of this world. Don't be afraid to play around with pork belly. I promise it'll be your new favorite meat.

INGREDIENTS

6 to 8 strips thick-cut raw pork belly (about 1 pound)

1 tablespoon smoked paprika

1 teaspoon granulated sweetener

1 teaspoon pink Himalayan salt

½ teaspoon ground black pepper

DIRECTIONS

1. Preheat the oven to 400°F.

2. Lay the strips of pork belly in a single layer in a 9 by 13-inch glass baking dish.

3. In a small bowl, mix together the paprika, sweetener, salt, and pepper. Sprinkle half of the mixture on the strips, then flip them over and sprinkle the other sides with the rest of the mixture.

4. Bake for 20 minutes, then turn the oven to the broil setting and broil for 6 to 8 minutes, until crispy. Remove from the oven and serve!

5. Store leftovers (psh, what leftovers?) in the refrigerator for up to 5 days. Reheat in a skillet with some butter or ghee.

Nutritional information (per serving)
Calories: 1173   Total Carbs: 1g
Fat: 120g   Fiber: 0g
Protein: 21g   Net Carbs: 1g

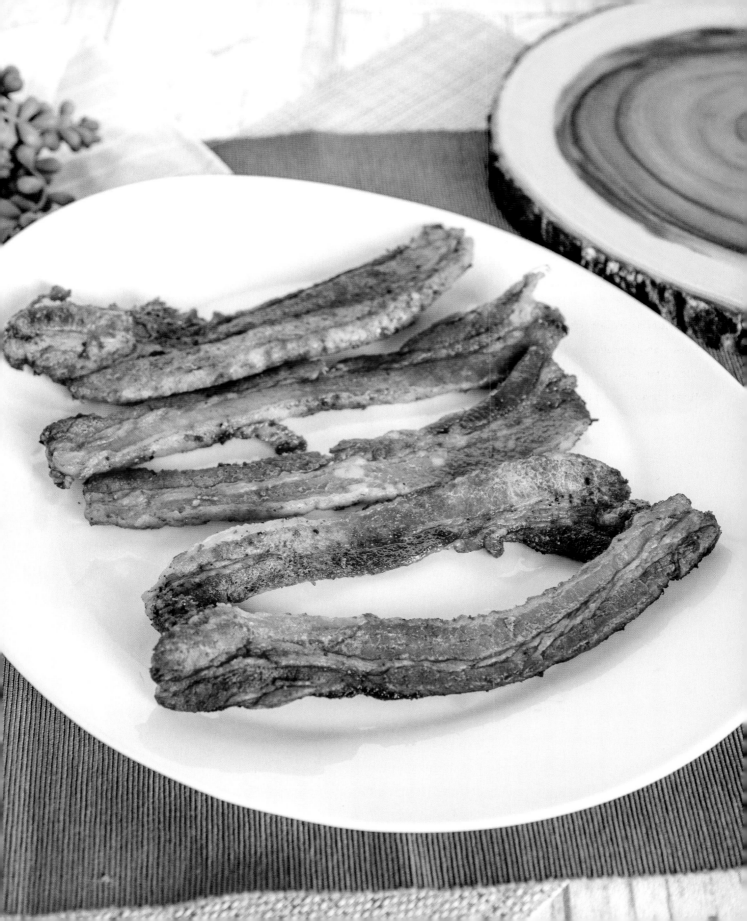

SPANAKOPITA BITES

MAKES 4 servings   **PREP TIME: 10 minutes**   **COOK TIME: 12 minutes**

I'll eat anything with feta cheese in it. I created these bad boys one day when I was trying to figure out a way to use up some kale we had in the fridge. I came up with these shockingly yummy and addicting bites! You could also use spinach in place of the kale for a more traditional take on this recipe.

INGREDIENTS

2 cups chopped kale

4 ounces Parmesan cheese, shredded or grated (about 1 cup)

6 ounces feta cheese, crumbled (about 1 cup)

½ teaspoon garlic powder

½ teaspoon onion powder

1 large egg

Special Equipment:
Food processor

DIRECTIONS

1. Preheat the oven to 400°F. Line a baking sheet with parchment paper or a silicone baking mat.

2. Place the kale, Parmesan, feta, garlic powder, and onion powder in a food processor and gently pulse until there are no large chunks.

3. Pour the mixture into a large bowl and add the egg. Stir until the egg is fully mixed in with everything else. The mixture will be crumbly at this point.

4. Place small clumps of the mixture, about the size of a cracker, on the lined baking sheet and form into rough circles. The clumps do not have to be perfectly formed into circles; rustic-looking clumps are just fine!

5. Bake for 10 to 12 minutes, until golden brown and the cheese is melted, then serve! Store leftovers in the refrigerator for up to 3 days. Reheat in the microwave or oven.

Nutritional information (per serving)

Calories: 250	Total Carbs: 5g
Fat: 18g	Fiber: 1g
Protein: 19g	Net Carbs: 4g

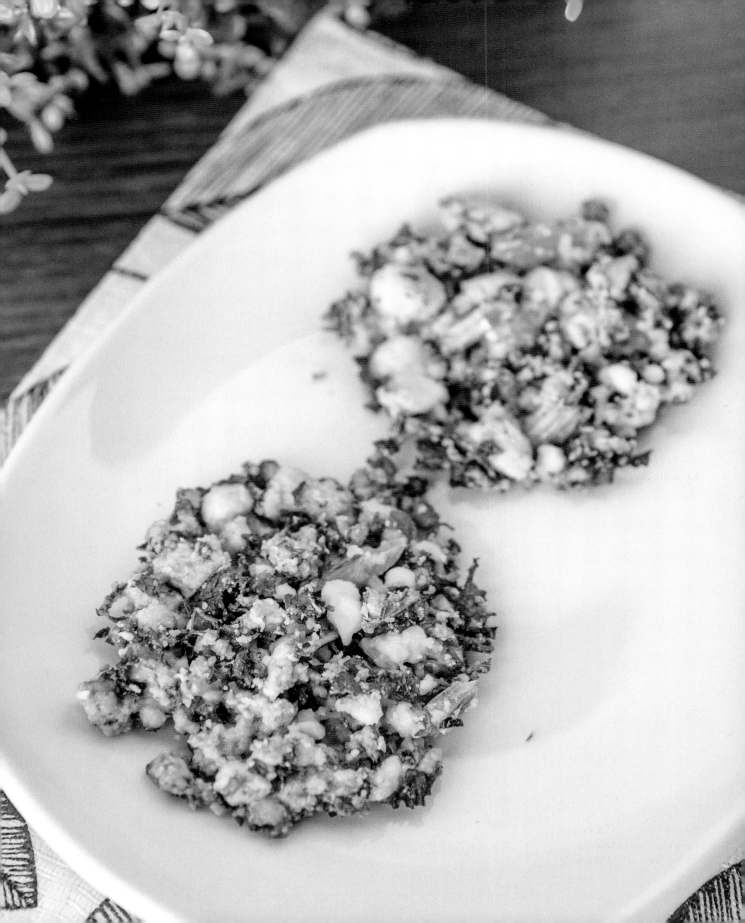

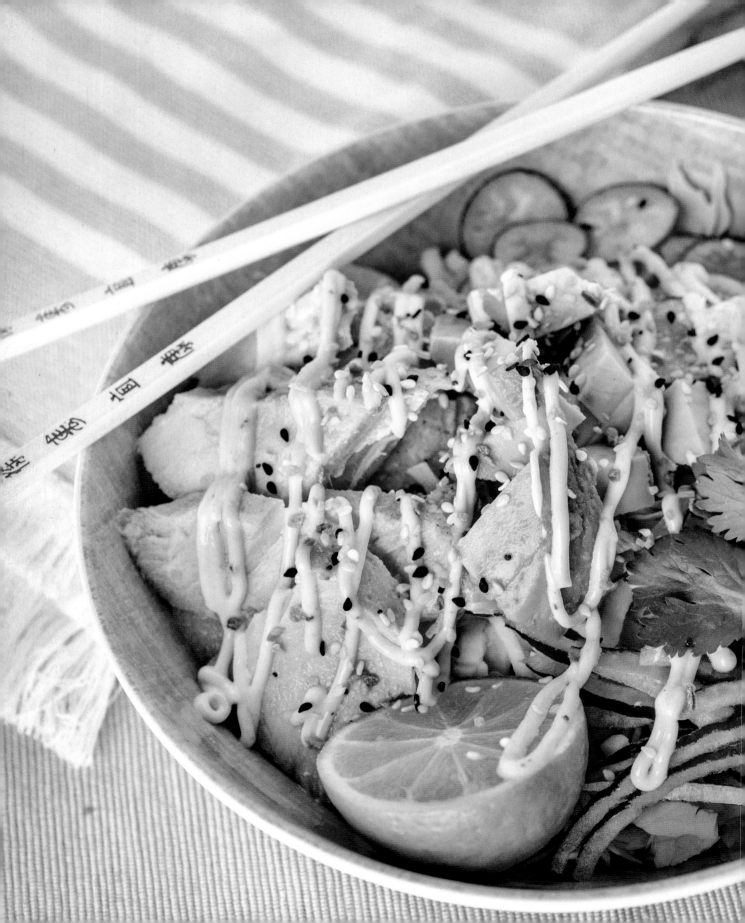

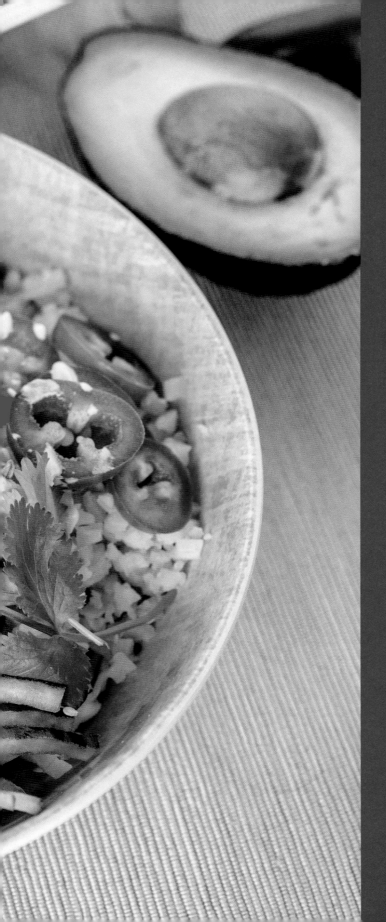

(3) SOUPS & SALADS

NET CARBS
6g

STRAWBERRY SPINACH SALAD

MAKES 4 servings   PREP TIME: 8 minutes   COOK TIME: —

This salad is a summer staple! It is not only beautiful and colorful, but also fresh and delicious. The dressing is tangy and sweet and an excellent way to add fats without being super heavy.

INGREDIENTS

1 (16-ounce) bag fresh spinach

6 to 8 fresh strawberries, sliced

¼ cup sliced or diced red onions

4 ounces feta cheese, crumbled (about ⅔ cup)

FOR THE DRESSING:

¼ cup extra-virgin olive oil

2 tablespoons unseasoned rice vinegar

¼ teaspoon garlic powder

¼ teaspoon granulated sweetener

Salt and ground black pepper

DIRECTIONS

1. Place the spinach, strawberries, onions, and feta cheese in a large bowl and toss to combine. Set aside.

2. Make the dressing: Place the oil, vinegar, garlic powder, and sweetener in a small bowl or dressing shaker. Sprinkle with salt and pepper and whisk together or shake until everything is mixed well.

3. Pour the dressing over the salad and eat immediately. (If you're making this dish in advance, wait to pour the dressing on top until you are ready to eat.) Store leftover salad and dressing in separate containers in the refrigerator for up to 1 week.

Nutritional information (per serving)

Calories: 242	Total Carbs: 9g
Fat: 21g	Fiber: 3g
Protein: 9g	Net Carbs: 6g

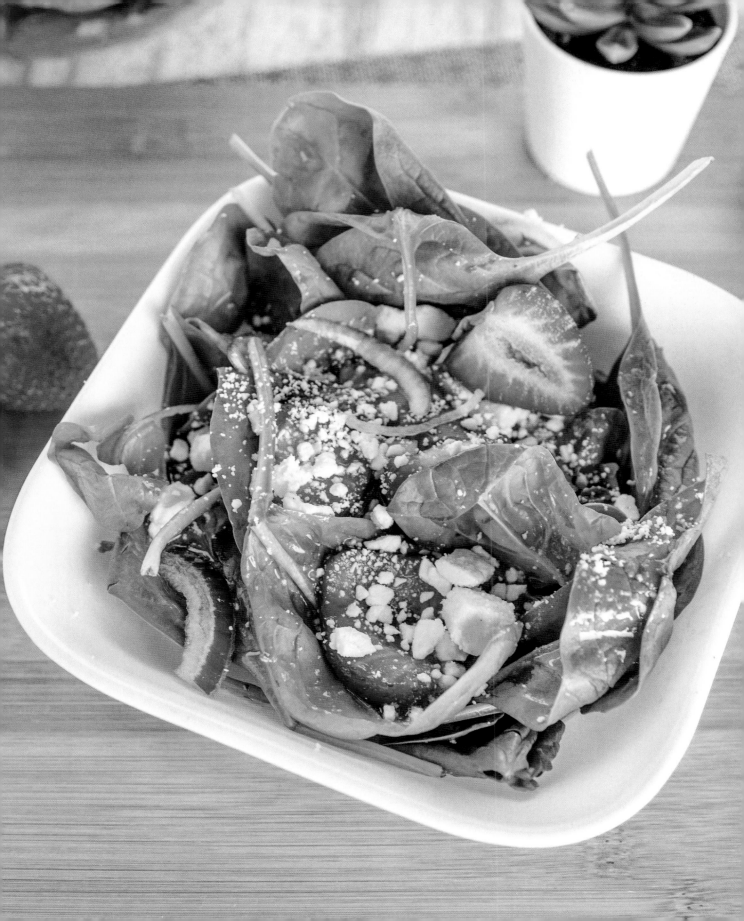

ZUPPA TOSCANA

NET CARBS
5g
OPTION OPTION

MAKES 6 servings   **PREP TIME: 10 minutes**   **COOK TIME: 35 minutes**

I've been using this recipe for years as a copycat version of Zuppa Toscana from the Olive Garden. (Best thing on their menu, if you ask me.) The only change I needed to make in order to make this soup keto-friendly was to replace the potatoes with cauliflower. This soup is so hearty and flavorful, and this is coming from someone who doesn't even like cauliflower!

INGREDIENTS

1 tablespoon unsalted butter or ghee

6 slices bacon, cut into bite-sized pieces

1 pound bulk (ground) hot or mild Italian sausage

1 medium yellow onion, diced

4 cloves garlic, minced

2 cups bite-sized fresh cauliflower florets

4 cups chicken bone broth

2 cups chopped kale

1 cup heavy whipping cream or coconut cream

½ teaspoon red pepper flakes (optional)

DIRECTIONS

1. In a 6-quart stockpot, melt the butter over medium-high heat. Add the bacon pieces and cook for 5 minutes, or until it reaches your desired doneness. Using a slotted spoon, remove the bacon to a paper towel–lined plate; leave as much bacon grease in the pan as possible. Set aside.

2. Add the sausage, onion, and garlic to the pot with the bacon grease and cook until the sausage is browned, about 10 minutes.

3. Add the cauliflower and broth. Simmer, uncovered, for 20 minutes, until the cauliflower has softened.

4. Add the kale and heavy cream and stir. Remove from the heat.

5. Top the soup with the bacon and red pepper flakes, if using, and serve immediately. Store leftovers in the refrigerator for up to 1 week. Reheat in a saucepan over medium heat.

Nutritional information (per serving)

Calories: 494	Total Carbs: 7g
Fat: 38g	Fiber: 2g
Protein: 25g	Net Carbs: 5g

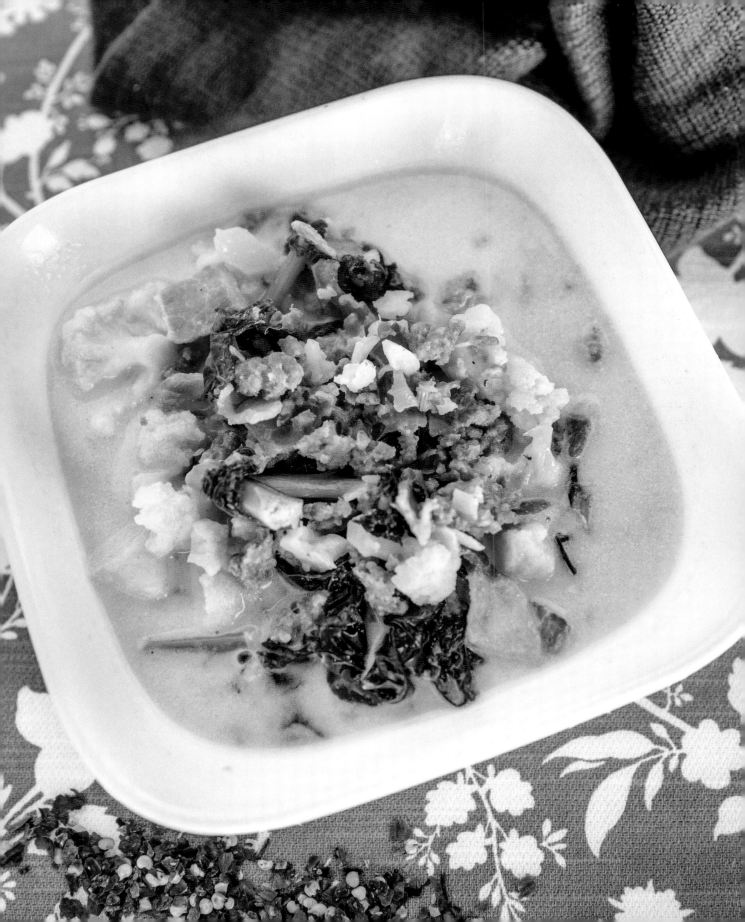

FRENCH ONION SOUP

MAKES 2 servings   PREP TIME: 10 minutes (not including time to make Caramelized Onions)   COOK TIME: 15 minutes

French onion soup was always one of my favorite things to order when dining out. If it weren't for that damn chunk of bread they put in it, I could probably still order it. Then again, I always trust homemade because I know exactly what I'm putting in the recipe. The flavors of this soup are perfect, and the cheesiness makes you forget that there's no bread! Although this version calls for provolone slices, you can use any cheese you like. I've made this with Gruyère, muenster, Brie, and Parmesan. All are amazing!

INGREDIENTS

2½ cups beef bone broth

2 tablespoons onion soup mix, store-bought or homemade (page 306)

1½ cups Caramelized Onions (page 298), divided

2 slices provolone cheese, plus extra shredded cheese for sprinkling

DIRECTIONS

1. Preheat the oven to the broil setting.

2. While the oven is heating, put the broth and soup mix in a medium-sized saucepan. Bring to a boil, then reduce the heat to low and simmer for 10 minutes.

3. Ladle the soup into two oven-safe mugs or bowls, filling them about three-fourths of the way to the top. Divide the caramelized onions evenly between the mugs, then top each with a sprinkle of shredded cheese.

4. Place a slice of provolone cheese on top of each mug so that it covers the opening. (It makes it look really pretty!) Then place the mugs on a rimmed baking sheet.

5. Broil for 3 to 5 minutes, until the cheese gets melty and bubbly. Serve immediately.

Nutritional information (per serving)

Calories: 369	Total Carbs: 10g
Fat: 30g	Fiber: 2g
Protein: 12g	Net Carbs: 8g

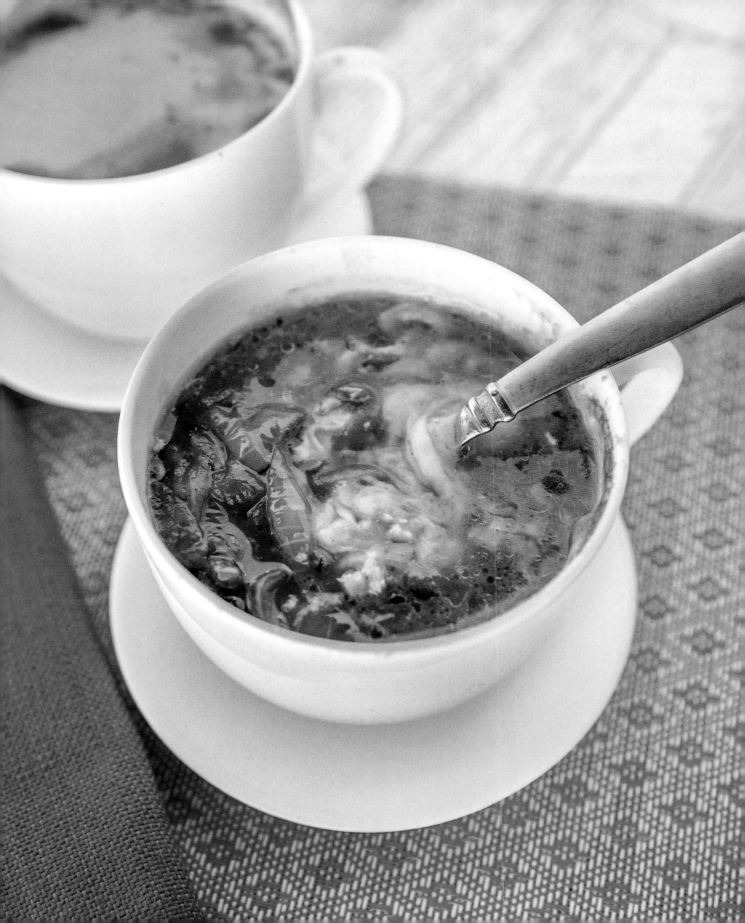

CLASSIC COLESLAW

MAKES 8 servings **PREP TIME: 10 minutes, plus 1 hour to chill** **COOK TIME: —**

This coleslaw quickly became a favorite around my house, as well as for my Instagram followers. We love it on pulled pork sandwiches made with Cheddar Cheese Buns (page 122), smothered in sugar-free BBQ sauce—SO GOOD! If you want to jazz up the flavor, please do. This is a great base for any type of coleslaw.

INGREDIENTS

1 (16-ounce) package coleslaw (or
1 large head cabbage, thinly chopped)

¼ cup diced yellow onions

FOR THE DRESSING:

½ cup mayonnaise

½ cup heavy whipping cream

2 tablespoons white vinegar

Juice of ½ lemon

1 teaspoon poppy seeds

½ teaspoon granulated sweetener

½ teaspoon celery salt

Salt and ground black pepper, to taste

DIRECTIONS

1. Place the coleslaw and onions in a large bowl and set aside.

2. Make the dressing: Place the dressing ingredients in a small bowl and whisk to combine. Pour the dressing over the coleslaw and onions and toss to coat the cabbage evenly.

3. Chill in the fridge for an hour before serving. Store leftovers in the refrigerator for up to 5 days.

Nutritional information (per serving)

Calories: 165	Total Carbs: 5g
Fat: 15g	Fiber: 1g
Protein: 1g	Net Carbs: 4g

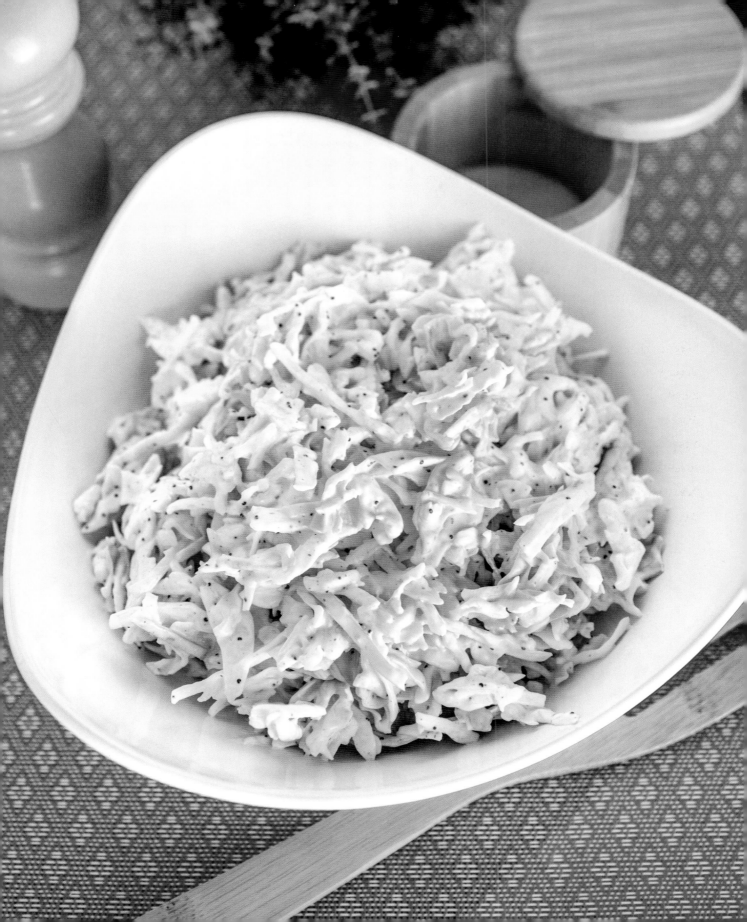

REUBEN IN A BOWL

MAKES 4 servings   **PREP TIME: 10 minutes (not including time to make dressing)**   **COOK TIME: —**

My mom is a New Yorker. When I was little, she would take me to these amazing New York delis to get Reuben sandwiches. I learned at a very early age that that combination of flavors is one of my very favorites. To me, this stuff is the ultimate comfort food. This dish instantly takes me back to my childhood.

Friendly tip: Don't add all the dressing if you're not going to eat the whole salad in one sitting. It's best to dress the salad just before you eat it. Otherwise, the salad will get soggy.

INGREDIENTS

1 (16-ounce) bag coleslaw, or 1 head cabbage, chopped

1 pound pastrami or corned beef

4 slices Swiss cheese

½ cup Thousand Island Dressing (page 284)

Salt and ground black pepper

DIRECTIONS

1. Place the coleslaw in a large salad bowl.

2. Cut the pastrami and Swiss cheese into bite-sized pieces and add to the bowl with the coleslaw.

3. Pour the dressing over the coleslaw mixture and toss to coat. Season with salt and pepper.

4. Serve! Store leftovers in the refrigerator for up to 4 days.

Nutritional information (per serving)

Calories: 650	Total Carbs: 8g
Fat: 53g	Fiber: 3g
Protein: 32g	Net Carbs: 5g

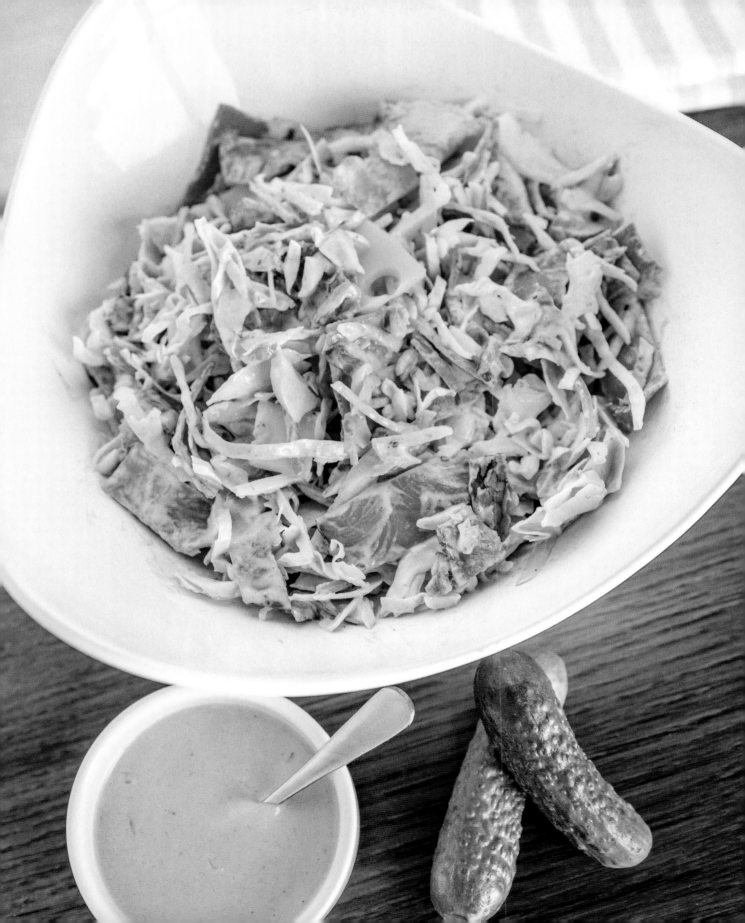

BUFFALO WING CHILI

MAKES 8 servings   PREP TIME: 10 minutes   COOK TIME: 35 minutes

Be ready to win your chili cook-off with this recipe! This is such a hearty, fresh, clean-tasting chili. My oldest child thinks I'm a rock star every time I make it. The best part is that we don't even miss the beans.

INGREDIENTS

2 tablespoons unsalted butter or ghee

1 large onion, diced

4 stalks celery, chopped

4 cloves garlic, minced

Salt and ground black pepper

2 pounds ground chicken

1 tablespoon smoked paprika

2 cups chicken bone broth

½ cup medium-hot hot sauce (such as Frank's RedHot) or Buffalo sauce

1 (14½-ounce) can diced tomatoes

1 (15-ounce) can low-sugar tomato sauce

1½ ounces blue cheese, crumbled (about ¼ cup), for serving (optional; omit for dairy-free)

DIRECTIONS

1. Melt the butter in a large pot over medium-high heat. Add the onion, celery, and garlic, sprinkle with salt and pepper, and sauté for 7 minutes, until the onion is translucent.

2. Add the ground chicken and smoked paprika and stir. Cook for 10 minutes, until the chicken is cooked all the way through, stirring occasionally to break up the clumps.

3. Add the broth, hot sauce, tomatoes, and tomato sauce and stir until well combined. Don't forget to scrape the bottom of the pan to remove all the browned bits. Let the chili simmer for about 20 minutes.

4. Serve topped with blue cheese crumbles, if desired. Store leftovers in the refrigerator for up to 5 days. Reheat in a saucepan over medium heat.

Nutritional information (per serving)

Calories: 263	Total Carbs: 8g
Fat: 15g	Fiber: 2g
Protein: 24g	Net Carbs: 6g

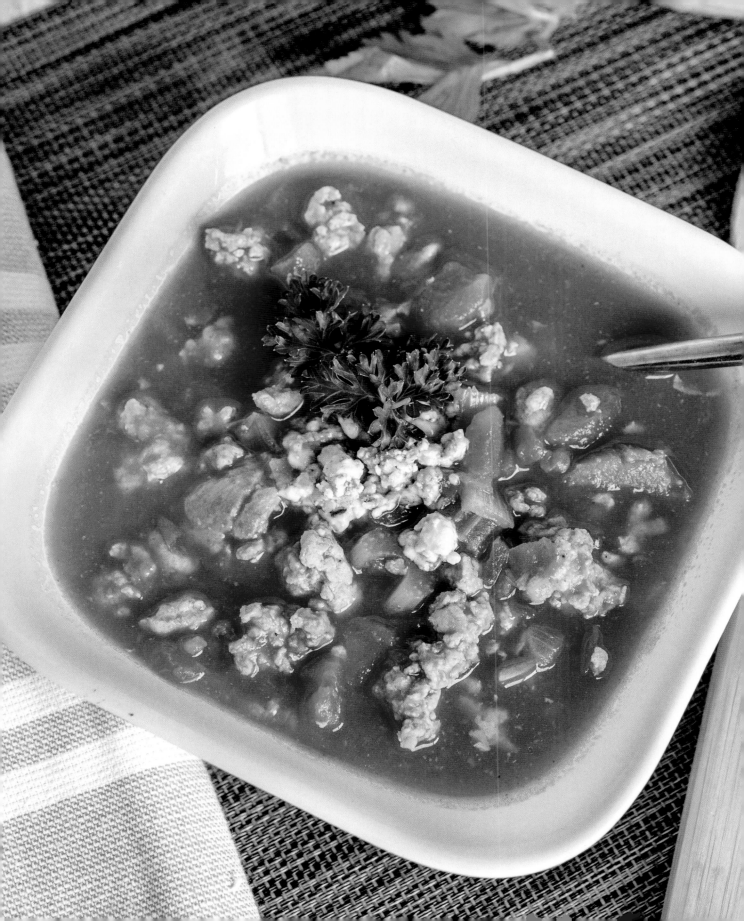

SALMON BOWLS

MAKES 4 servings   **PREP TIME: 10 minutes (not including time to cook salmon)**   **COOK TIME: 5 minutes**

Bowls like these are some of the greatest gifts known to keto. They're the perfect balance of proteins, veggies, and fats. Consider this recipe as a guideline because you can use any amounts of these ingredients, depending on your tastes. Don't be afraid to get creative!

INGREDIENTS

1 (10-ounce) bag frozen riced cauliflower

1 (16-ounce) bag shredded cabbage or coleslaw mix

1 small red onion, thinly sliced or chopped

3 to 4 radishes, thinly sliced

1 medium avocado, pitted and sliced or chopped

1 jalapeño pepper, sliced

¼ cup fresh cilantro leaves

1 (1-pound) salmon fillet, cooked and chilled

1 cup Chipotle Mayo (page 272), for serving

Juice of 1 lime, for serving

DIRECTIONS

1. Microwave the riced cauliflower according to the package directions (usually 4 to 6 minutes on high). Set aside to cool.

2. In a large bowl, toss the cabbage, onion, radishes, avocado, jalapeño, and cilantro. When the cauliflower has cooled, add it to the bowl. Then place the salmon on top.

3. Drizzle the salad with the chipotle mayo and lime juice before serving. Store leftover salad undressed in the refrigerator for up to 5 days.

> *Tip:* To cook the salmon for this recipe, simply salt and pepper both sides of the fillet and bake, covered in foil, in a preheated 450°F oven for 12 to 15 minutes, until the fish flakes easily.

Nutritional information (per serving)

Calories: 868	Total Carbs: 14g
Fat: 78g	Fiber: 5g
Protein: 28g	Net Carbs: 9g

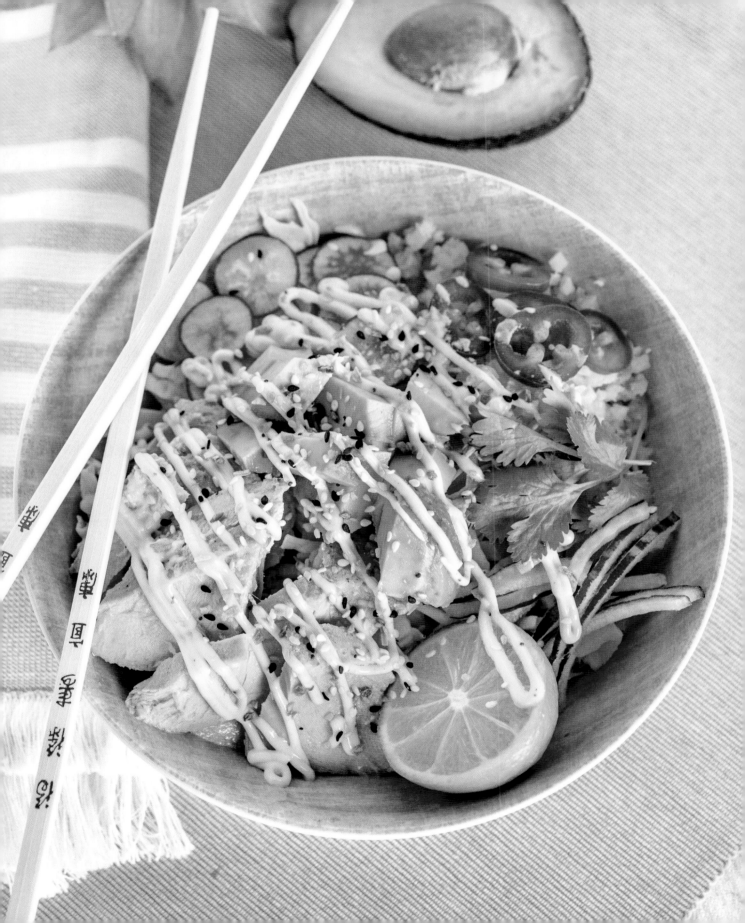

TOMATO CUCUMBER SALAD

MAKES 4 servings   **PREP TIME: 10 minutes**   **COOK TIME:** —

This is the perfect summer salad, and I don't even like tomatoes! Feel free to play around with this recipe. If you love cucumbers, add more. Not an onion fan? Leave it out! Use this recipe as a guide to make your perfect veggie salad. It would also be great with olives, avocados, or artichoke hearts—endless possibilities.

INGREDIENTS

1 cucumber, diced

2 large heirloom tomatoes, diced

1 medium red onion, diced or sliced

3 ounces feta cheese, crumbled (about ½ cup)

FOR THE DRESSING:

¼ cup extra-virgin olive oil

2 tablespoons red wine vinegar

1½ teaspoons lemon juice

½ teaspoon garlic powder

½ teaspoon Italian seasoning

Salt and ground black pepper

DIRECTIONS

1. Place the cucumber, tomatoes, onion, and feta in a large bowl and toss to combine. Set aside.

2. Make the dressing: Place the oil, vinegar, lemon juice, garlic powder, and Italian seasoning in a small bowl or dressing shaker. Sprinkle with salt and pepper and whisk or shake until well combined.

3. Pour the dressing over the veggies and toss until well coated. Store leftovers in the refrigerator for up to 5 days.

Nutritional information (per serving)

Calories: 209	Total Carbs: 8g
Fat: 19g	Fiber: 1g
Protein: 4g	Net Carbs: 7g

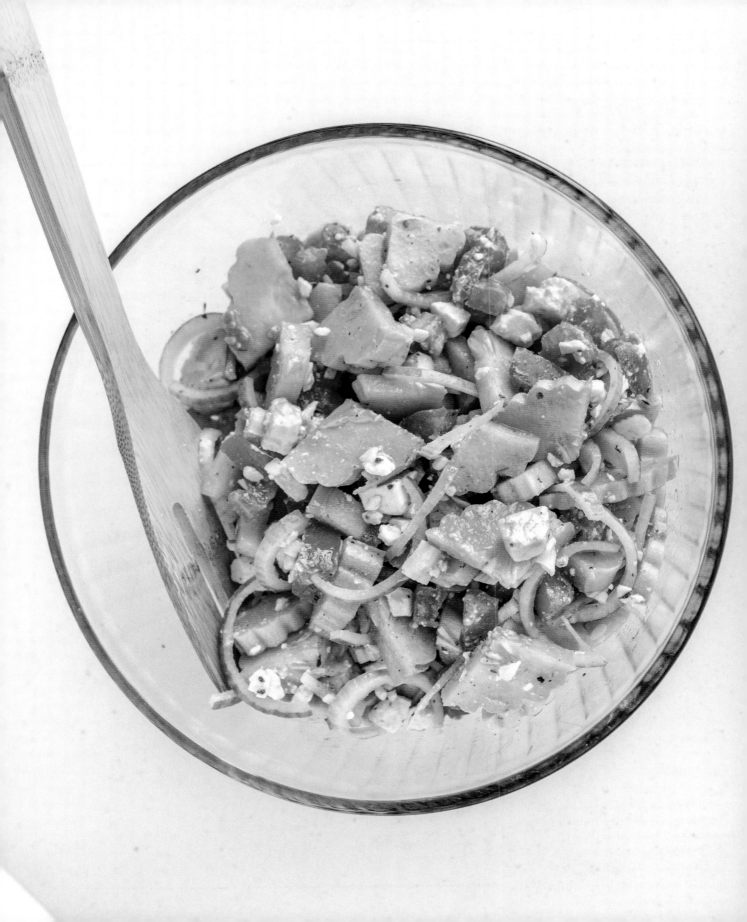

CHICKEN CABBAGE SALAD

NET CARBS
5g

MAKES 8 servings   **PREP TIME:** 15 minutes, plus 1 hour to chill   **COOK TIME:** 5 minutes

Another crowd-pleaser here! This cabbage salad is so quick and so easy; you could make a batch and live off of it for a few days. It's perfect for packing in lunches for work or school. And don't worry about the dressing making it soggy. It doesn't. In fact, I think the longer this salad chills in the refrigerator, the better it gets, dressing and all!

INGREDIENTS

2 (12½-ounce) cans chunk chicken breast, drained, or 2 cups shredded cooked chicken

1 medium head cabbage, thinly sliced or chopped

¼ cup chopped green onions

⅔ cup sliced almonds

FOR THE DRESSING:

¾ cup extra-virgin olive oil

¼ cup unseasoned rice vinegar

2 teaspoons granulated sweetener

½ teaspoon garlic powder

½ teaspoon onion powder

½ teaspoon poppy seeds

Salt and ground black pepper, to taste

DIRECTIONS

1. In a large bowl, toss the chicken, cabbage, and green onions together. Set aside.

2. Make the dressing: Place all the ingredients for the dressing in a small mixing bowl, dressing shaker, or jar with a lid. Whisk together or shake until everything is well mixed.

3. Pour the dressing over the cabbage mixture and toss to coat. Set aside.

4. Toast the sliced almonds in a small skillet over medium-high heat, about 5 minutes. Stir constantly so the almonds don't burn.

5. Add the toasted almonds to the salad and mix together.

6. Serve right away or chill in the fridge for at least 1 hour before serving to enhance the flavor. Store leftovers in the refrigerator for up to 5 days.

Nutritional information (per serving)

Calories: 319	**Total Carbs:** 9g
Fat: 26g	**Fiber:** 4g
Protein: 17g	**Net Carbs:** 5g

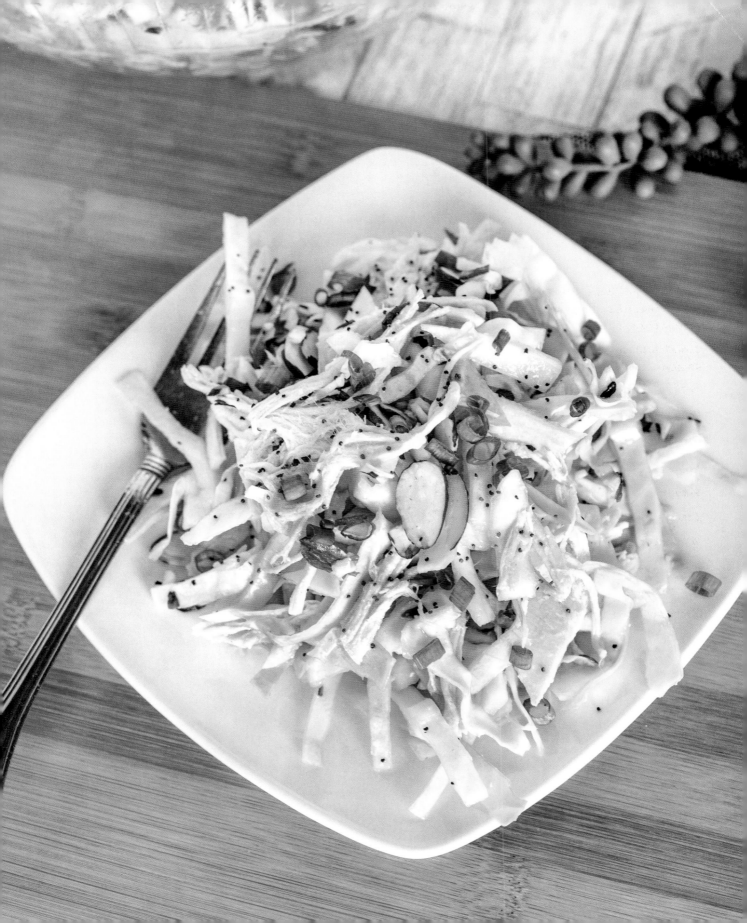

BROCCOLI CHEESE SOUP

MAKES 10 servings **PREP TIME: 5 minutes** **COOK TIME: 35 minutes**

When I was a little girl, I remember going to the mall with my mom in Chicago. We would shop and then eat at this restaurant that served baked potatoes with your favorite toppings. I always topped mine with broccoli cheese soup. It wasn't something we ever ate at home, so it always felt like the biggest, heartiest treat. Every time I eat broccoli cheese soup, I am immediately taken back to my childhood and those cozy days of shopping with my mom. I don't even miss the baked potato!

INGREDIENTS

2 tablespoons extra-virgin olive oil or unsalted butter

½ yellow onion, diced

4 cloves garlic, minced

4 cups chicken bone broth

1 cup heavy whipping cream

½ teaspoon xanthan gum

4 cups frozen broccoli

12 ounces cheddar cheese, shredded (about 3 cups)

Salt and ground black pepper

Special Equipment:
Food processor

DIRECTIONS

1. Place a 6-quart stockpot over medium-high heat and coat the bottom of the pan with the oil. Add the onion and garlic and cook for 5 minutes, until the onion becomes translucent. Stir often so the garlic doesn't burn.

2. Add the broth, heavy cream, and xanthan gum and whisk until the xanthan gum is fully incorporated. Bring to a boil.

3. Meanwhile, place the broccoli in a medium-sized bowl or dish and microwave for 1 minute 30 seconds to thaw slightly. Place half of the broccoli in a food processor and pulse into tiny bits. (You can process all the broccoli if you like, but we like our soup with some big broccoli chunks in it.)

4. Add all the broccoli to the soup and simmer for another 20 minutes.

5. Reduce the heat to low and add the cheddar cheese ½ cup at a time, stirring after each addition so that the cheese fully melts into the soup before adding the next ½ cup.

6. Season with salt and pepper and serve. Store leftovers in the refrigerator for up to 5 days. Reheat in the microwave or in a saucepan over medium heat.

Nutritional information (per serving)

Calories: 273	Total Carbs: 4g
Fat: 22g	Fiber: 1g
Protein: 12g	Net Carbs: 3g

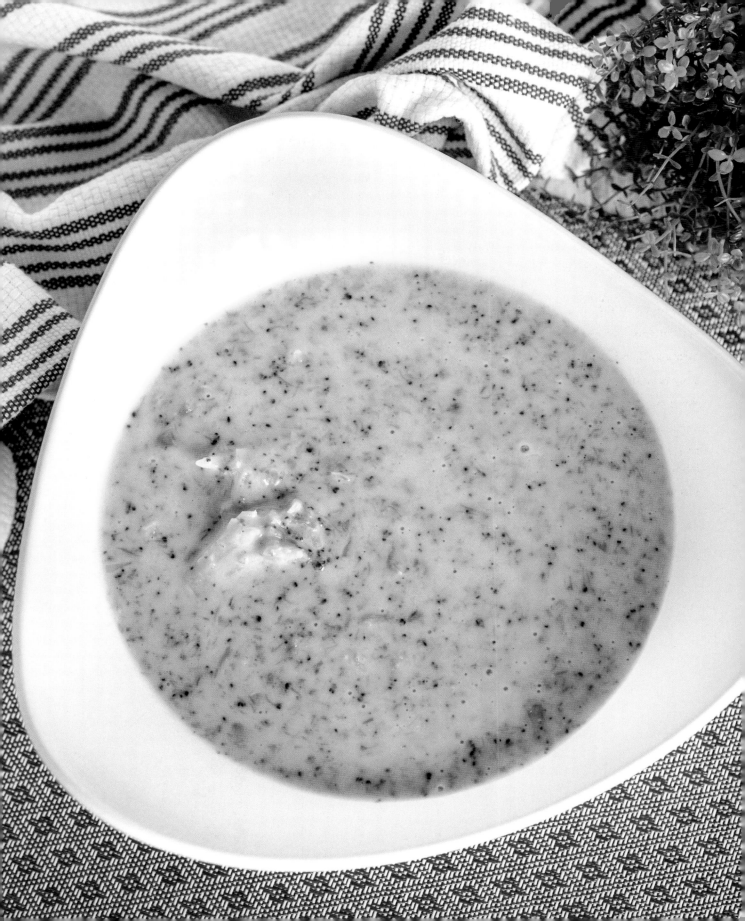

EGG DROP SOUP

MAKES 4 servings   **PREP TIME:** 2 minutes   **COOK TIME:** 20 minutes

I was never a fan of egg drop soup growing up, but it has quickly become a keto favorite of mine. The flavor is so light and clean-tasting, yet it fills your belly on a cold winter day. It's also a fantastic way to incorporate any veggies in your fridge that need to be used. This soup would be great with mushrooms, bell peppers, and even chicken, beef, or shrimp!

INGREDIENTS

4 cups chicken bone broth

1 teaspoon xanthan gum

¼ teaspoon garlic powder

2 large eggs

2 large egg whites

1 teaspoon toasted sesame oil

3 green onions, chopped, plus more for garnish

DIRECTIONS

1. In a large saucepan, whisk together the broth, xanthan gum, and garlic powder. Turn the heat to medium-high and bring the mixture to a boil.

2. Meanwhile, whisk together the eggs and egg whites in a small bowl. Set aside.

3. Once the broth mixture is at a boil, swirl it in a circle to create a whirlpool. Slowly pour the eggs into the pan.

4. Remove from the heat and stir in the sesame oil and green onions. Serve garnished with extra green onions. Store leftovers in the refrigerator for up to 5 days. Reheat in the microwave or in a saucepan over medium heat.

Nutritional information (per serving)

Calories: 110	Total Carbs: 2g
Fat: 5g	Fiber: 1g
Protein: 11g	Net Carbs: 1g

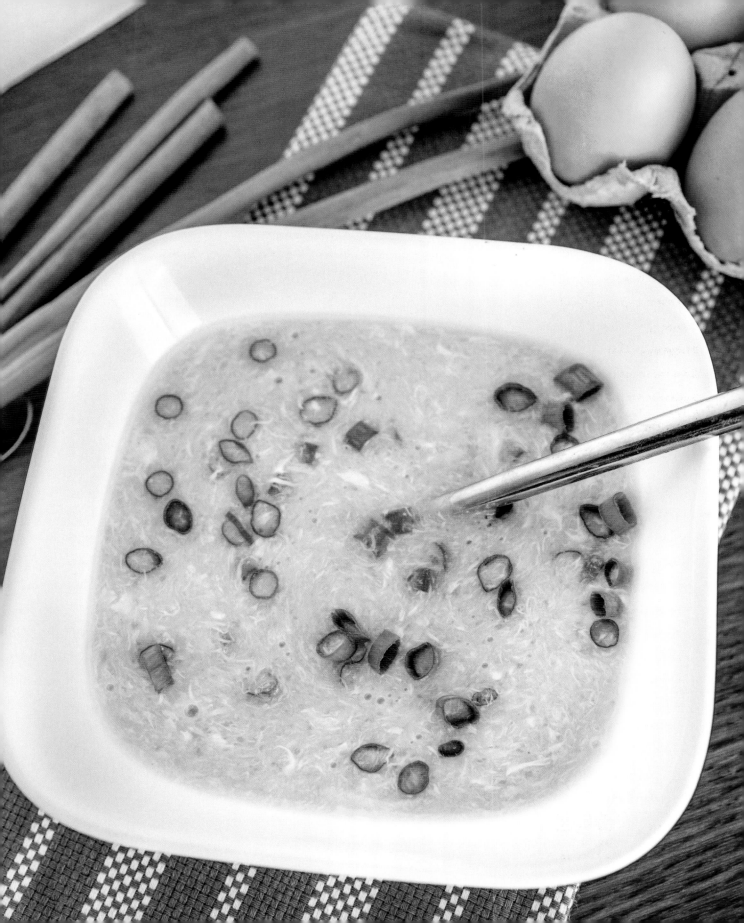

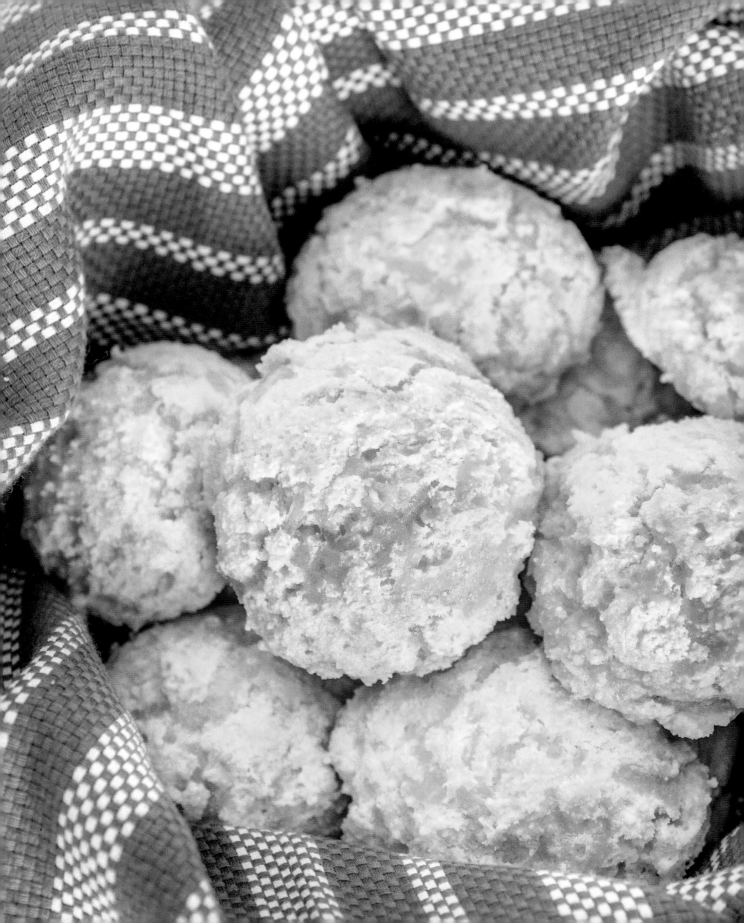

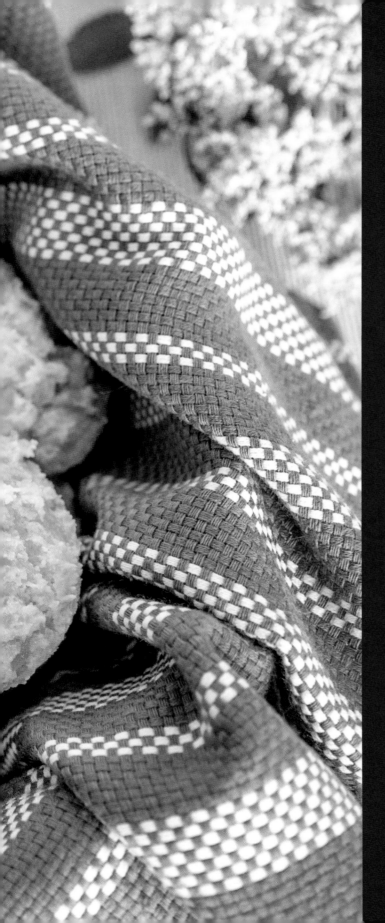

4 ON THE SIDE

CREAMED SPINACH

MAKES 5 servings (½ cup per serving)   PREP TIME: 30 minutes   COOK TIME: 10 minutes

When I was five or six years old, we went to my uncle's house for Thanksgiving. I don't remember much, but I do remember the creamed spinach! It was the first time I actually liked something with spinach in it—probably because it was loaded with all the good stuff, like butter, cheese, and cream. But still...I loved it then and I love it now. Guilt-free!

INGREDIENTS

1 (10-ounce) package frozen spinach

1 tablespoon unsalted butter

1 clove garlic, minced

⅔ cup heavy whipping cream

4 ounces shredded Parmesan cheese (about 1 cup)

⅓ cup mascarpone cheese

Salt and ground black pepper

DIRECTIONS

1. Thaw the spinach in the microwave according to the package directions (usually 4 to 6 minutes on high). When the spinach is done, empty the contents into a clean dish towel and squeeze out the excess liquid.

2. Melt the butter in a medium-sized skillet over medium heat. Add the garlic and cook for 1 minute, until fragrant.

3. Add the spinach, heavy cream, Parmesan, and mascarpone and stir until well combined. Season with salt and pepper.

4. Cook for about 5 minutes to allow the flavors to marry. Serve immediately. Store leftovers in the refrigerator for up to 5 days. Reheat in the microwave or in a skillet.

Nutritional information (per serving)

Calories: 292	Total Carbs: 4g
Fat: 25g	Fiber: 1g
Protein: 10g	Net Carbs: 3g

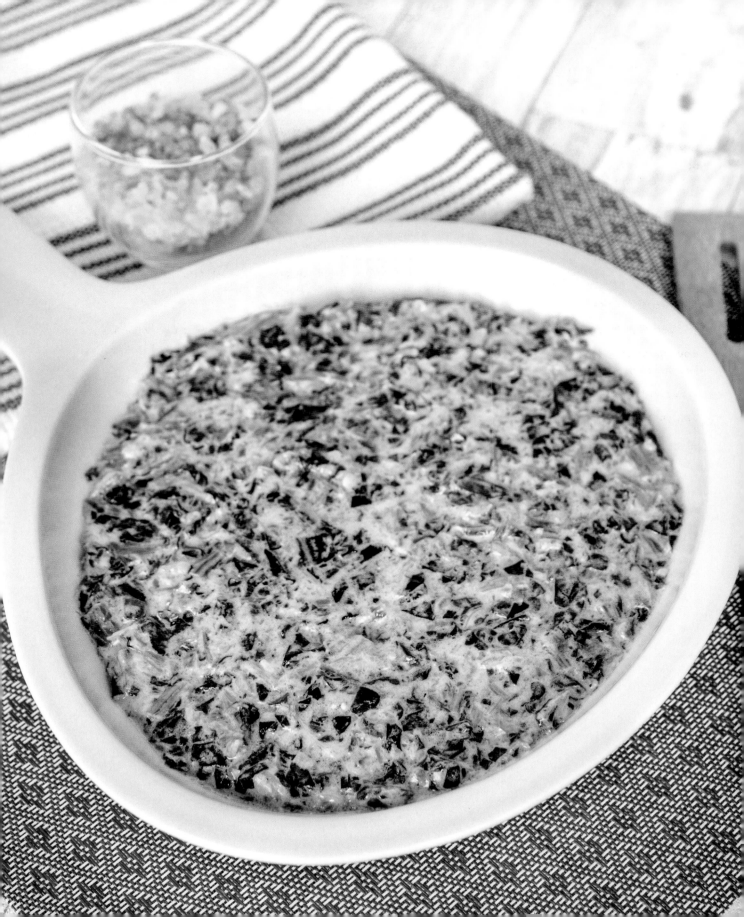

CHEDDAR CHEESE BUNS

MAKES 4 buns (2 per serving)   PREP TIME: 5 minutes   COOK TIME: 15 minutes

This recipe was inspired by fellow Instagrammer Christina (@cheeseisthenewbread). I've modified her version a bit to give these buns the perfect texture. Cameron loves them—he makes them a couple times a week for sandwiches or burgers, or just eats them as a side. Feel free to get creative by using different cheeses. The possibilities are endless!

INGREDIENTS

4½ ounces cheddar cheese, shredded (about 1 heaping cup), plus more if needed

1⅓ ounces grated Parmesan cheese (about ⅓ cup)

2 large eggs

½ teaspoon baking powder

¼ teaspoon xanthan gum

¼ teaspoon garlic powder

¼ teaspoon onion powder

DIRECTIONS

1. Preheat the oven to 400°F. Line a baking sheet with parchment paper or a silicone baking mat.

2. Place all the ingredients in a medium-sized bowl and mix well with a fork. Then divide the dough into four equal portions.

3. Take one portion of dough, form it into a ball, and place it on the lined baking sheet. If the dough is too runny to form into balls, simply mix in a little more cheddar cheese. Repeat until you have four balls.

4. Bake for 15 minutes, until golden brown. Allow to cool slightly. Serve on their own or use as sandwich or hamburger buns. Store leftovers in the refrigerator for up to 5 days. Reheat in the microwave for about 30 seconds.

Nutritional information (per serving)

Calories: 411	Total Carbs: 3g
Fat: 32g	Fiber: 0g
Protein: 29g	Net Carbs: 3g

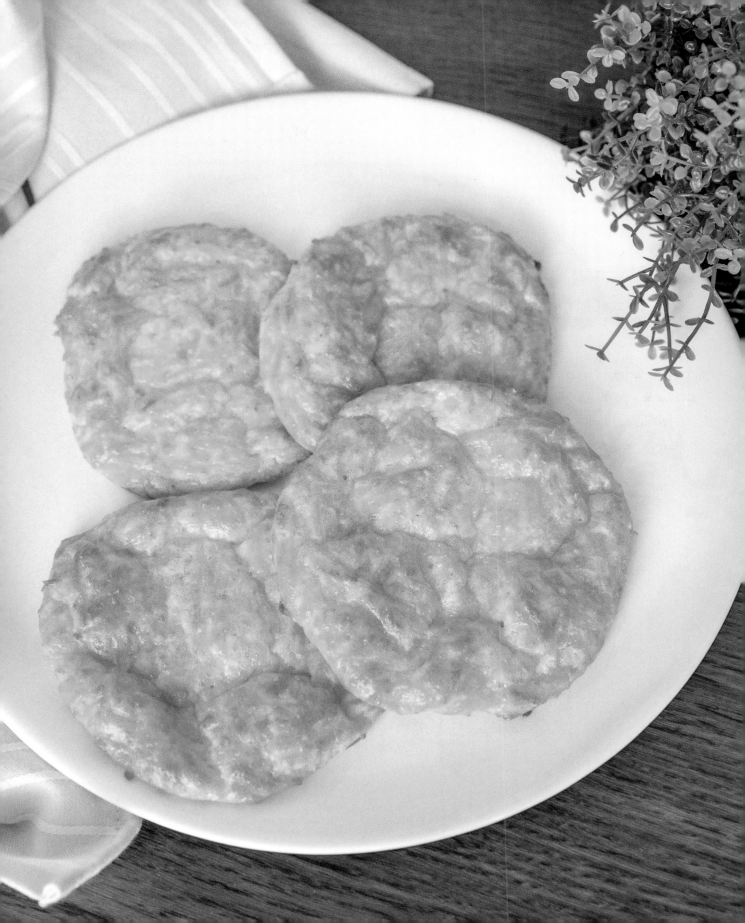

ROASTED EGGPLANT

MAKES 4 servings   PREP TIME: 8 minutes   COOK TIME: 22 minutes

My mom made this dish all the time when I was growing up. It was one of those vegetables that I always looked forward to eating. I mean, it's smothered in cheese! Cheese always makes vegetables more appealing. If you've never cooked eggplant, give this recipe a try!

INGREDIENTS

1 large eggplant

¼ cup extra-virgin olive oil or avocado oil, divided

Salt and ground black pepper

1 (1-pound) log fresh mozzarella cheese, cut into 16 slices

1 teaspoon Italian seasoning

DIRECTIONS

1. Preheat the oven to 375°F. Line a rimmed baking sheet with aluminum foil.

2. Cut the ends off the eggplant and discard. Cut the eggplant crosswise into ¼- to ½-inch slices and place on the lined baking sheet. You should have 8 to 12 slices.

3. Drizzle the eggplant slices with half of the oil, then season with salt and pepper. Flip the slices over and repeat on the other side.

4. Roast for 15 minutes, or until the eggplant is soft. Remove from the oven and turn the oven to the broil setting.

5. While the broiler heats up, place 2 slices of cheese on top of each eggplant slice, then sprinkle with the Italian seasoning.

6. Broil the eggplant for 5 to 7 minutes, until the cheese is lightly golden and bubbly.

7. Serve as a side dish or make a meal out of it! Store leftovers in the refrigerator for up to 3 days. Best reheated under the oven broiler until the cheese is bubbly.

Nutritional information (per serving)

Calories: 166   Total Carbs: 7g
Fat: 15g   Fiber: 3g
Protein: 2g   Net Carbs: 4g

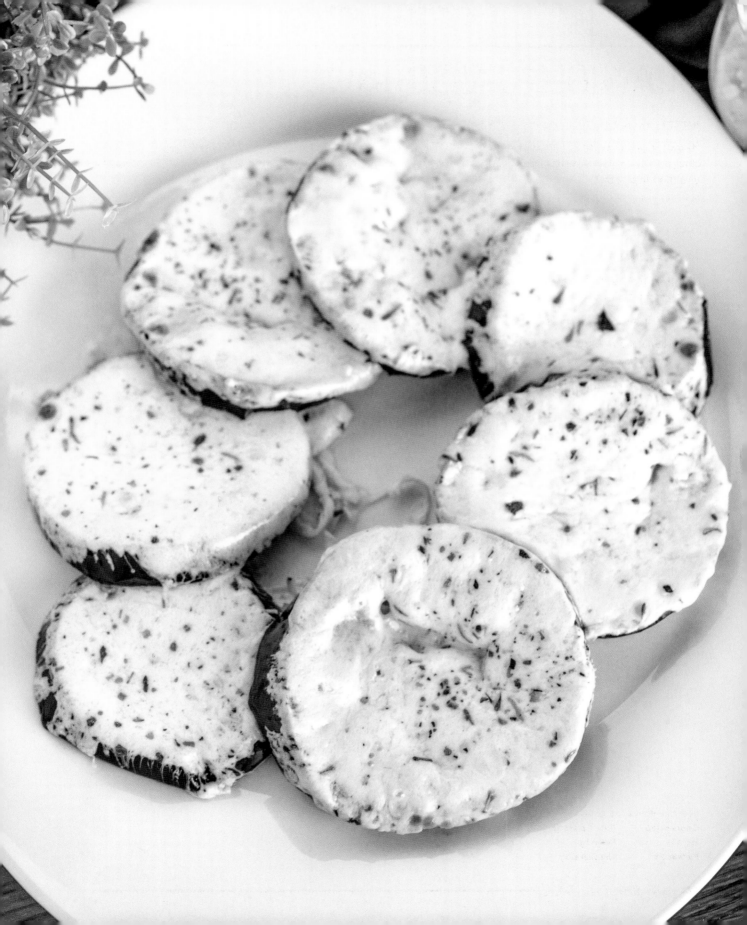

SPANISH CAULI-RICE

NET CARBS
9g

MAKES 2 servings PREP TIME: 4 minutes COOK TIME: 11 minutes

This Spanish rice is KILLER. If you love spicy foods, this dish is for you! My mouth is always on fire when I eat this stuff, yet I can't get enough. Also, did I mention that I absolutely loathe cauliflower? That should tell you how delicious this rice is! I use El Pato brand tomato sauce for this recipe. It's found in the Mexican food aisle, and if you've never tried it, now's the time. It's similar to regular tomato sauce, but it's packed with flavor and spice—such a beautiful addition to Mexican dishes. We love this rice with carne asada and Gavin's Guac (page 68)!

INGREDIENTS

1 (10-ounce) bag frozen riced cauliflower

1 (7¾-ounce) can El Pato brand tomato sauce

2 tablespoons unsalted butter or ghee

Juice of 1 lime, plus more for serving if desired

½ teaspoon ground cumin

Chopped fresh cilantro leaves, for garnish

DIRECTIONS

1. Microwave the riced cauliflower according to the package directions (usually 4 to 6 minutes on high). When the cauliflower is done, empty it into a medium-sized saucepan.

2. Place the saucepan over medium-high heat. Add the tomato sauce, butter, lime juice, and cumin and stir until well combined. Cook for about 5 minutes, stirring constantly, until the rice is soft and the flavors have had a chance to soak into the cauliflower.

3. Remove from the heat and top with the cilantro and more lime juice, if desired, before serving.

Nutritional information (per serving)

Calories: 178	Total Carbs: 12g
Fat: 14g	Fiber: 3g
Protein: 4g	Net Carbs: 9g

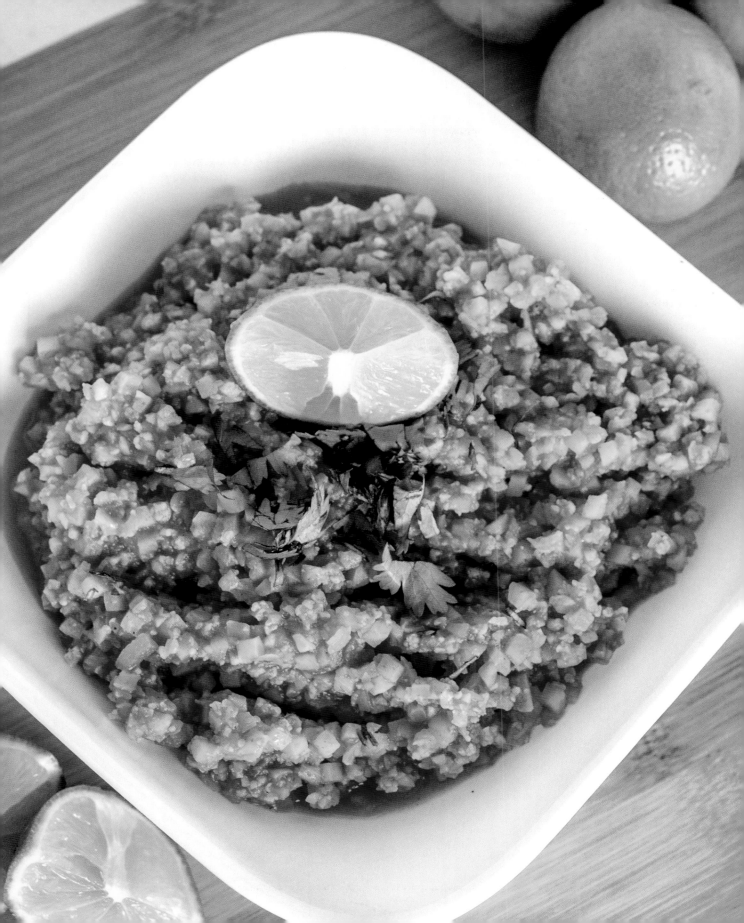

SOUR CREAM AND CHEDDAR BISCUITS

MAKES 12 biscuits (2 per serving) PREP TIME: 7 minutes   COOK TIME: 18 minutes

Yes, it's possible to have biscuits on keto! These things are the perfect addition to any meal. They are fluffy and full of flavor—everything you want in a good biscuit!

INGREDIENTS

2 cups blanched almond flour

2 teaspoons baking powder

½ teaspoon salt

3 large eggs

½ cup (1 stick) unsalted butter or ghee, melted but not hot

2⅔ ounces cheddar cheese, shredded (about ⅔ cup)

¼ cup sour cream

DIRECTIONS

1. Preheat the oven to 350°F. Line a baking sheet with parchment paper or a silicone baking mat.

2. Place all the ingredients in a large mixing bowl and mix well with a fork until evenly combined.

3. Use a cookie scoop or spoon to scoop out a portion of the dough (about the size of a golf ball) and place on the lined baking sheet. (If using a spoon, form the biscuit dough into a ball with your hands.) Repeat with the remaining dough. You should get 12 biscuits.

4. Bake for 18 minutes, or until cooked through and no longer doughy in the center. Serve warm. Store leftovers in a resealable plastic bag in the refrigerator for up to 5 days. Reheat in the microwave or in a toaster oven.

Nutritional information (per serving)

Calories: 493	Total Carbs: 8g
Fat: 47g	Fiber: 4g
Protein: 17g	Net Carbs: 4g

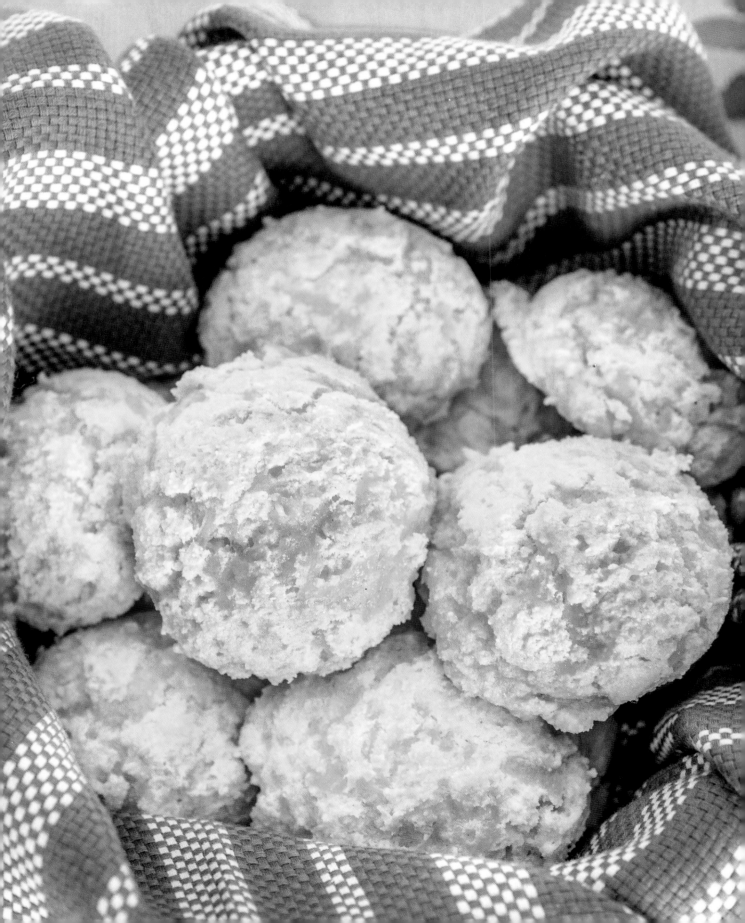

FAUX-TATOES

MAKES 4 servings   PREP TIME: 8 minutes   COOK TIME: 30 minutes

I was skeptical about substituting radishes for potatoes, but honestly, they are such a pleasant surprise. Give these a try!

INGREDIENTS

1 pound radishes

Extra-virgin olive oil, for drizzling

1 teaspoon Italian seasoning

1 teaspoon garlic powder

1 teaspoon onion powder

1 teaspoon paprika

½ teaspoon xanthan gum

Pinch of salt

Pinch of ground black pepper

DIRECTIONS

1. Preheat the oven to 400°F. Line a rimmed baking sheet with aluminum foil or a silicone baking mat.

2. Remove any stems from the radishes and discard. Rinse the radishes until they are clean, then dry with paper towels.

3. Cut the radishes into bite-sized pieces (in quarters if large, or in half if small). Place the radishes on the lined baking sheet and heavily drizzle with olive oil. Toss them with your hands so the radishes are evenly coated.

4. Put the remaining ingredients in a small bowl, include a sprinkle of salt and pepper, and mix together. Sprinkle the spice mixture on top of the radishes. Toss them again with your hands to evenly distribute the spice mixture.

5. Bake for 15 minutes, then flip the radishes over. Return the pan to the oven and bake for an additional 10 to 15 minutes, until golden brown.

6. Serve immediately. Store leftovers in the refrigerator for up to 3 days. Reheat in a skillet with some butter or olive oil.

Nutritional information (per serving)

Calories: 56	Total Carbs: 5g
Fat: 4g	Fiber: 2g
Protein: 1g	Net Carbs: 3g

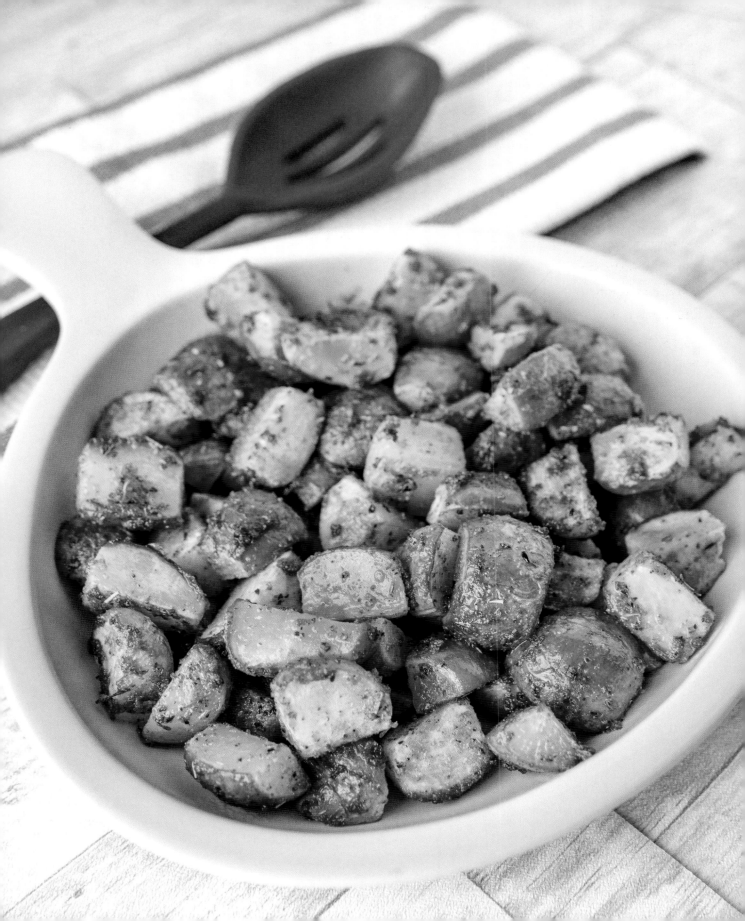

BACON PARMESAN BRUSSELS SPROUTS

MAKES 4 servings   PREP TIME: 15 minutes   COOK TIME: 22 minutes

I never liked Brussels sprouts until keto came along. They've always gotten such a bad rap, but they are severely underrated. Throw in some bacon and cheese, and they can't get any better! In fact, in my early keto days, I ate these things for lunch and dinner—sometimes a few days in a row.

INGREDIENTS

1 pound Brussels sprouts

8 ounces bacon

½ yellow onion, diced

1 teaspoon minced garlic

1 tablespoon balsamic vinegar (see Note)

1 ounce Parmesan cheese, shredded (about ¼ cup) (omit for dairy-free)

Variation: Add some unsweetened dried cranberries for a sweeter version.

DIRECTIONS

1. Cut the stems off the Brussels sprouts and discard. Then cut the sprouts into bite-sized pieces. (I usually quarter mine, depending on the size.) Rinse and drain in a colander and set aside.

2. Set a large skillet over medium-high heat. While the pan is heating, cut the bacon into bite-sized pieces. Once the pan is hot, add the bacon and cook until it reaches your desired doneness, about 10 minutes for crispy bacon.

3. Using a slotted spoon, remove the bacon from the pan, keeping as much of the grease in the pan as possible, and set on a paper towel–lined plate.

4. Add the onion and garlic to the pan. Cook for about 2 minutes, until the onion is translucent, stirring constantly so the garlic doesn't burn.

5. Turn the heat to high and add the Brussels sprouts and balsamic vinegar. Stir to coat the sprouts in the bacon grease. Cook until the sprouts are soft on the inside and crispy on the outside, about 10 minutes.

6. Sprinkle the Parmesan cheese and bacon on top and serve. Store leftovers in the refrigerator for up to 5 days. Reheat in the microwave or in a skillet.

> *Note:* *Choose the balsamic vinegar with the least amount of sugar. If you can't find a low-sugar one, you can eliminate the balsamic from this dish completely.*

Nutritional information (per serving)

Calories: 327	Total Carbs: 11g
Fat: 21g	Fiber: 4g
Protein: 25g	Net Carbs: 7g

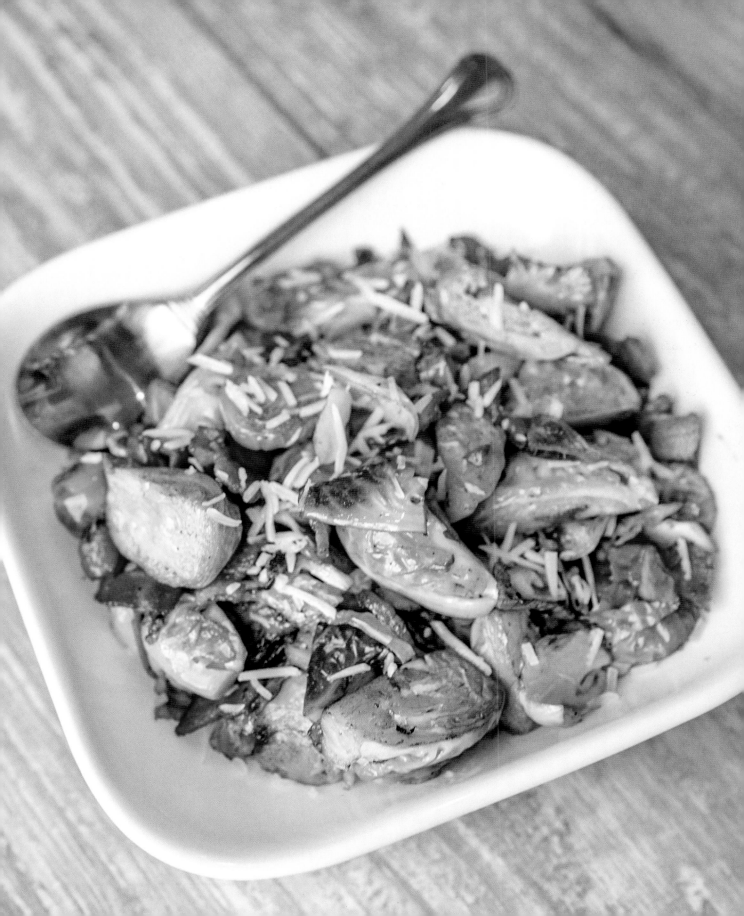

DINNER ROLLS

MAKES 6 rolls (1 per serving)   PREP TIME: 10 minutes, plus 30 minutes to chill   COOK TIME: 17 minutes

You don't have to give up dinner rolls when switching to a ketogenic lifestyle. You just need to swap out the ingredients for better, keto-friendly ones. These beautiful rolls definitely hit the spot when you're dying for some bread.

INGREDIENTS

3 ounces mozzarella cheese, shredded (about ¾ cup)

2 ounces cream cheese (¼ cup)

¾ cup blanched almond flour

1 large egg

½ teaspoon garlic powder

½ teaspoon onion powder

DIRECTIONS

1. Preheat the oven to 425°F. Line a baking sheet with parchment paper or a silicone baking mat.

2. Place the mozzarella and cream cheese in a large microwave-safe bowl; there's no need to stir yet. Microwave on high for 1 minute. Stir with a fork, then microwave for another minute. At this point, the cheeses should be smooth. If necessary, microwave for another 30 seconds.

3. Add the almond flour, egg, garlic powder, and onion powder to the bowl with the melted cheeses and mix with your hands. The dough will be hot, so you may need to let it cool for a minute before mixing. If the dough is too sticky, simply wet your hands and continue kneading until the dough is well combined.

4. Roll the dough into a ball, wrap in plastic wrap, and chill in the refrigerator for 20 to 30 minutes.

5. Take the dough out of the refrigerator and divide it into 6 equal portions. Using your hands, take one portion of the dough and roll it into a ball. Place on the parchment paper and repeat with the remaining dough.

6. Bake for 15 minutes, or until golden brown.

7. Serve as a side dish or use as buns for sandwiches. Store leftovers in the refrigerator for up to 1 week. Reheat in the microwave for about 30 seconds.

Nutritional information (per serving)

Calories: 129   Total Carbs: 3g
Fat: 11g   Fiber: 1g
Protein: 7g   Net Carbs: 2g

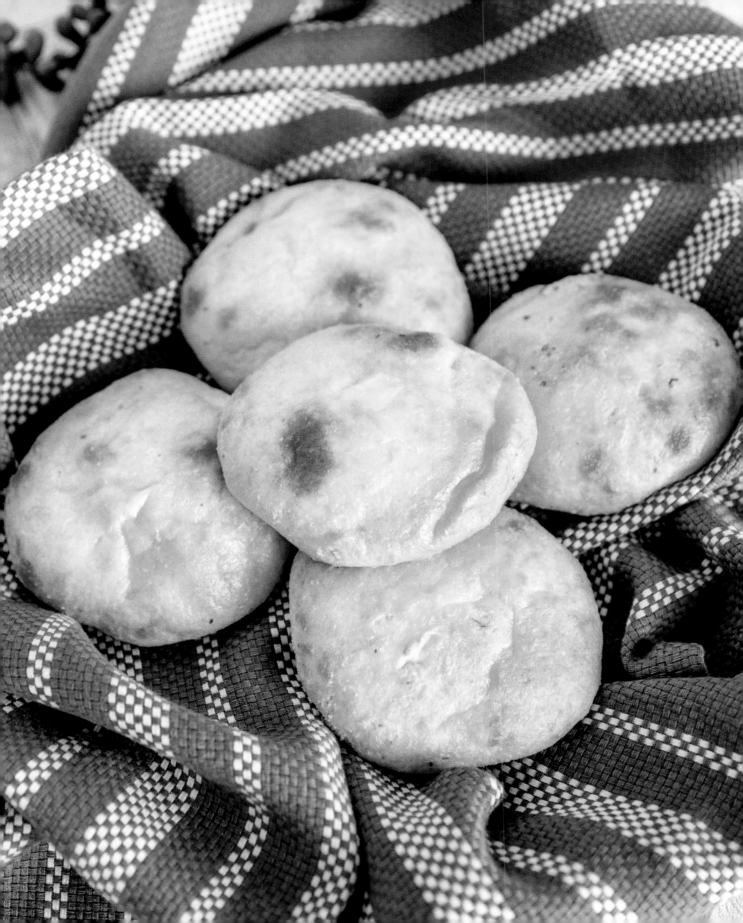

SIMPLE ASPARAGUS

MAKES 4 servings   **PREP TIME:** 5 minutes   **COOK TIME:** 30 minutes

My kids aren't super veggie lovers, but they all love asparagus. When you bake asparagus this way, it makes the tips crispy and almost gives the asparagus a nutty flavor. Keto made simple, for sure.

INGREDIENTS

2 (1-pound) bundles asparagus

½ cup extra-virgin olive oil

Salt and ground black pepper

1 ounce Parmesan cheese, grated (about ¼ cup)

DIRECTIONS

1. Preheat the oven to 425°F. Line a baking sheet with aluminum foil.

2. Rinse the asparagus and lay on a paper towel to dry. Take one stalk of asparagus and snap it in two. This will naturally remove the tough end. Line up the remaining asparagus and chop off the tough ends, using the broken one as a guideline for where to cut.

3. Line up the asparagus on the lined baking sheet in a single layer and drizzle with the oil. Use your hands to toss so that the asparagus is evenly coated. Sprinkle with salt and pepper.

4. Bake for 25 to 30 minutes, until the asparagus is crisp-tender.

5. Remove from the oven and sprinkle the Parmesan cheese on top. Serve hot. Store leftovers in the refrigerator for up to 4 days. Reheat in the microwave.

Nutritional information (per serving)

Calories: 316	Total Carbs: 9g
Fat: 30g	Fiber: 5g
Protein: 8g	Net Carbs: 4g

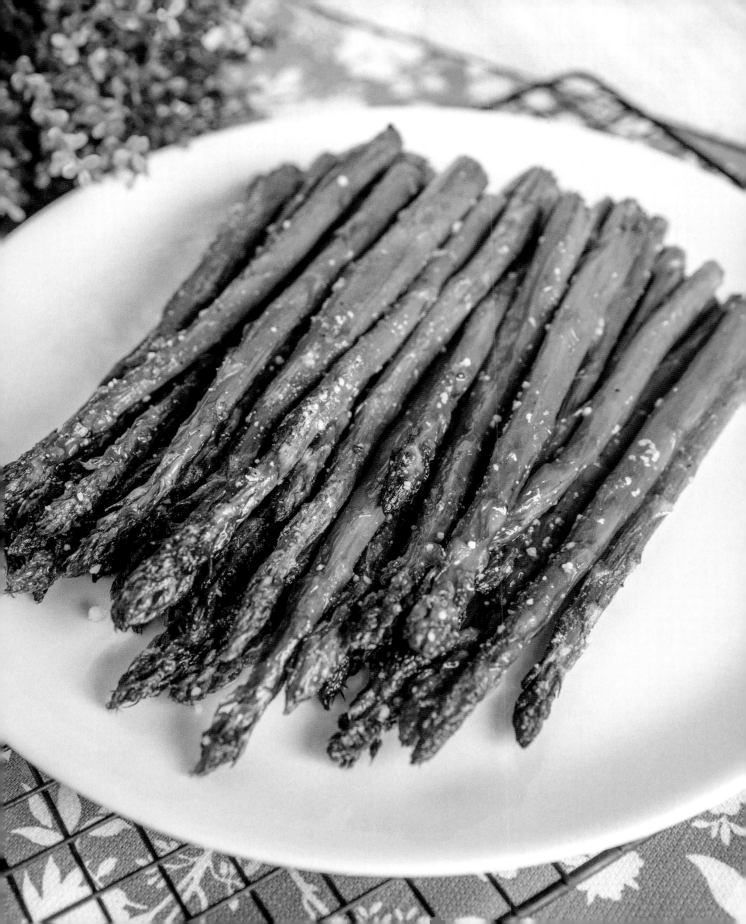

PORK RIND STUFFING

MAKES 4 servings   PREP TIME: 10 minutes   COOK TIME: 45 minutes

Thanksgiving doesn't have to be a day when you feel deprived of the traditional foods you love. This pork rind stuffing has been a hit at our keto Thanksgivings. I know it sounds super weird to use pork rinds, but you'll be pleasantly surprised at how well they take on traditional stuffing flavors. This will be a staple at all your Thanksgivings from now on!

INGREDIENTS

2 tablespoons unsalted butter, ghee, or extra-virgin olive oil

1 small yellow onion, diced

4 stalks celery, chopped

1 (3-ounce) bag plain pork rinds

1 large egg, beaten

¾ cup chicken bone broth

1 teaspoon poultry seasoning

½ teaspoon dried thyme leaves

DIRECTIONS

1. Preheat the oven to 375°F.

2. Melt the butter in a medium-sized saucepan over medium heat. Add the onion and celery and sauté until soft. Remove the pan from the heat and set aside.

3. Crush the pork rinds until they reach your desired consistency. I like a few large chunks but the majority crushed (not powdered). Add the crushed pork rinds to the onion and celery mixture and stir.

4. Pour the beaten egg into the pork rind mixture and toss until thoroughly mixed.

5. Place the broth, poultry seasoning, and thyme in a small bowl. Stir until the seasonings are mixed in, then pour over the pork rind mixture in the saucepan. Stir to thoroughly combine.

6. Spoon the stuffing mixture into a 9-inch square or smaller glass or ceramic baking dish and bake for 40 to 45 minutes, until golden.

7. Serve! Store leftovers in the refrigerator for up to 5 days. Reheat in the oven or microwave.

Nutritional information (per serving)

Calories: 209	Total Carbs: 2g
Fat: 15g	Fiber: 1g
Protein: 17g	Net Carbs: 1g

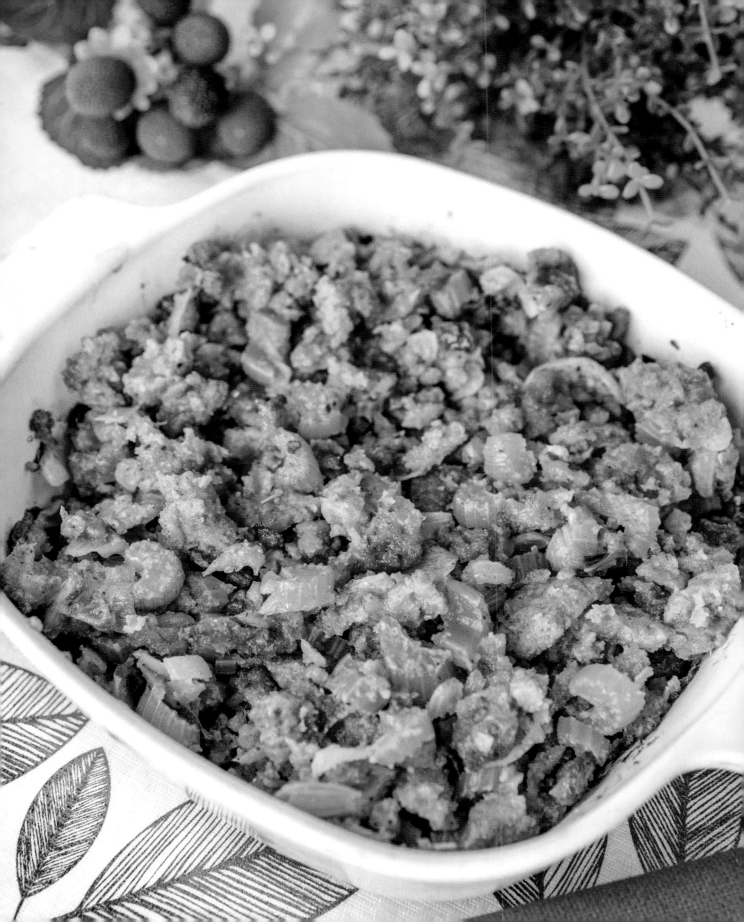

DAMN GOOD BISCUITS

MAKES 12 biscuits (2 per serving)   **PREP TIME: 5 minutes**   **COOK TIME: 15 minutes**

These biscuits are such a classic! They are the perfect side dish to any meal—breakfast, lunch, or dinner. So. Damn. Good.

INGREDIENTS

2 cups blanched almond flour

2 teaspoons baking powder

¼ teaspoon salt

¼ teaspoon xanthan gum

⅓ cup unsalted butter, melted but not hot

2 large eggs

1 teaspoon sour cream

DIRECTIONS

1. Preheat the oven to 350°F. Line a baking sheet with parchment paper or a silicone baking mat.

2. Mix together the almond flour, baking powder, salt, and xanthan gum in a large bowl.

3. Add the melted butter, eggs, and sour cream, then mix with a fork until well combined. Use a spoon or cookie scoop to scoop about 2 tablespoons of the dough onto the lined baking sheet. (If using a spoon, form the biscuit dough into a ball with your hands.) Repeat to make a total of 12 biscuits. Shape the dough into rounded biscuit shapes.

4. Bake for 13 to 15 minutes, until firm and golden.

5. Serve! Store leftovers in the refrigerator for up to 1 week or in the freezer for up to 1 month. Reheat in the microwave, if desired.

Nutritional information (per serving)

Calories: 342	Total Carbs: 7g
Fat: 32g	Fiber: 4g
Protein: 13g	Net Carbs: 3g

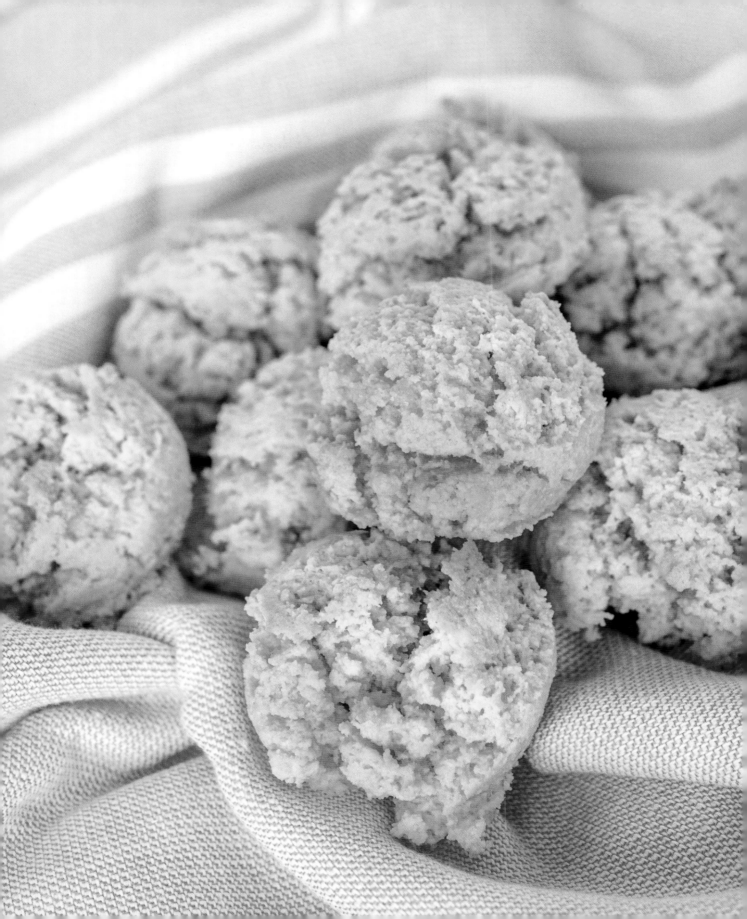

CHEESY GARLIC FLATBREAD

MAKES 4 servings **PREP TIME: 5 minutes** **COOK TIME: 15 minutes**

Calling all cheese lovers—this one's for you! This recipe couldn't be any easier to make. You can use the dough to make flatbread, pizza crust, rolls, or buns. I love to brush mine with melted butter when it's fresh outta the oven, then top it with some more Parmesan cheese, or even dipped in some low-carb marinara. Yum!

INGREDIENTS

4 ounces mozzarella cheese, shredded (about 1 cup)

1 ounce Parmesan cheese, shredded or grated (about ¼ cup)

2 large eggs

½ teaspoon xanthan gum

¼ teaspoon garlic powder

¼ teaspoon Italian seasoning

DIRECTIONS

1. Preheat the oven to 400°F. Line a baking sheet with parchment paper or a silicone baking mat.

2. Put the mozzarella, Parmesan, eggs, xanthan gum, and garlic powder in a medium-sized bowl. Mix well with a fork.

3. Transfer the cheese mixture to the lined baking sheet. Form the dough into a circle and gently press into an even layer. You can make it as thin or as thick as you'd like—there are no rules here. Sprinkle the Italian seasoning on top.

4. Bake until the bread is golden brown and has reached the desired crispness, 15 to 18 minutes. (The exact baking time will depend on how thick you make the dough and how crispy you want the bread to be.)

5. If desired, slice into strips, then enjoy! Store leftovers in the refrigerator for up to 1 week. Reheat in the microwave for about 30 seconds.

Nutritional information (per serving)

Calories: 122   Total Carbs: 2g

Fat: 8g   Fiber: 0g

Protein: 10g   Net Carbs: 2g

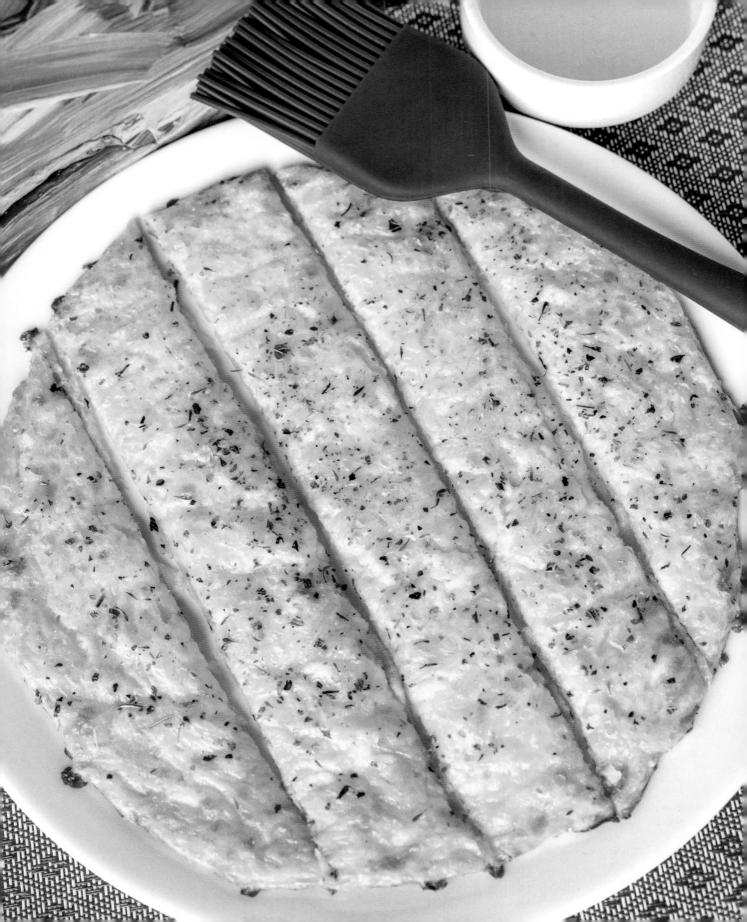

GARLICKY GREEN BEANS

MAKES 4 servings   **PREP TIME:** 5 minutes   **COOK TIME:** 10 minutes

One day after school, my kids and their friends came home to these beans sitting on the counter. They asked if they could try them, and of course I said yes. I walked back into the kitchen to find them all standing around the island, devouring the entire plate. It made my soul happy to see that these little kids were chomping on green beans like they were chips. That's a win in my book!

INGREDIENTS

1 tablespoon unsalted butter or ghee

1 to 2 cloves garlic, minced

1 pound fresh green beans

Salt and ground black pepper

¼ teaspoon red pepper flakes

¼ cup gluten-free soy sauce (tamari)

2 tablespoons unseasoned rice vinegar

1 tablespoon medium-hot hot sauce (such as Frank's RedHot) or Buffalo sauce

1 tablespoon toasted sesame oil

3 tablespoons brown sugar substitute

½ teaspoon xanthan gum

¼ cup sesame seeds, for topping (optional)

DIRECTIONS

1. Place the butter and garlic in a large skillet over medium-high heat and sauté until the garlic becomes fragrant, about 1 minute.

2. Add the green beans and stir to coat with the buttery garlic. Sprinkle with salt and pepper and the red pepper flakes.

3. Add the soy sauce, rice vinegar, hot sauce, sesame oil, brown sugar substitute, and xanthan gum and stir until the ingredients are well incorporated. Continue to cook the beans until the sauce forms a glaze, about 5 minutes.

4. Top with the sesame seeds, if desired, and serve! Store leftovers in the refrigerator for up to 4 days. Reheat in a skillet with some butter, or in the microwave.

Nutritional information (per serving)

Calories: 117   Total Carbs: 10g

Fat: 7g   Fiber: 3g

Protein: 5g   Net Carbs: 7g

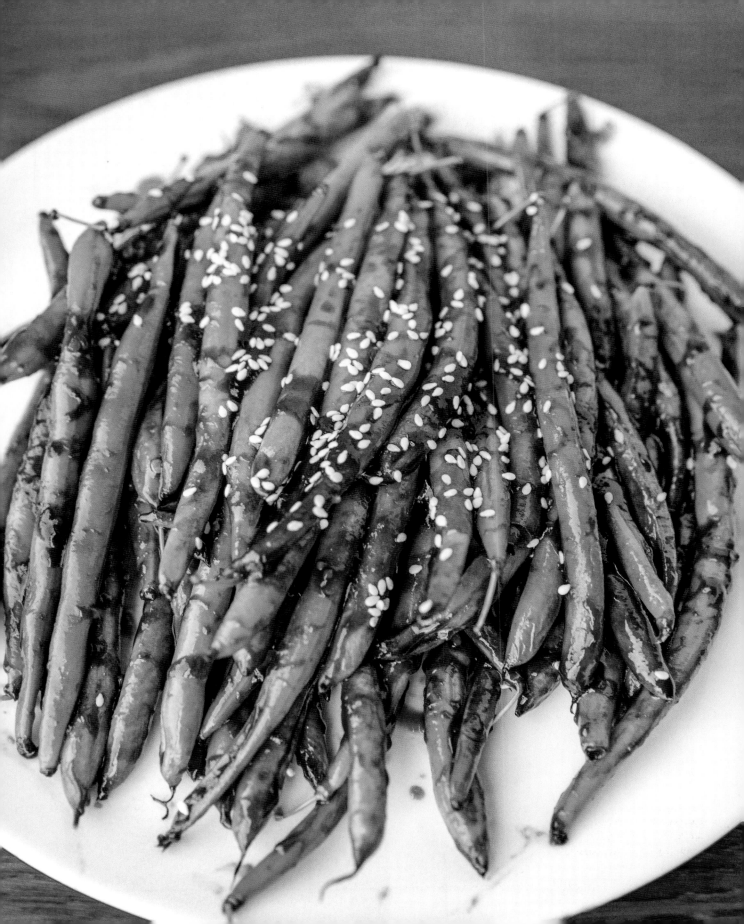

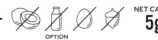

NET CARBS
5g

OPTION

SIMPLE SPAGHETTI SQUASH

MAKES 4 servings   **PREP TIME:** 8 minutes   **COOK TIME:** 15 minutes

Yes, you can microwave spaghetti squash. So easy! This is a super quick technique that you can jazz up any way you like. We love to serve spaghetti squash hot with butter and Parmesan cheese. You could also use it as a pasta substitute.

INGREDIENTS

1 large spaghetti squash (2 to 3 pounds)

Salt and ground black pepper

DIRECTIONS

1. Using a large sharp knife, cut the squash in half lengthwise. If the skin is too thick or is difficult to cut, poke a few holes in the squash with a fork and microwave the squash on high for 20 seconds. Once it is cut in half, use a spoon to scoop out the seeds.

2. Place the squash halves, cut sides up, in a 9 by 13-inch glass baking dish. Cover the dish with plastic wrap and secure all the edges tightly.

3. Microwave on high for 13 to 15 minutes, until fork-tender.

4. Drag a fork up and down the flesh of the squash so that it creates spaghetti-like strings. Continue until all the flesh is removed.

5. Season with salt and pepper and serve! Store leftovers in the refrigerator for up to 1 week. Reheat in the microwave or in a skillet.

Nutritional information (per serving)

Calories: 31	Total Carbs: 7g
Fat: 1g	Fiber: 2g
Protein: 1g	Net Carbs: 5g

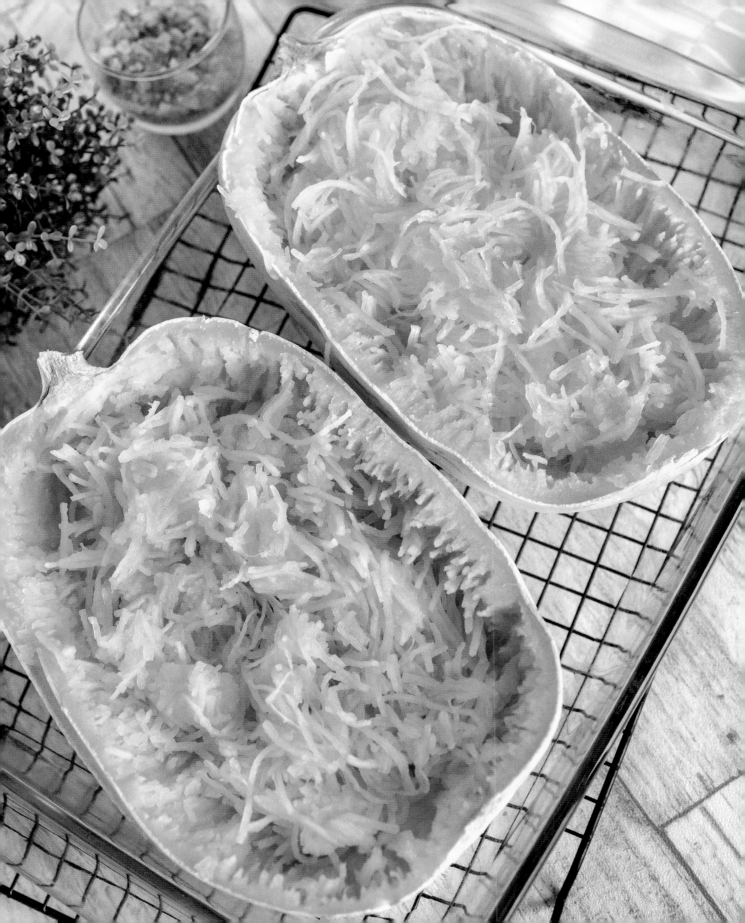

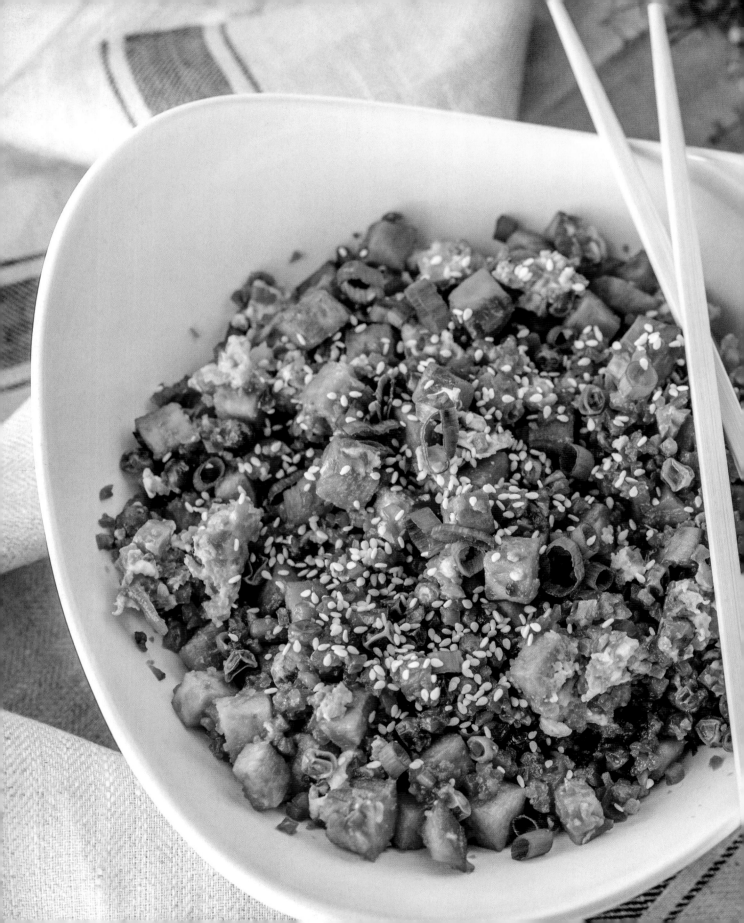

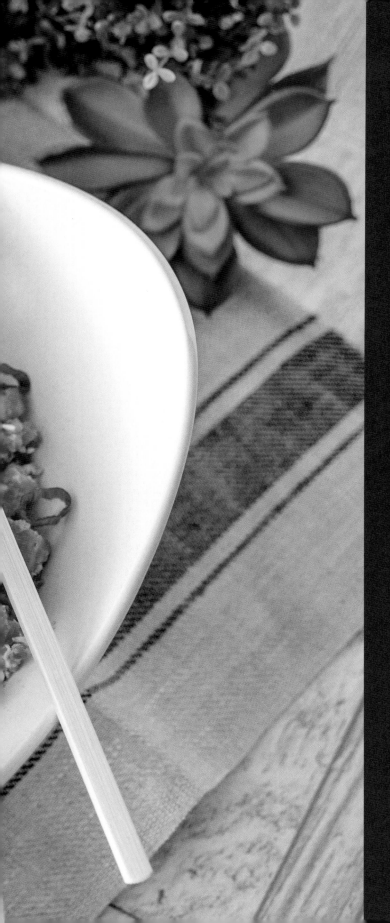

(5) MAIN DISHES

BBQ CHICKEN PIZZA

MAKES 8 servings   PREP TIME: 5 minutes (not including time to cook bacon)   COOK TIME: 12 minutes

BBQ chicken pizza will always be one of my favorite meals. The combination of sweet and savory is tough to beat. This combination of toppings would also be amazing on my Chicken Pizza Crust (page 294).

INGREDIENTS

1 par-baked Fathead Pizza Crust (page 288)

¾ cup sugar-free BBQ sauce

1½ cups shredded fiesta-blend cheese (or your favorite cheese) (about 6 ounces)

1 (12½-ounce) can chunk chicken breast, drained

4 slices bacon, cooked and chopped into bite-sized pieces

½ cup diced red onions

Chopped fresh cilantro leaves, for garnish

DIRECTIONS

1. Preheat the oven to 425°F. Line a baking sheet with parchment paper or a silicone baking mat, then place the par-baked crust on top.

2. Pour the BBQ sauce on top of the crust and spread it in an even layer, then sprinkle the cheese on top of the sauce. Scatter the chicken, bacon, and red onions over the sauce.

3. Bake for 12 minutes, or until the crust is golden brown.

4. Garnish with cilantro and serve hot!

Nutritional information (per serving)

Calories: 381	Total Carbs: 8g
Fat: 29g	Fiber: 2g
Protein: 26g	Net Carbs: 6g

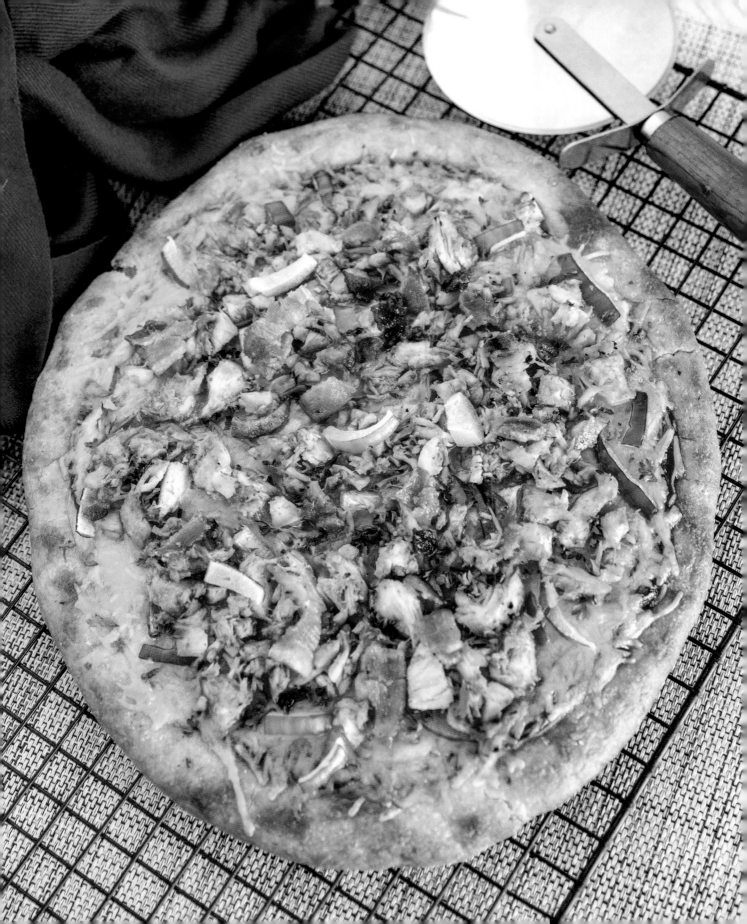

EGG ROLL IN A BOWL

MAKES 4 servings   PREP TIME: 5 minutes   COOK TIME: 18 minutes

One of my earliest childhood memories is of going to this incredible Chinese takeout joint near my grandma's house in New York. They had the best egg rolls I've ever eaten in my entire life. I swear if I close my eyes, I can still taste them! This recipe does not disappoint. Eat this dish alone in a bowl, or stuff it inside my empanada dough (page 164) for a heartier meal.

INGREDIENTS

½ cup diced yellow onions

2 cloves garlic, minced

1 pound bulk (ground) pork sausage

1 (16-ounce) bag coleslaw mix

½ teaspoon freshly grated ginger

2 tablespoons toasted sesame oil

2 tablespoons gluten-free soy sauce (tamari)

1 green onion, chopped

FOR GARNISH (OPTIONAL):

¼ teaspoon red pepper flakes

1 tablespoon chili garlic sauce

1 tablespoon Sriracha sauce

Everything bagel seasoning

DIRECTIONS

1. Place the onions, garlic, and sausage in a large skillet and cook until the sausage is browned, about 10 minutes.

2. Add the coleslaw, ginger, sesame oil, and soy sauce. Toss until well combined.

3. Transfer the egg roll mixture to a large serving bowl, then top with the chopped green onion and garnish with any of the optional ingredients: red pepper flakes, chili garlic sauce, Sriracha, and everything bagel seasoning.

4. Serve immediately. Store leftovers in the refrigerator for up to 5 days. Reheat in a skillet or in the microwave.

Nutritional information (per serving)

Calories: 486	Total Carbs: 8g
Fat: 39g	Fiber: 3g
Protein: 23g	Net Carbs: 5g

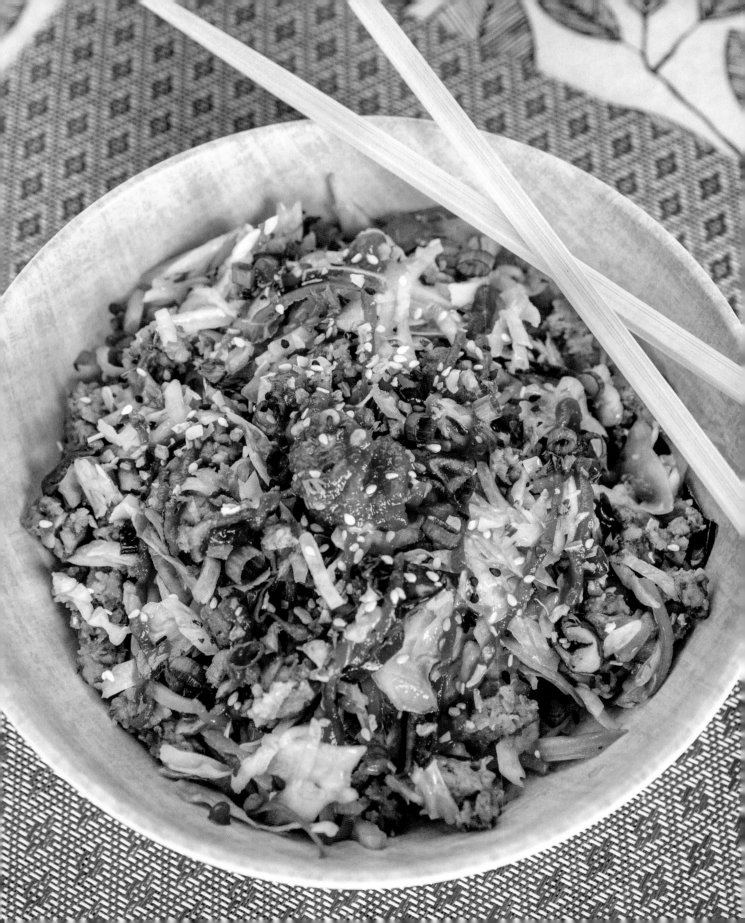

HAM FRIED RICE

MAKES 4 servings   PREP TIME: 10 minutes   COOK TIME: 18 minutes

Early on in my adult life, I would implement a meatless dinner once a week to cut down on the cost of groceries. A version of this fried rice dish was always on my list of meatless meals. Yes, there is meat in here, but a ham steak costs far less than chicken or beef, and you're still getting some protein. Added bonus: the flavors in this dish completely drown out the "nasty cauliflower rice taste." Those are Cameron's words, and let me just tell you, if I can get my husband to eat cauliflower and actually enjoy it, I know it's good.

INGREDIENTS

1 (10-ounce) bag frozen riced cauliflower

Extra-virgin olive oil, for the pan

½ cup diced yellow onions

2 cloves garlic, minced

1 (12-ounce) bag frozen peas and carrots

1 ham steak (about 1 pound)

¼ cup gluten-free soy sauce (tamari)

1 tablespoon toasted sesame oil

2 tablespoons brown sugar substitute

1 tablespoon granulated sweetener

2 large eggs

Sliced green onions, for garnish (optional)

Sesame seeds, for garnish (optional)

DIRECTIONS

1. Microwave the riced cauliflower according to package directions (usually 4 to 6 minutes on high). Set aside.

2. Place a large skillet over high heat and drizzle with olive oil to thinly coat the bottom of the pan. Add the onions and garlic and sauté until fragrant, about 5 minutes.

3. Meanwhile, chop the ham into ¼-inch pieces. When the onions and garlic are fragrant, add the ham and continue to sauté for 3 minutes, until the ham turns golden brown.

4. Place the peas and carrots in a small strainer and rinse with room-temperature water just to take the chill off. Then add the peas and carrots to the skillet.

5. Empty the riced cauliflower into the skillet and stir until all the ingredients are mixed well.

6. Add the soy sauce, sesame oil, and sweeteners to the skillet and stir to combine. Move the cauli-rice mixture to one side of the pan, then add the eggs to the empty side. Scramble the eggs and slowly merge them into the cauli-rice mixture. Stir to make sure all the flavors are well combined.

7. Garnish each serving of fried rice with green onions and sesame seeds, if desired, and enjoy! Store leftovers in the refrigerator for up to 5 days. Reheat in a skillet with some olive oil or butter.

Nutritional information (per serving)

Calories: 217	Total Carbs: 15g
Fat: 12g	Fiber: 5g
Protein: 14g	Net Carbs: 10g

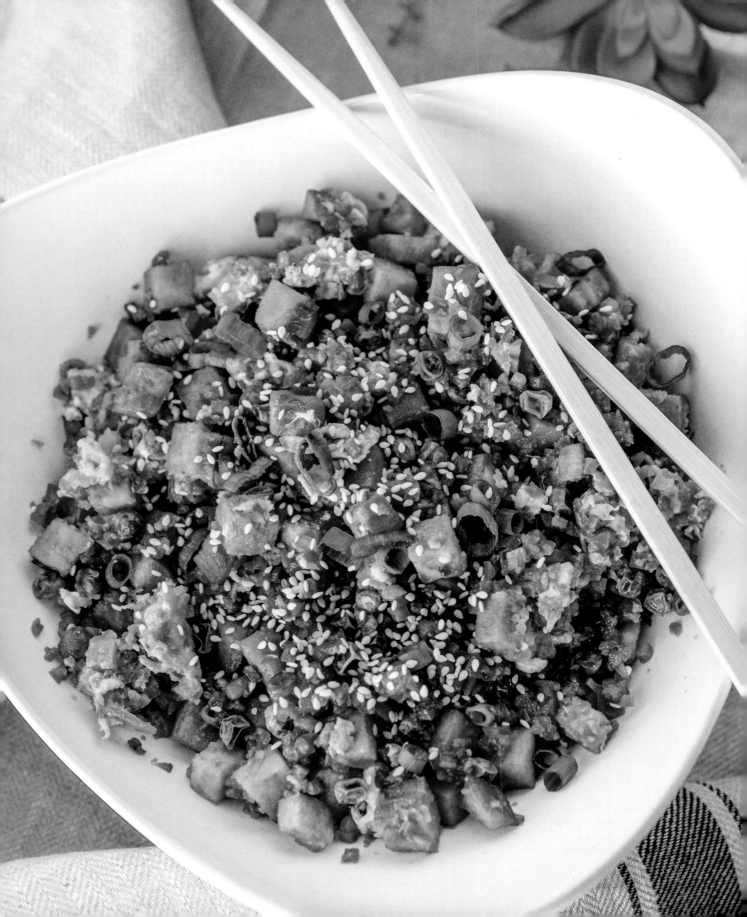

ONE-POT MUSTARD CHICKEN

MAKES 4 servings **PREP TIME: 5 minutes** **COOK TIME: 35 minutes**

If you're a mustard lover, this chicken dish is so up your alley! Even if you're not, you should still give it a try. My whole family loves this dish, and we have a few picky eaters around here!

INGREDIENTS

8 ounces bacon

4 boneless, skinless chicken breast halves (about 4 ounces each)

1 teaspoon smoked paprika

Salt and ground black pepper

1 cup chicken bone broth

¾ cup heavy whipping cream

½ cup Dijon mustard

1 to 2 tablespoons stone-ground mustard

2 tablespoons fresh thyme leaves

DIRECTIONS

1. Place a large skillet over medium-high heat. While the skillet is heating, cut the bacon into bite-sized pieces. Once the skillet is hot, add the bacon and cook for 7 minutes, or until it reaches your desired doneness.

2. Remove the bacon to a paper towel–lined plate and set aside; leave as much of the bacon grease in the pan as possible.

3. Cut each chicken breast in half horizontally to make two thinner layers. Place the breasts between two pieces of plastic wrap and pound to an even thickness. If you don't have a meat mallet, a rolling pin works like a charm!

4. Place the chicken in the skillet with the bacon grease, still over medium-high heat. Sprinkle with the paprika and season with salt and pepper. Cook on each side for 4 to 6 minutes; the chicken does not need to be cooked all the way through at this point. Remove the chicken from the pan and set aside.

5. Add the broth, heavy cream, and mustards to the skillet and stir to combine. Make sure to scrape up all the bits stuck to the bottom of the pan—that's where all the good stuff is hiding! Bring to a boil.

6. Once the sauce is boiling, reduce the heat to low. Return the chicken to the pan and simmer for another 15 minutes, or until the chicken is cooked all the way through.

7. Return the bacon to the skillet and stir to incorporate into the sauce. Sprinkle with the fresh thyme and serve. Store leftovers in the refrigerator for up to 5 days. Reheat in the microwave.

Nutritional information (per serving)

Calories: 496	Total Carbs: 1g
Fat: 37g	Fiber: 0g
Protein: 32g	Net Carbs: 1g

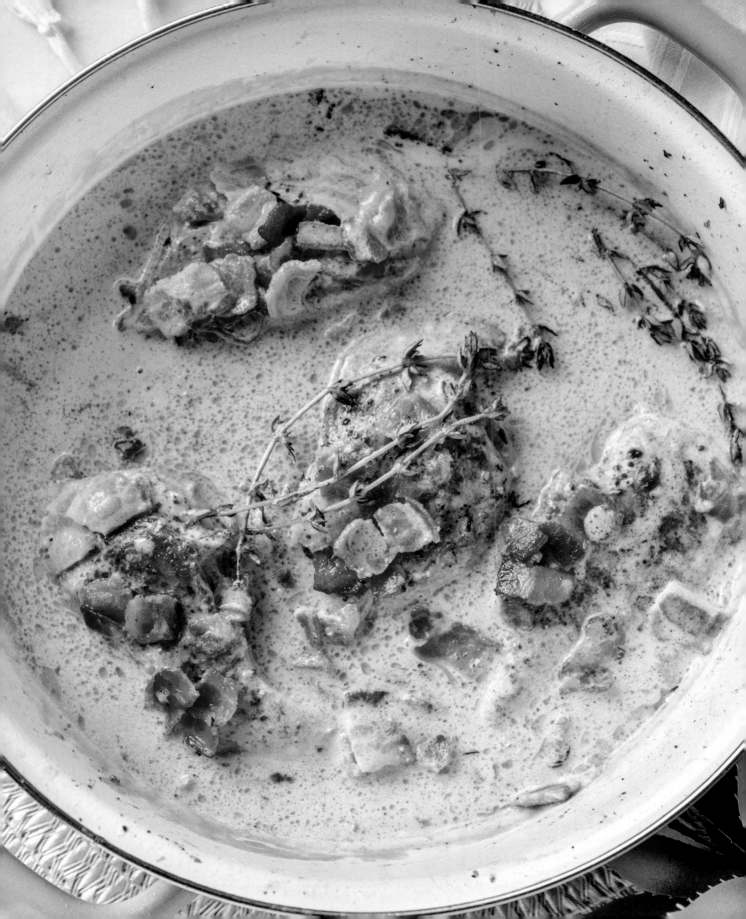

SHEET PAN KIELBASA AND VEGGIES

MAKES 4 servings   PREP TIME: 10 minutes   COOK TIME: 30 minutes

We love easy dinners around our house—mainly because I'm lazy, but also because we are an incredibly busy family. This sheet pan dish is so quick to make, and the cleanup is even quicker! Just roll up that foil and toss it!

INGREDIENTS

8 ounces fresh green beans

2 cups fresh broccoli florets

5 to 7 cloves garlic, peeled

½ cup extra-virgin olive oil

Salt and ground black pepper

1 pound kielbasa

Lemon wedges, for serving

DIRECTIONS

1. Preheat the oven to 425°F. Line a rimmed baking sheet with aluminum foil.

2. Place the green beans and broccoli in a colander and rinse with cold water. Set the veggies on a clean kitchen towel to dry.

3. Scatter the dry veggies and garlic on the lined baking sheet. Drizzle the oil over the veggies and toss with your fingers to evenly coat the veggies in the oil. Sprinkle with salt and pepper.

4. Bake for 20 minutes, or until the veggies are golden brown.

5. Remove the baking sheet from the oven and turn the oven setting to broil.

6. While the oven is heating, cut the kielbasa into ½-inch slices and scatter on the baking sheet with the veggies.

7. Return the baking sheet to the oven and broil for 5 to 10 minutes, depending on how crispy you like your veggies. Serve with lemon wedges. Store leftovers in the refrigerator for up to 1 week. Reheat in a skillet with some butter or olive oil.

Nutritional information (per serving)

Calories: 525   Total Carbs: 9g

Fat: 39g   Fiber: 3g

Protein: 19g   Net Carbs: 6g

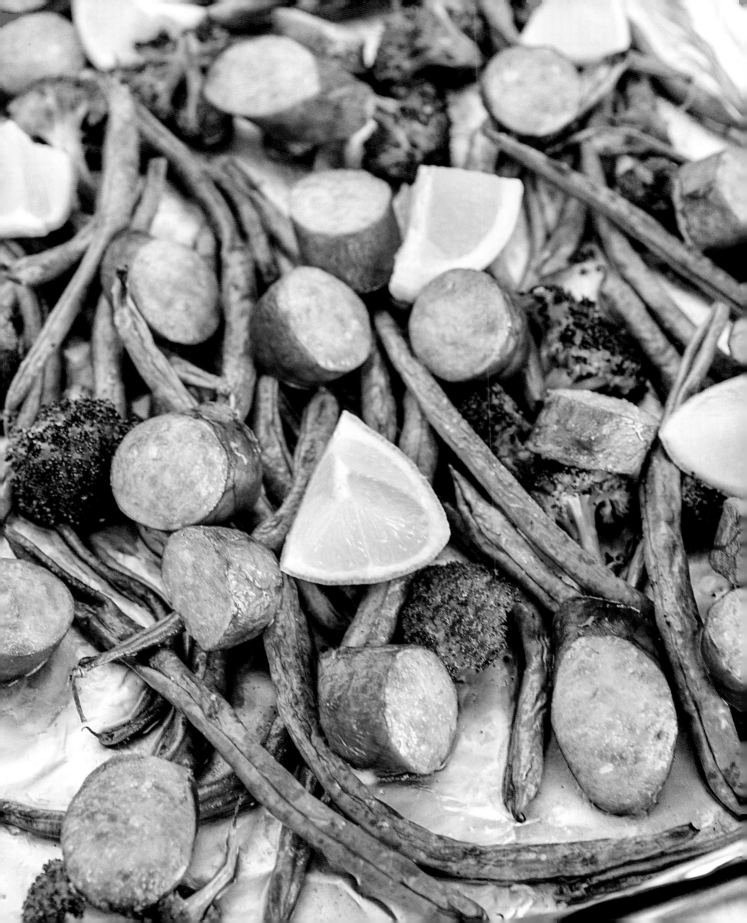

JALAPEÑO POPPER CHICKEN BAKE

MAKES 4 servings   PREP TIME: 25 minutes   COOK TIME: 55 minutes

This may be my favorite dinner in the whole book. It's creamy and hearty, and the freshness of the jalapeños is incredible. You could certainly use jarred jalapeños if you don't have fresh ones on hand. Either way, I hope this becomes a family favorite for you as well!

INGREDIENTS

4 boneless, skinless chicken breast halves (about 4 ounces each)

Salt and ground black pepper

6 slices bacon, cut into bite-sized pieces

1 or 2 jalapeño peppers

¼ cup diced yellow onions

2 cloves garlic, minced

½ cup mayonnaise

4 ounces cheddar cheese, shredded (about 1 cup)

1½ ounces Parmesan cheese, grated (about ½ cup)

2 ounces cream cheese (¼ cup), softened

FOR THE BREADING:

4 cups plain pork rinds

1 ounce Parmesan cheese, grated (about ¼ cup)

2 tablespoons unsalted butter, softened

DIRECTIONS

1. Preheat the oven to 425°F. Place the chicken breasts in a 9 by 13-inch glass baking dish and sprinkle with salt and pepper. Bake for 30 minutes.

2. Meanwhile, set a large skillet over medium-high heat. Place the chopped bacon in the skillet and cook for 5 minutes, or until it reaches your desired doneness. (We love crispy bacon!) Remove the bacon to a paper towel–lined plate and set aside; leave as much of the bacon grease in the skillet as possible.

3. While wearing gloves (trust me on this!), cut the jalapeño(s) in half lengthwise. Scoop out the seeds and veins. (That's where all the heat is, so if you don't like heat, make sure to get them all out!) Then chop the jalapeño(s). If desired, cut a couple of slices and reserve them for garnish.

4. Add the onions, garlic, and jalapeños to the skillet. Sauté for 5 minutes, or until the onions are translucent.

5. Place the mayonnaise, cheddar, Parmesan, and cream cheese in a medium-sized bowl and mix well. Then add the bacon and the onion mixture to the cheese mixture and stir until well combined.

6. Remove the chicken from the oven and reduce the temperature to 350°F. Spoon a thick layer of the bacon and cheese mixture on top of each chicken breast. Don't be shy! The chicken should be smothered in a thick layer. Return the baking dish to the oven and cook for another 10 minutes.

7. While the chicken is baking, place the pork rinds in a gallon-sized resealable plastic bag. Let all the air out of the bag and seal, then crush the pork rinds with a rolling pin. You want them to be very fine, like breadcrumbs. Add the Parmesan cheese and butter and shake the bag until the breading ingredients are well combined.

Nutritional information (per serving)

Calories: 493	Total Carbs: 3g
Fat: 43g	Fiber: 0g
Protein: 25g	Net Carbs: 3g

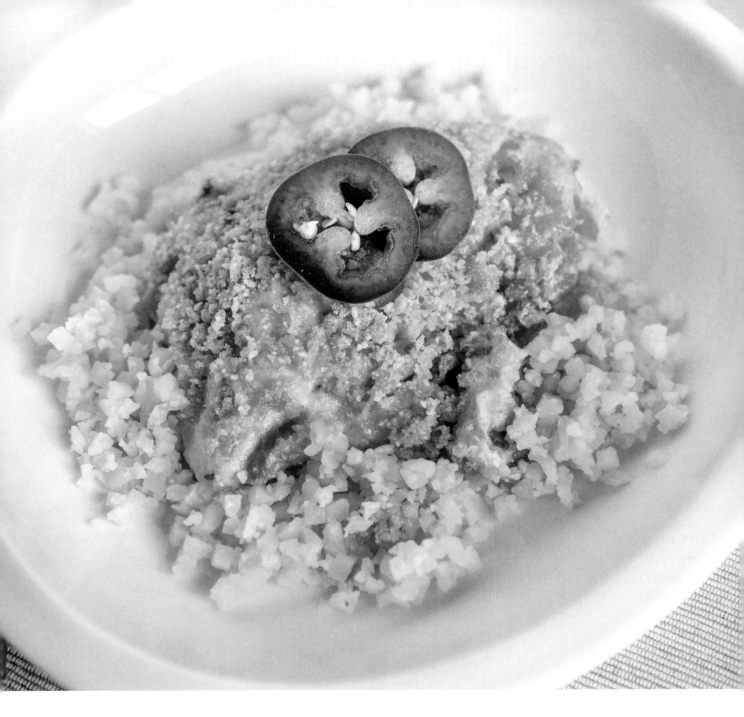

8. Remove the chicken from the oven and shake the breading mixture on top of the chicken until each breast is fully covered. Place back in the oven for 5 minutes, or until the topping is golden brown.

9. Top the chicken with the reserved jalapeño slices and serve! Store leftovers in the refrigerator for up to 5 days. Reheat in the oven.

MAPLE-GLAZED SALMON

MAKES 2 servings   PREP TIME: 15 minutes   COOK TIME: 27 minutes

This is one of those dishes that makes you look like a rock star in the kitchen. Even if you think you have zero kitchen skills, I promise you can make this. Salmon will always be a favorite of mine, and this dish hits all parts of your palate—sweet, savory, tart, rich, and delicious.

INGREDIENTS

1 (1-pound) salmon fillet, or 2 (8-ounce) salmon fillets

Salt and ground black pepper

1 lemon, thinly sliced

¼ cup (½ stick) unsalted butter or ghee, melted

4 tablespoons sugar-free maple syrup, store-bought or homemade (page 269), divided

2 cloves garlic, minced

½ teaspoon Italian seasoning

¼ teaspoon chopped fresh dill, for garnish

DIRECTIONS

1. Preheat the oven to 375°F. Line a rimmed baking sheet with aluminum foil.

2. Place the salmon on the lined baking sheet. Sprinkle with salt and pepper. Place a couple of lemon slices under the salmon. (It will soak up the lemon juice as it cooks.)

3. In a medium-sized bowl, whisk together the melted butter, 2 tablespoons of the maple syrup, the garlic, and Italian seasoning.

4. Lift up the sides of the foil to create a bowl to hold the sauce. Pour the sauce over the salmon, then fold the foil over the top of the salmon to cover.

5. Bake for 15 to 17 minutes, until the edges are golden brown.

6. Remove the baking sheet from the oven and turn the oven to the broil setting. Unwrap the salmon so the top is exposed. Baste the salmon with the remaining maple syrup. Bake for another 8 to 10 minutes, until it becomes crispy, watching closely so it doesn't burn.

7. Garnish the salmon with the remaining lemon slices and the dill and serve immediately!

Nutritional information (per serving)

Calories: 681	Total Carbs: 5g
Fat: 41g	Fiber: 0g
Protein: 58g	Net Carbs: 5g

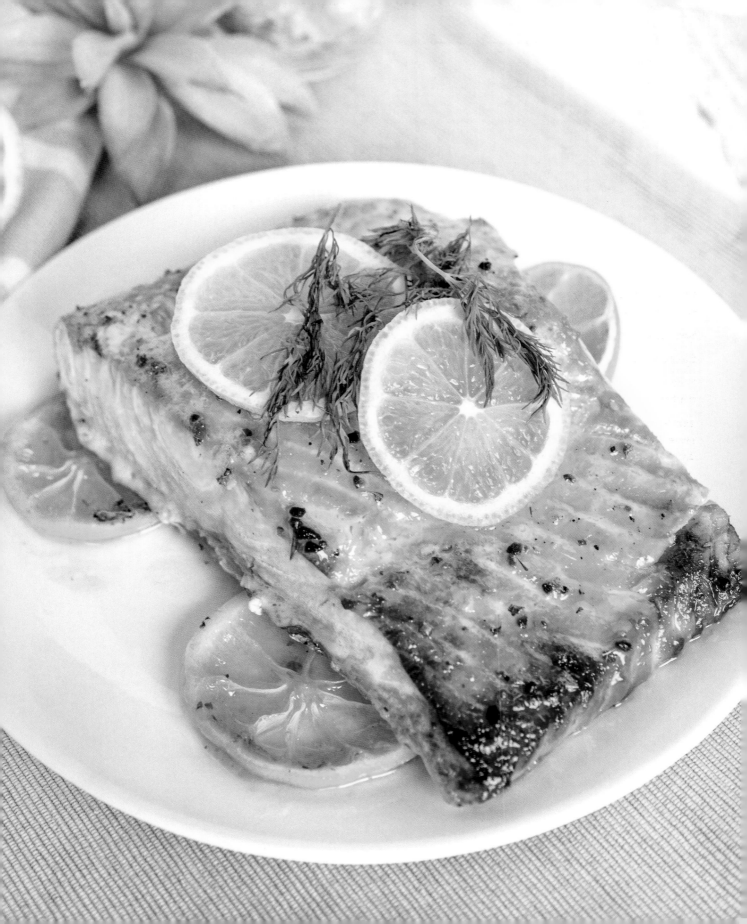

BEEF EMPANADAS

MAKES 6 empanadas (2 per serving)   PREP TIME: 35 minutes   COOK TIME: 16 minutes

The beauty of keto is that you can re-create almost anything from your old way of eating. Empanadas are one of those comfort foods that leave me feeling full and happy. This keto version does the exact same thing, and I don't feel guilty eating it! Try serving these empanadas with apple cider vinegar for dipping—it sounds weird but tastes amazing!

INGREDIENTS

FOR THE BEEF FILLING:

1 tablespoon unsalted butter, plus more if needed

¼ cup diced white onions

8 ounces ground beef

Salt and ground black pepper

1 teaspoon apple cider vinegar, plus more for dipping if desired

2 ounces cheddar cheese, shredded (½ cup)

FOR THE DOUGH:

6 ounces mozzarella cheese, shredded (about 1½ cups)

2 ounces cream cheese (¼ cup)

¾ cup blanched almond flour

1 large egg

½ teaspoon garlic powder

½ teaspoon onion powder

½ teaspoon salt

Lime wedges, for garnish (optional)

DIRECTIONS

1. Place the butter in a medium-sized skillet over medium-high heat. When the butter begins to bubble, add the onions. Sauté for 5 minutes, until the onions become translucent.

2. Add the ground beef to the skillet and sprinkle with salt and pepper. Cook for 10 minutes, stirring occasionally, until the beef is browned and cooked all the way through.

3. Once the beef is browned, stir in the vinegar. Remove from the heat and set aside.

4. Make the dough: Place the mozzarella and cream cheese in a large microwave-safe bowl; there is no need to stir at this point. Microwave on high for 1 minute. Remove from the microwave and stir the cheeses with a fork. You may need to heat again for an additional 20 to 30 seconds to make sure the cheeses are well combined.

5. Add the remaining dough ingredients to the bowl with the melted cheeses. Wet your hands and mix the dough together. The dough will be hot, so you may need to let it cool for a minute before mixing. It may take some time to get it all incorporated. If the dough starts to stick to your hands, wet your hands again and continue working the dough until all the ingredients are thoroughly combined. Microwave the dough for 15 seconds, if necessary.

6. Preheat the oven to 425°F. Line a baking sheet with parchment paper or a silicone baking mat.

7. Lay a sheet of parchment paper on a large cutting board or a clean countertop. Put the dough on the parchment, then place another sheet of parchment paper on top of the dough. Roll out the dough with a rolling pin until it is about ⅛ inch thick.

8. Use a 3-inch circular cookie cutter (or a 3-inch bowl or cup) to cut the dough into 6 circles; lay the circles of dough on the lined baking sheet.

9. Top each circle with about a tablespoon of the beef mixture. Sprinkle about a teaspoon of cheddar cheese on top of the beef mixture on each empanada. You don't want to stuff the empanadas too full or they will break open when baked.

Nutritional information (per serving)

Calories: 654	Total Carbs: 9g
Fat: 54g	Fiber: 3g
Protein: 40g	Net Carbs: 6g

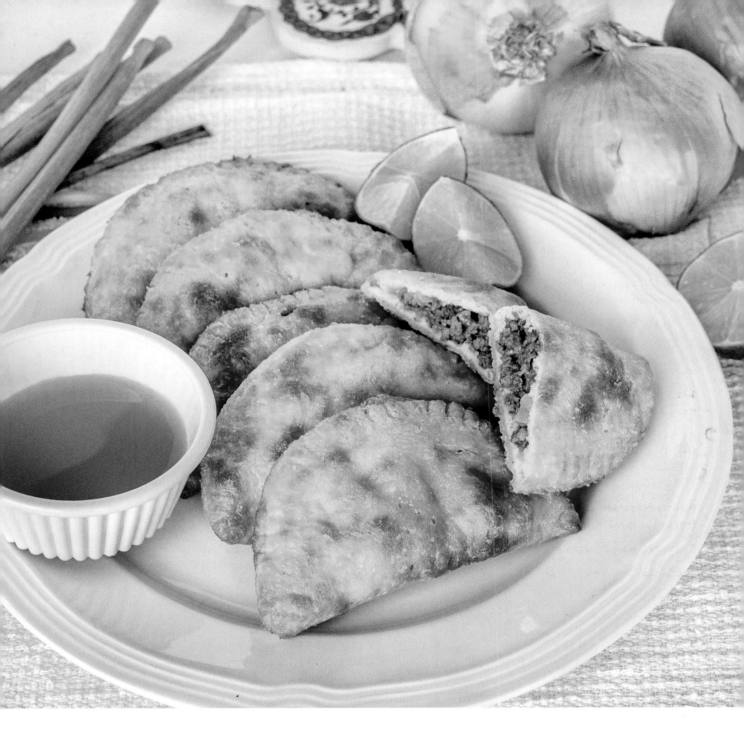

10. To seal the empanadas, fold one side of the circle over the beef and cheese and pinch the edges together, then use a fork to press down the edges so the filling is completely sealed inside.

11. Bake for 14 to 16 minutes, until the empanadas are golden brown.

12. Garnish with lime wedges and serve with a side of apple cider vinegar for dipping, if desired.

CARAMELIZED ONION TART

MAKES 6 servings   PREP TIME: 20 minutes   COOK TIME: 26 minutes

I created this recipe very early on in my keto journey, and I honestly thought I had died and gone to heaven when I tasted it. This thing hits all areas of your taste buds! The sugar-free maple syrup is optional, but please try it! It sounds insane, but I promise it'll be a very pleasant surprise. This recipe has been a huge hit with my Instagram followers, and I know you'll love it, too!

INGREDIENTS

FOR THE DOUGH:

6 ounces mozzarella cheese, shredded (about 1½ cups)

2 ounces cream cheese (¼ cup)

¾ cup blanched almond flour

1 large egg

1 teaspoon garlic salt

TOPPINGS:

4 ounces Brie cheese, shredded (1 cup) (see Note)

2 ounces mozzarella cheese, shredded (about ½ cup)

1½ cups Caramelized Onions (page 298)

3 tablespoons balsamic vinegar

3 tablespoons sugar-free maple syrup, store-bought or homemade (page 269) (optional)

Fresh basil leaves, cut into ribbons (optional)

Variation: For a nut-free tart, use a Chicken Pizza Crust (page 294).

DIRECTIONS

1. Preheat the oven to 400°F. Line a baking sheet with parchment paper or a silicone baking mat.

2. Make the dough: Place the mozzarella and cream cheese in a large microwave-safe bowl; there is no need to stir at this point. Microwave on high for 1 minute. Remove from the microwave and stir the cheeses with a fork. Then microwave for another 30 seconds, stirring again until the cheeses are well combined and form a gummy consistency. Stir in almond flour and egg.

3. Wet your hands and knead the dough until all the ingredients are well incorporated. If the dough becomes too sticky, simply wet your hands again and continue kneading. Form the dough into a ball.

4. Lay a sheet of parchment paper on a large cutting board or clean countertop. Put the dough on the parchment and place another sheet of parchment paper on top of the dough. Roll out the dough with a rolling pin to a thickness of ½ to ⅓ inch.

5. Roll the edge of the dough toward the center so it forms a "crust." (This step is optional, but it makes the tart look pretty and gives the toppings a barrier to keep them from oozing over the side.)

6. Using a fork, poke holes in the dough to prevent bubbling. Sprinkle the dough with the garlic salt.

7. Par-bake for 12 to 14 minutes, until slightly browned on top.

8. Remove the crust from the oven and sprinkle with the Brie and mozzarella. Spread the caramelized onions evenly over the cheeses.

9. Bake for an additional 10 to 12 minutes, until the cheeses are fully melted.

10. Top with the balsamic vinegar, maple syrup, and basil ribbons, if desired. Serve immediately. Store leftovers in the refrigerator for up to 5 days. Reheat in the oven.

Nutritional information (per serving)

Calories: 514	Total Carbs: 10g
Fat: 44g	Fiber: 3g
Protein: 26g	Net Carbs: 7g

> *Note:* It's nearly impossible to find preshredded Brie, so plan on shredding it yourself.

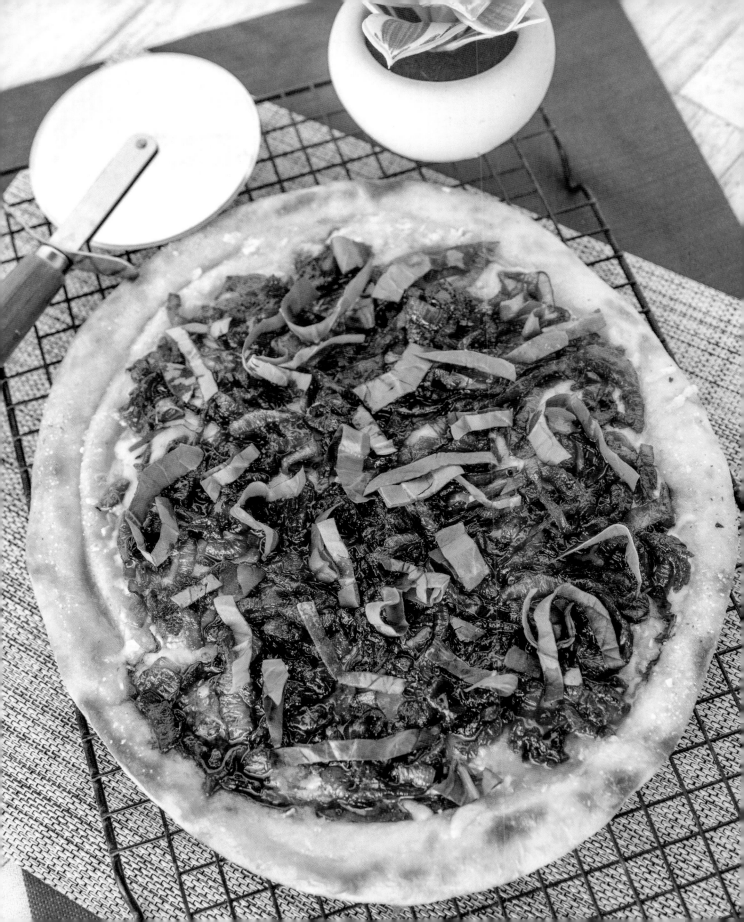

BLTA WRAPS

NET CARBS 2g

MAKES 8 wraps (2 per serving)   **PREP TIME: 5 minutes**   **COOK TIME: 25 minutes**

This is probably my family's favorite lazy meal. We prefer lettuce wraps over sandwiches any day—such a fresh and guilt-free meal that everyone enjoys! The best part is that there are no limits to how you can prepare these wraps. Want more bacon? Add more bacon!

INGREDIENTS

1 pound bacon

8 teaspoons mayonnaise

8 romaine or butter lettuce leaves

2 Roma tomatoes, diced

1 medium avocado, cubed

¼ cup diced red onions (optional)

Salt and ground black pepper

DIRECTIONS

1. Cook the bacon until it reaches your desired doneness. (We love bacon cooked in the oven on a foil–lined baking sheet for 20 to 25 minutes at 400°F.) Let the bacon cool, then crumble it.

2. Assemble the wraps: Spread about a teaspoon of mayonnaise on a lettuce leaf, then add some bacon, tomatoes, avocado, and diced onions. Repeat with the remaining ingredients, making a total of 8 wraps. Season with salt and pepper and serve!

Nutritional information (per serving)

Calories: 633	Total Carbs: 5g
Fat: 50g	Fiber: 3g
Protein: 39g	Net Carbs: 2g

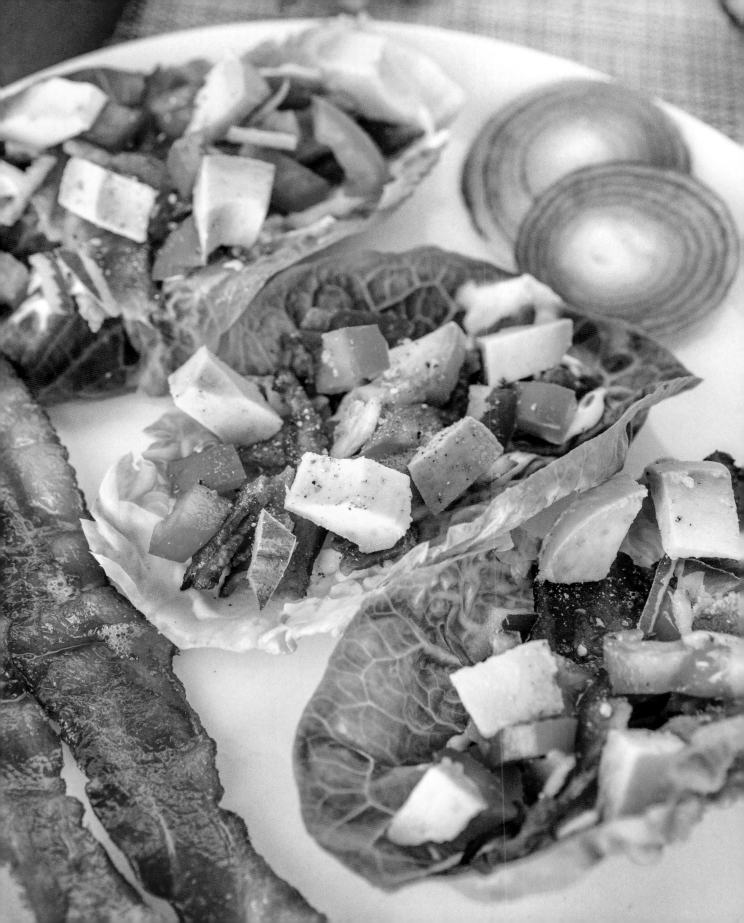

CHEESY TACO BAKE

MAKES 6 servings   PREP TIME: 3 minutes   COOK TIME: 22 minutes

This taco bake is another family favorite. It reminds me of the insides of a bean and cheese burrito, minus the beans, obviously. The salsa and cream cheese give this dish an amazing creamy texture that melts in your mouth. It is also a great one to make ahead and freeze for later. Then you can just whip it out of the freezer and bake it when you're ready to eat. Serve as a casserole or as a dip with sliced veggies.

INGREDIENTS

1 pound ground beef

½ cup diced yellow onions

2 tablespoons taco seasoning, store-bought or homemade (page 308)

¼ cup sugar-free ketchup

1 (8-ounce) package cream cheese, softened, or 1 cup full-fat cottage cheese

¾ cup salsa (see Note)

4 ounces cheddar cheese, shredded (about 1 cup)

DIRECTIONS

1. Preheat the oven to 350°F.

2. Cook the ground beef and onions in a medium-sized skillet over medium-high heat for 10 minutes, or until the beef is fully browned.

3. Add the taco seasoning and ketchup and stir until everything is well incorporated. Add the cream cheese and salsa and stir again until the mixture is combined.

4. Transfer the ground beef mixture to a 9-inch square glass baking dish. Top with the cheddar cheese.

5. Bake for 5 to 7 minutes, until the cheese is melted. Serve hot.

6. Store leftovers in the refrigerator for up to 5 days. Reheat in the oven or microwave.

> *Note:* *When purchasing salsa, try to find the one with the lowest amounts of carbs and sugars. Fiesta-blend cheese would be yummy, too!*

Nutritional information (per serving)

Calories: 364	Total Carbs: 7g
Fat: 28g	Fiber: 1g
Protein: 23g	Net Carbs: 6g

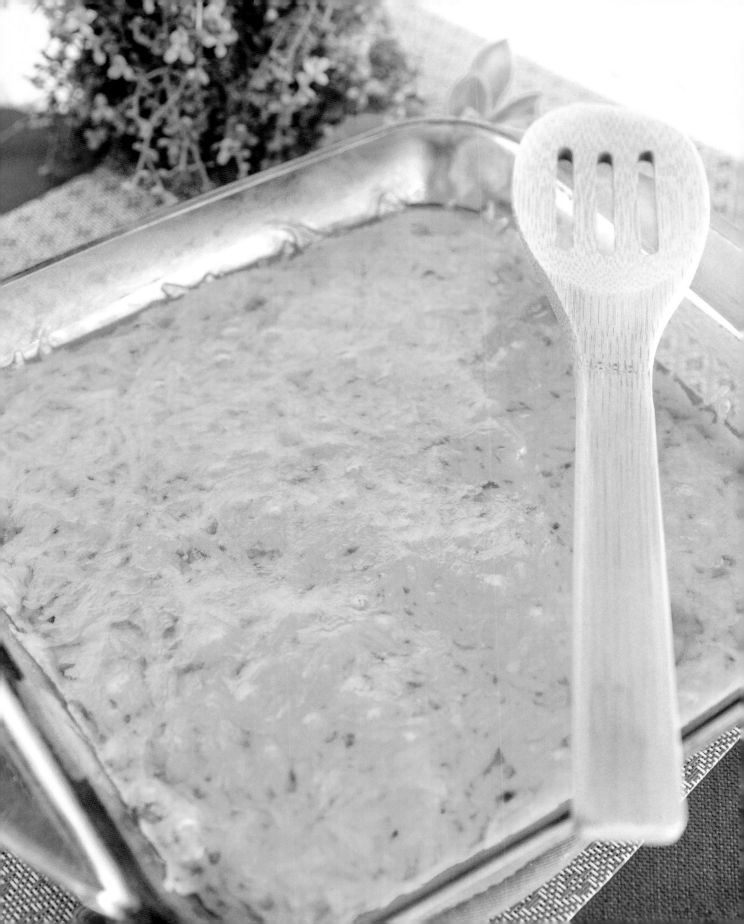

GREEN CHILI SAUSAGE CASSEROLE

MAKES 4 servings **PREP TIME: 10 minutes** **COOK TIME: 25 minutes**

This casserole is so hearty! It would also be an amazing filling for stuffed peppers or even a dip for hot-and-spicy pork rinds. It's up to you on how you'd like to devour it. I prefer just a spoon.

INGREDIENTS

1 pound bulk (ground) breakfast sausage

¼ teaspoon red pepper flakes

Salt and ground black pepper

1 (8-ounce) package cream cheese, softened

1 (7-ounce) can diced green chilis, with liquid

¾ cup Savory Breadcrumbs (page 304)

DIRECTIONS

1. Preheat the oven to 350°F.

2. Place the sausage in a medium-sized skillet over medium-high heat. Add the red pepper flakes and sprinkle with salt and pepper. Cook for 10 minutes, until the sausage is cooked all the way through.

3. Add the cream cheese and green chilis to the seasoned sausage. Stir to fully incorporate the cream cheese.

4. Transfer the sausage mixture to an 8-inch square or smaller baking dish. Sprinkle the breadcrumbs on top.

5. Bake for 10 to 15 minutes, until the breadcrumbs turn golden brown. Serve hot!

6. Store leftovers in the refrigerator for up to 5 days. Reheat in the oven or microwave.

Nutritional information (per serving)

Calories: 667	Total Carbs: 5g
Fat: 53g	Fiber: 1g
Protein: 32g	Net Carbs: 4g

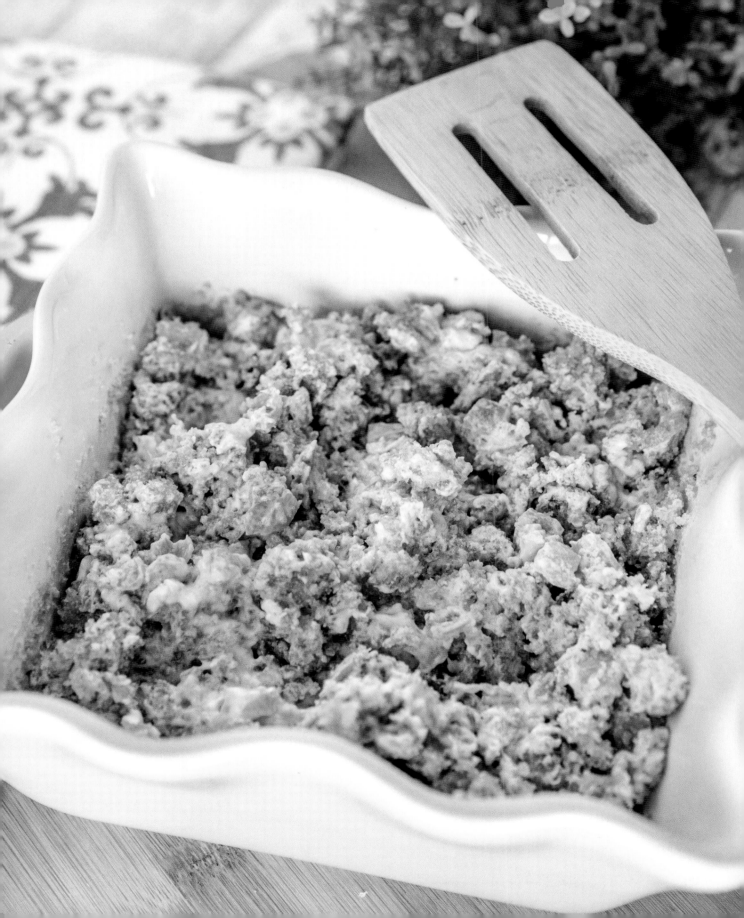

CHICKEN NUGGETS

MAKES 4 servings   PREP TIME: 30 minutes, plus 4 hours to marinate   COOK TIME: 24 minutes

One of my favorite places to eat with the kids when they were little was Chick-fil-A, especially during the winter months here in Utah. It gave us all the chance to get out of the house and eat delicious food, and the kids could burn off some energy in the play place. I was bummed when I started keto and realized I couldn't have their breaded nuggets anymore. I knew I had to create my own keto version, and this one does not disappoint! Even the kids agree that these nuggets taste like the real thing. There's just something amazing about marinating the chicken in pickle juice. Give these a try—and don't forget the Copycat Chick-fil-A Sauce for dipping!

INGREDIENTS

4 boneless, skinless chicken thighs

1 cup dill pickle juice

2 large eggs

2 tablespoons water

1½ cups Savory Breadcrumbs (page 304)

1 tablespoon paprika

1 tablespoon garlic powder

Avocado oil, for frying

½ cup Copycat Chick-fil-A Sauce, for dipping (page 290)

DIRECTIONS

1. Cut the chicken thighs into bite-sized pieces.

2. Place the chicken and pickle juice in a gallon-sized resealable bag, seal, and marinate in the refrigerator for a minimum of 4 hours; overnight is best.

3. When ready to cook the chicken, place the eggs and water in a small shallow bowl, whisk together, and set aside. Put the breadcrumbs, paprika, and garlic powder in another gallon-sized resealable plastic bag and shake to combine.

4. Remove the chicken from the pickle juice and dip a piece in the egg wash, then place in the bag with the breading mixture and toss to coat. Repeat until all the chicken is breaded.

5. Coat the bottom of a large skillet with avocado oil and place over high heat. When the oil is shimmering, carefully place a few of the chicken pieces in the hot oil. (You don't want to overcrowd the pan.) Fry until golden brown on one side, 3 to 4 minutes. Flip the chicken over and cook the other side until the breading is golden brown and the chicken is cooked all the way through, another 2 to 3 minutes. Remove the finished nuggets to a paper towel–lined plate. Repeat until all the chicken is cooked.

6. Serve immediately with the dipping sauce. Store leftovers in the refrigerator for up to 5 days. Reheat in the microwave or oven.

Nutritional information (per serving)

Calories: 310	Total Carbs: 4g
Fat: 13g	Fiber: 0g
Protein: 32g	Net Carbs: 4g

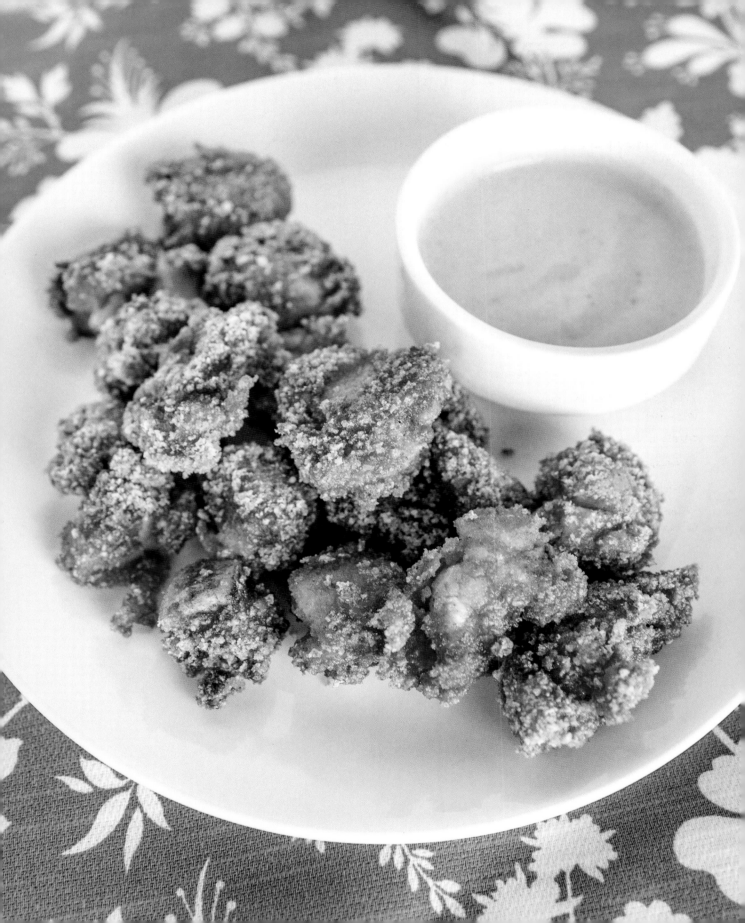

AVOCADO AND FETA TACOS

MAKES 4 tacos (2 per serving)   PREP TIME: 5 minutes   COOK TIME: 24 minutes

If you've never had avocado and feta together, you're missing out BIG TIME! It is such an amazing combination. The first time I tried it was at a local Mexican restaurant. I was crushed when the restaurant closed down, so I had to figure out a way to re-create those flavors.

INGREDIENTS

1 batch Cheese Shells (page 276)

1 medium avocado, diced

1½ ounces crumbled feta cheese (about ¼ cup)

1 large radish, thinly sliced

Extra-virgin olive oil, for drizzling

Lime wedges, for serving

Salt and ground black pepper (optional)

Variation: Add some shredded beef for a heartier meal!

DIRECTIONS

1. Preheat a griddle or a large nonstick skillet over medium-high heat (about 350°F if using an electric griddle). Place about ¾ cup of the cheddar cheese in a clump in the center of the griddle or skillet. Let the cheese melt and harden, about 3 minutes on each side. Hang the cheese over a wooden spoon suspended over two glasses or cups to make the shape of a taco shell. Repeat with the remaining cheese to make three more shells, then allow the shells to cool.

2. Assemble the tacos with the avocado, feta, and radish slices. Drizzle the tacos with olive oil and squeeze lime juice over the top. Season with salt and pepper, if desired. Serve immediately!

Nutritional information (per serving)

Calories: 920	Total Carbs: 12g
Fat: 79g	Fiber: 5g
Protein: 43g	Net Carbs: 7g

176   5: MAIN DISHES

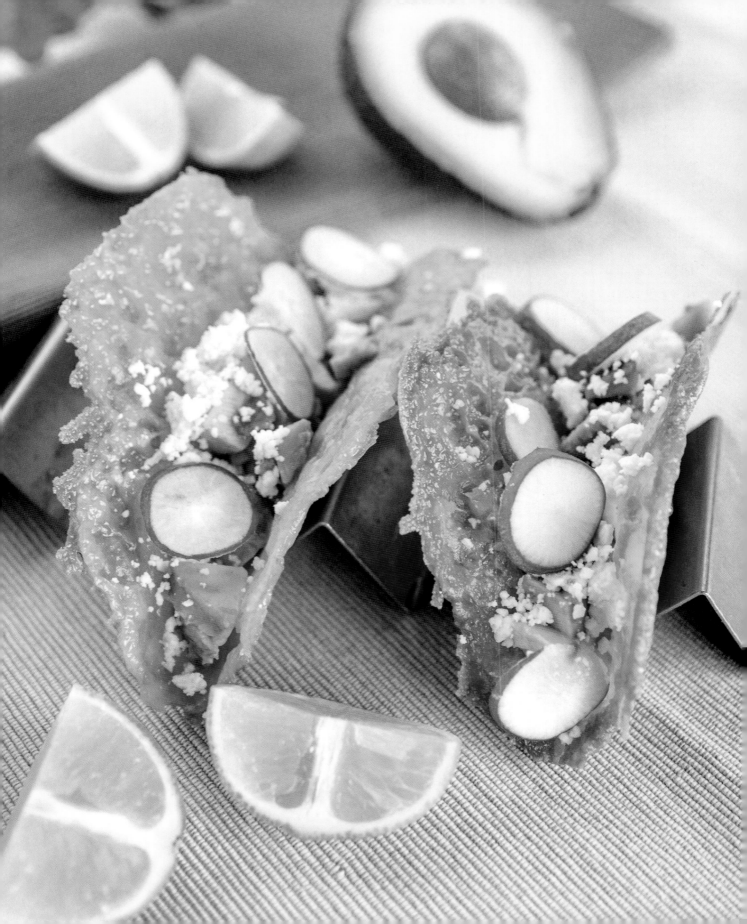

BACON CHICKEN ALFREDO PIZZA

MAKES 8 servings   **PREP TIME: 5 minutes**   **COOK TIME: 12 minutes**

Sometimes it blows my mind that I've been able to lose over 60 pounds by eating amazing dishes like this rich, fatty, and filling pizza. Pizza is a comfort food, right? Yes, yes it is. Although this recipe calls for the Fathead Pizza Crust, these toppings would also be amazing on my Chicken Pizza Crust (page 294).

INGREDIENTS

1 par-baked Fathead Pizza Crust (page 288)

¾ cup Alfredo sauce, store-bought or homemade (page 280)

6 ounces mozzarella cheese, shredded (about 1½ cups)

1 (12½-ounce) can chunk chicken breast, drained

5 slices bacon, cooked and chopped into bite-sized pieces

½ cup diced red onions

Chopped green onions, for garnish

DIRECTIONS

1. Preheat the oven to 425°F. Line a baking sheet with parchment paper or a silicone baking mat, then place the par-baked crust on top.

2. Assemble the pizza: Pour the Alfredo sauce over the crust. Spread it in an even layer, then sprinkle the cheese on top of the sauce. Scatter the chicken, bacon, and red onions over the sauce.

3. Bake for 12 minutes, or until the crust is golden brown and the cheese is melted.

4. Garnish with green onions and serve!

Nutritional information (per serving)

Calories: 434	Total Carbs: 7g
Fat: 34g	Fiber: 2g
Protein: 30g	Net Carbs: 5g

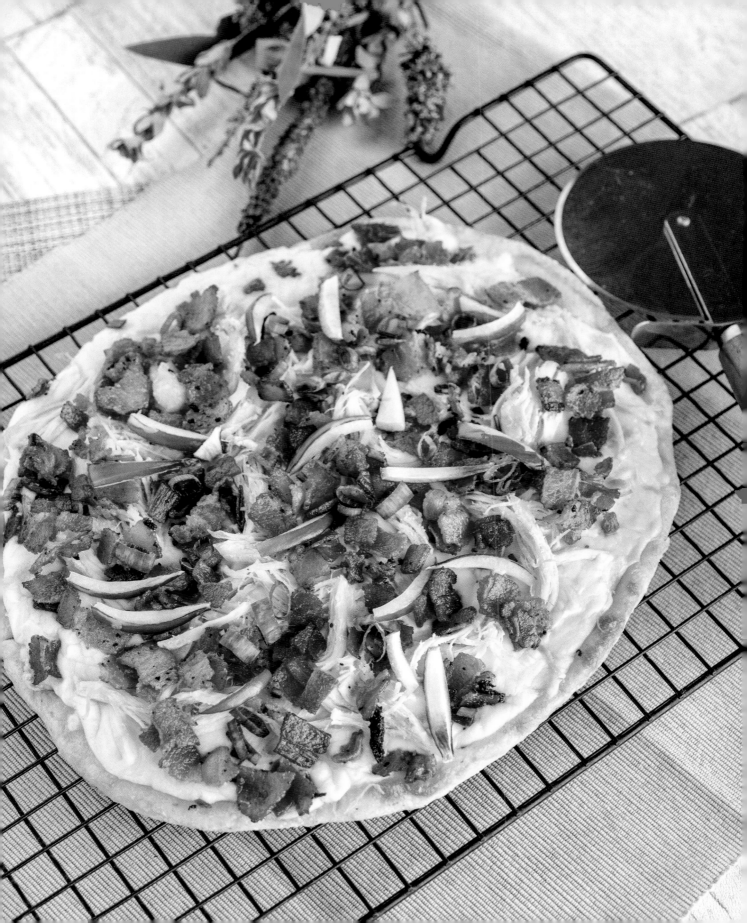

GREEK CHICKEN

MAKES 4 servings   **PREP TIME: 10 minutes, plus 30 minutes to marinate**   **COOK TIME: 10 minutes**

Chicken thighs are one of the most underrated meats out there, in my opinion. They tend to be fattier than breasts, which results in more flavor. I also find that chicken thighs have more moisture than breasts. This is one of my favorite chicken dishes, and it's perfect for a ketogenic lifestyle.

INGREDIENTS

4 boneless, skinless chicken thighs

1 cup mayonnaise

1 teaspoon garlic powder

Pink Himalayan salt and ground black pepper, to taste

Avocado oil or extra-virgin olive oil, for frying

FOR SERVING:

12 black olives, pitted

12 cucumber slices

6 ounces feta cheese, crumbled (about 1 cup)

½ cup sliced red onions

½ cup Tzatziki Sauce (page 300) (optional)

DIRECTIONS

1. Cut the chicken thighs into bite-sized chunks.

2. Place the chicken in a gallon-sized resealable plastic bag. To the bag, add the mayonnaise, garlic powder, and salt and pepper. Let all the excess air out of the bag and then seal. Mix the ingredients together in the bag so the mayo mixture coats all the chicken pieces. Place the bag in the refrigerator to marinate for 30 minutes.

3. After the chicken has marinated, heat a large skillet over medium-high heat. Coat the bottom of the pan with oil.

4. Place the marinated chicken in the pan and fry until cooked all the way through, about 10 minutes. Stir occasionally, making sure to scrape all the good bits from the bottom of the pan.

5. Serve immediately with black olives, cucumber slices, feta cheese, red onion slices, and tzatziki sauce. Store leftovers in the refrigerator for up to 4 days. Reheat in a skillet with some olive oil or butter.

Nutritional information (per serving, without Tzatziki Sauce)

Calories: 678	Total Carbs: 4g
Fat: 64g	Fiber: 1g
Protein: 26g	Net Carbs: 3g

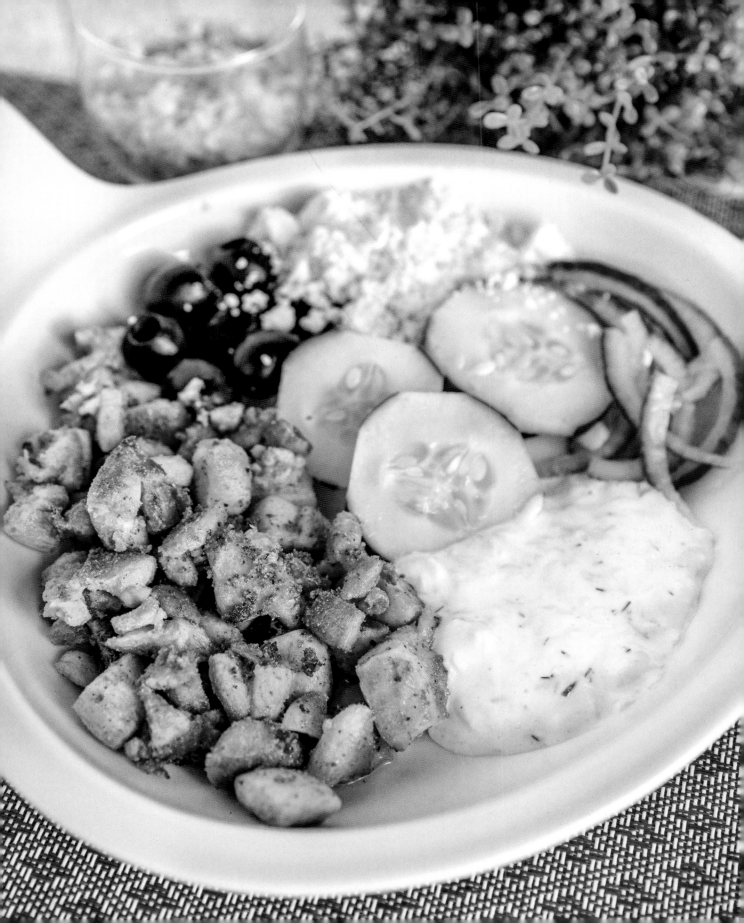

ZUCCHINI LASAGNA

MAKES 6 servings   PREP TIME: 25 minutes   COOK TIME: 1 hour 10 minutes

If you ask my kids what lasagna is, their answer is, "Garfield's favorite food." This just goes to show how often I make lasagna. I find it super time-consuming. However, every time I make it, I'm reminded of why it's so worth the effort! This dish is a modified version of the lasagna my mom used to make while I was growing up. I have replaced the noodles with zucchini, and the flavors are so wonderful that you won't even miss them. My kids love this recipe, too, except they just call it "that cheesy zucchini mush stuff." Serve it with a green salad or your favorite veggie.

INGREDIENTS

2 tablespoons extra-virgin olive oil or unsalted butter

½ yellow onion, diced

2 cloves garlic, minced

1 pound ground beef

1 teaspoon Italian seasoning

Salt and ground black pepper (optional)

1 (15-ounce) can low-sugar tomato sauce, divided

1 (32-ounce) tub ricotta cheese

1 large egg

½ teaspoon ground nutmeg

2 large zucchini

1 pound fresh mozzarella cheese, sliced

2¼ ounces grated or shredded Parmesan cheese (about ¾ cup)

DIRECTIONS

1. Preheat the oven to 375°F.

2. Heat the oil in a large saucepan over medium-high heat. Add the onion and garlic and sauté until the onion is translucent, about 5 minutes. Add the ground beef and Italian seasoning and sprinkle with salt and pepper, if desired. Cook for 10 minutes, or until the meat is fully browned.

3. Add the tomato sauce, reserving about ¼ cup for the bottom of the baking dish, and reduce the heat to low. Let the meat sauce simmer while you prepare the remaining ingredients.

4. Place the ricotta cheese, egg, and nutmeg in a medium-sized mixing bowl. Stir until everything is thoroughly mixed and set aside.

5. Cut the ends off of the zucchini and discard. Using a mandoline or knife, cut the zucchini lengthwise into ⅛-inch-thick slices.

6. Pour the reserved tomato sauce into a 9-inch square glass or ceramic baking dish. Add an even layer of the zucchini slices. Scatter the ricotta mixture on top of the zucchini, then add a layer of mozzarella slices and a layer of the meat mixture. Repeat until you have two or three layers. Top the last layer with the Parmesan cheese. (You might end up with leftover zucchini slices.)

7. Cover the dish with aluminum foil and bake for 30 minutes, then uncover and bake for an additional 20 minutes, until the cheese on top is fully melted and the edges are golden brown.

8. Store leftovers in the refrigerator for up to 1 week. Reheat in the microwave or oven.

Nutritional information (per serving)

Calories: 770	Total Carbs: 14g
Fat: 52g	Fiber: 5g
Protein: 63g	Net Carbs: 9g

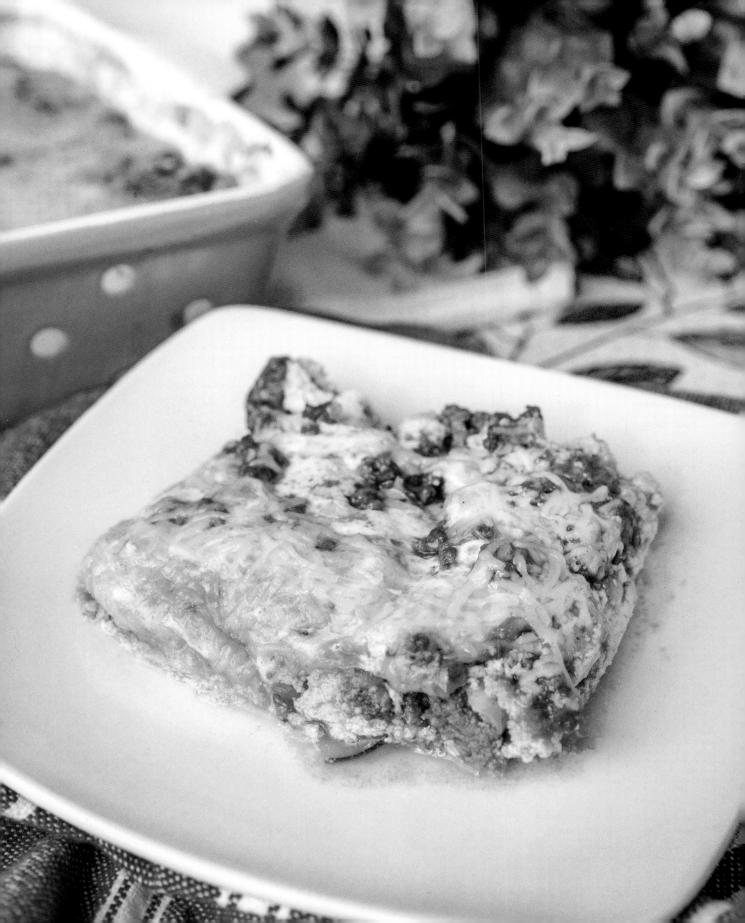

MAPLE-GLAZED DIJON CHICKEN

MAKES 4 servings   PREP TIME: 12 minutes, plus 30 minutes to marinate   COOK TIME: 30 minutes

I love cooking with Dijon mustard. It's sweet but has zero carbs, so you're getting the best of both worlds. Although the coconut flakes on this are not necessary, I highly recommend using them! The flavors of this dish come together so beautifully. Serve the chicken and sauce over a bed of cauliflower rice if you're into that sort of thing.

INGREDIENTS

4 boneless, skinless chicken breast halves (about 3 ounces each)

½ cup sugar-free maple syrup, store-bought or homemade (page 269)

½ cup Dijon mustard

2 tablespoons gluten-free soy sauce (tamari)

2 cloves garlic, minced

1 (10-ounce) bag frozen riced cauliflower

Pink Himalayan salt and ground black pepper

FOR GARNISH (OPTIONAL):

2 green onions, chopped

¼ cup unsweetened coconut flakes (omit for coconut-free)

DIRECTIONS

1. Place the chicken in a 9 by 13-inch glass baking dish. Cut a few slits in each breast and set aside.

2. In a small bowl, whisk together the maple syrup, mustard, soy sauce, and garlic. Transfer about ¼ cup to a separate bowl for serving.

3. Brush the rest of the sauce onto the chicken, making sure it gets into the slits. Cover and place in the refrigerator to marinate for 30 minutes.

4. Preheat the oven to 350°F. Remove the pan with the chicken and marinade from the refrigerator.

5. Bake for 30 minutes, or until the juices run clear and the chicken is crispy on the edges.

6. When the chicken is nearly done baking, microwave the riced cauliflower according to the package directions (usually 4 to 6 minutes on high). Season to taste with salt and pepper.

7. Serve the chicken and sauce from the baking dish over the cauliflower rice. Top with the reserved sauce. Garnish with the green onions and coconut flakes, if desired.

8. Store leftovers in the refrigerator for up to 5 days. Reheat in the microwave.

Nutritional information (per serving)

Calories: 282	Total Carbs: 6g
Fat: 8g	Fiber: 3g
Protein: 42g	Net Carbs: 3g

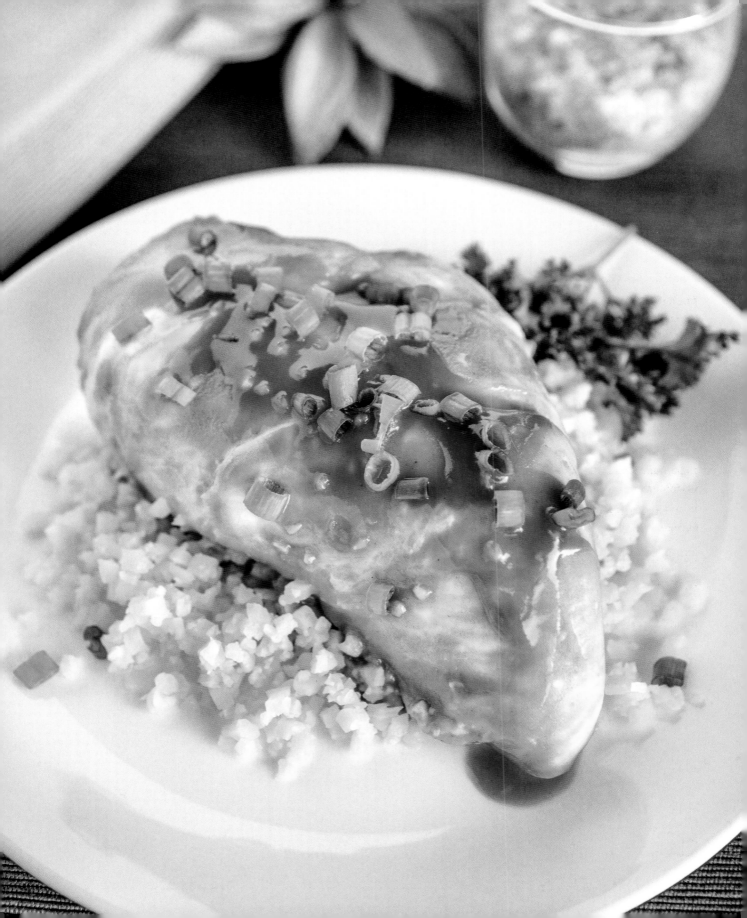

ONE-PAN CHICKEN FAJITAS

MAKES 6 servings   PREP TIME: 15 minutes (not including time to cook tortillas)   COOK TIME: 27 minutes

As a busy mom, and a busy human in general, there's nothing better than a super-easy one-pan meal. This is a great recipe to make if you're into meal prepping. Make it once and eat it for days! It doesn't get much simpler.

INGREDIENTS

2 tablespoons coconut oil

3 to 4 cloves garlic, minced

2 pounds boneless, skinless chicken breasts, cut into bite-sized pieces

3 tablespoons taco seasoning, store-bought or homemade (page 308)

1 large yellow onion, sliced

1 green bell pepper, sliced

1 orange bell pepper, sliced

1 red bell pepper, sliced

1 lime, halved

FOR SERVING/GARNISH:

Guacamole, store-bought or homemade (page 68)

Sour cream (omit for dairy-free, or use dairy-free sour cream)

12 Savory Tortillas (page 282) (omit for dairy/egg-free)

Fresh cilantro (optional)

DIRECTIONS

1. Heat the coconut oil in a large skillet over high heat. Add the garlic and cook until fragrant, 30 to 60 seconds. Be careful not to burn the garlic; otherwise, it'll turn bitter.

2. Add the chicken and sprinkle with the taco seasoning. Cook, stirring often, until the chicken is cooked all the way through, 12 to 15 minutes.

3. Add the onion and peppers to the skillet and stir so the seasonings from the chicken mix into the vegetables. Cook for 5 minutes, or until the peppers are tender.

4. Squeeze the lime halves over the fajita mixture and serve with guacamole, sour cream, and tortillas. Garnish with cilantro, if desired.

5. Store leftovers in the refrigerator for up to 4 days. Reheat in a skillet with butter or olive oil.

Nutritional information (per serving)

Calories: 218	Total Carbs: 6g
Fat: 9g	Fiber: 1g
Protein: 30g	Net Carbs: 5g

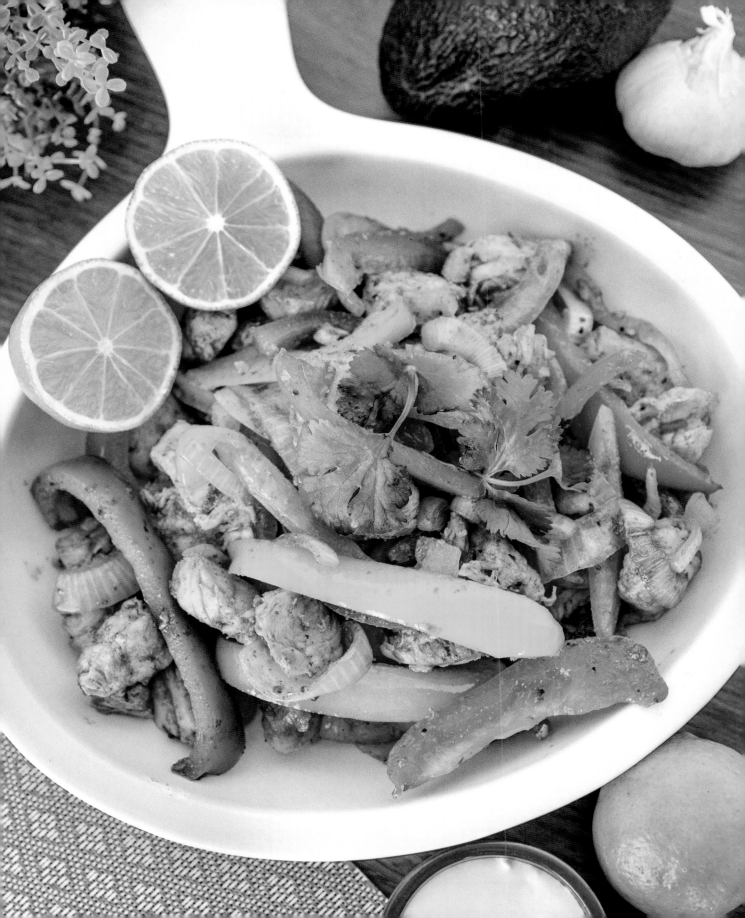

GREEN CHILI CHICKEN ENCHILADAS

MAKES 6 servings   PREP TIME: 25 minutes   COOK TIME: 10 minutes

This recipe is a bit labor-intensive, but I swear it's worth it! These enchiladas are filling and full of flavor, and if you close your eyes, they taste exactly like the real thing.

INGREDIENTS

1 cup shredded cooked chicken (see Note)

1 (8-ounce) package cream cheese, softened, divided

2 (4-ounce) cans diced green chilis, with liquid

4 ounces mozzarella cheese, shredded (about 1 cup)

6 Savory Tortillas (page 282)

DIRECTIONS

1. Preheat oven to 400°F. Grease an 8-inch square baking dish.

2. Place the chicken, half of the cream cheese, and one can of green chilis in a large bowl. Stir until everything is mixed well.

3. Put the remaining cream cheese and the other can of green chilis in a separate small bowl and mix to combine. Set aside.

4. Fill a tortilla with 2 tablespoons of the chicken mixture and 1 teaspoon of mozzarella. Roll up the tortilla and place it in the greased baking dish. Repeat with the remaining tortillas and filling ingredients.

5. Top the enchiladas in the baking dish with the cream cheese and green chili mixture. Then cover the enchiladas with the remaining mozzarella cheese.

6. Bake for 7 to 10 minutes, until the cheese is completely melted. Serve immediately.

7. Store leftovers in the refrigerator for up to 4 days. Reheat in the oven or microwave.

> NOTE: *Canned chicken works great in this recipe. I like Costco brand canned chicken.*

Nutritional information (per serving)

Calories: 321	Total Carbs: 4g
Fat: 25g	Fiber: 1g
Protein: 18g	Net Carbs: 3g

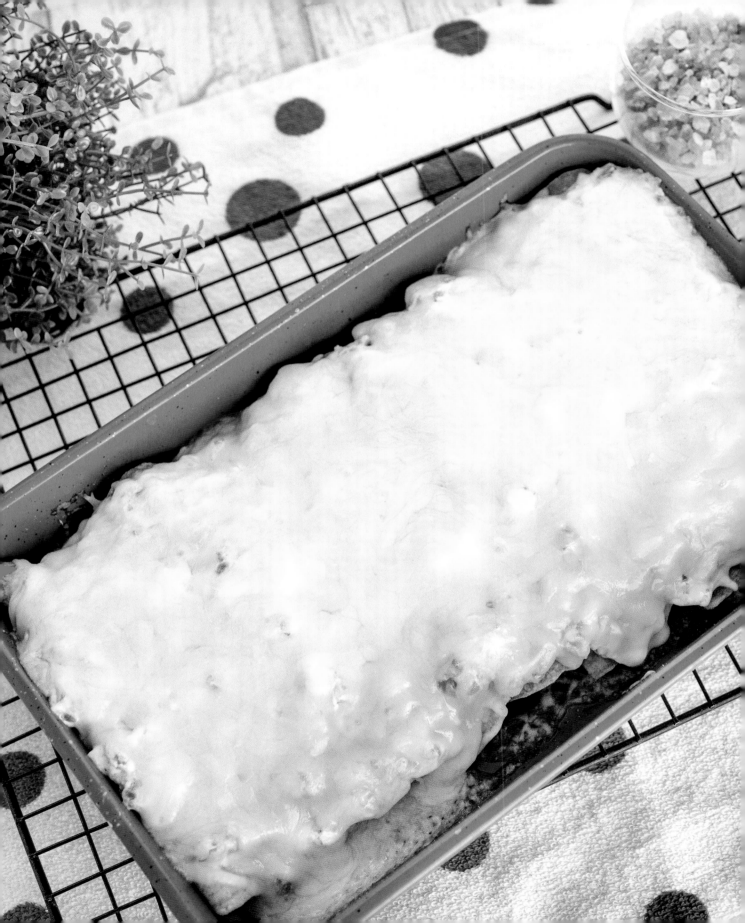

MISSISSIPPI POT ROAST

NET CARBS
6g
OPTION

MAKES 6 servings   PREP TIME: 5 minutes   COOK TIME: 10 hours

This pot roast is a family favorite. It doesn't get much easier than throwing ingredients into a slow cooker and letting it do all the work for you. Plus, it makes the house smell amazing as it cooks. Comfort food at its finest! Serve over cauliflower rice with dinner rolls (page 134) and a green salad, if desired.

INGREDIENTS

1 (4- to 6-pound) boneless beef chuck roast

2 tablespoons ranch seasoning mix, store bought or homemade (page 310)

1 batch onion soup mix, store-bought or homemade (page 306)

½ cup (1 stick) unsalted butter or ghee

8 to 10 pepperoncini

Variation: Oven Cooking Method. Preheat the oven to 200°F, or the lowest possible setting. Place the roast in a roasting pan and top with the remaining ingredients. Bake, covered, for 8 to 10 hours, until the beef is fork-tender.

DIRECTIONS

1. Turn your slow cooker to low.

2. Place the roast in the slow cooker, then top with the remaining ingredients. (No water or stirring is necessary.) Place the lid on the slow cooker and cook on low for 8 to 10 hours, until the beef is fork-tender.

3. Shred the beef with two forks. Transfer to a serving dish and top with the pepperoncini.

4. Store leftovers in the refrigerator for up to 5 days. Reheat in the oven or on the stovetop.

Nutritional information (per serving)

Calories: 595	Total Carbs: 6g
Fat: 49g	Fiber: 0g
Protein: 33g	Net Carbs: 6g

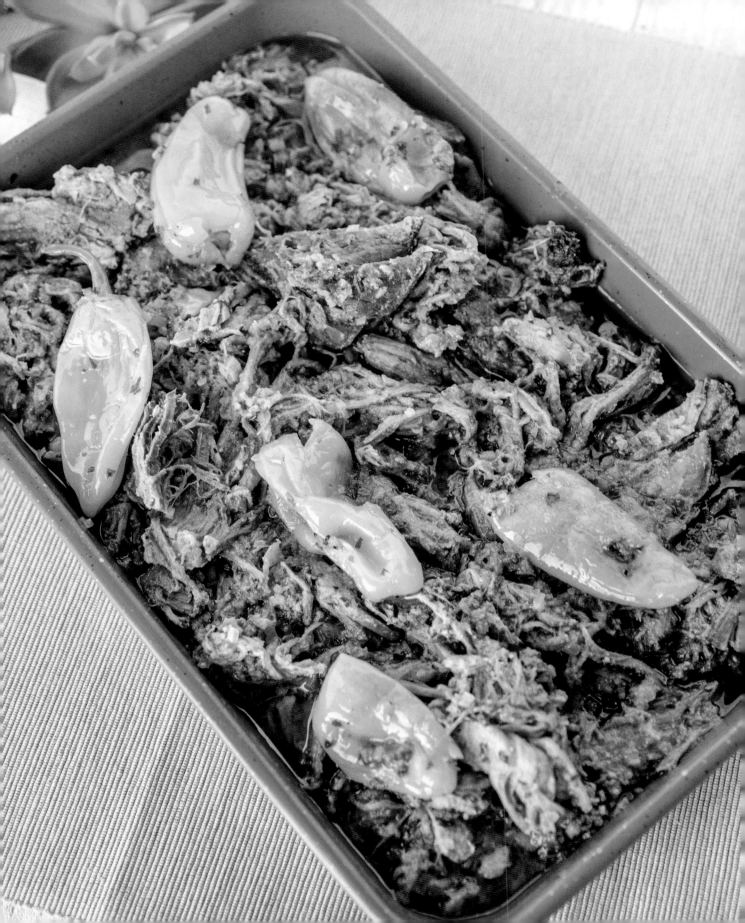

MINI MEATLOAVES

MAKES 12 mini loaves (3 per serving) **PREP TIME: 15 minutes** **COOK TIME: 25 minutes**

These tasty and flavorful mini meatloaves are great for meal prep. Make a large batch at the beginning of the week and pack them for lunches the rest of the week!

INGREDIENTS

Cooking spray

1 pound ground beef

⅓ cup Savory Breadcrumbs (page 304)

1 large egg

½ teaspoon garlic powder

½ teaspoon onion powder

½ teaspoon Italian seasoning

2 tablespoons Worcestershire sauce

2 tablespoons sugar-free ketchup, divided

DIRECTIONS

1. Preheat the oven to 350°F. Spray a standard-size 12-well muffin pan with cooking spray.

2. Place all the ingredients, except the ketchup, in a large mixing bowl. Using your hands, mix the ingredients until the spices and breadcrumbs are evenly distributed throughout the meat.

3. Form the meat mixture into 12 small balls, about the size of golf balls, and place them in the greased wells of the muffin tin. Top each ball with ½ teaspoon of ketchup.

4. Bake for 20 to 25 minutes, until the meatloaves are cooked all the way through. Serve warm with your favorite veggies!

5. Store leftovers in the refrigerator for up to 5 days. Reheat in the microwave or oven.

Nutritional information (per serving)

Calories: 233	Total Carbs: 3g
Fat: 13g	Fiber: 0g
Protein: 25g	Net Carbs: 3g

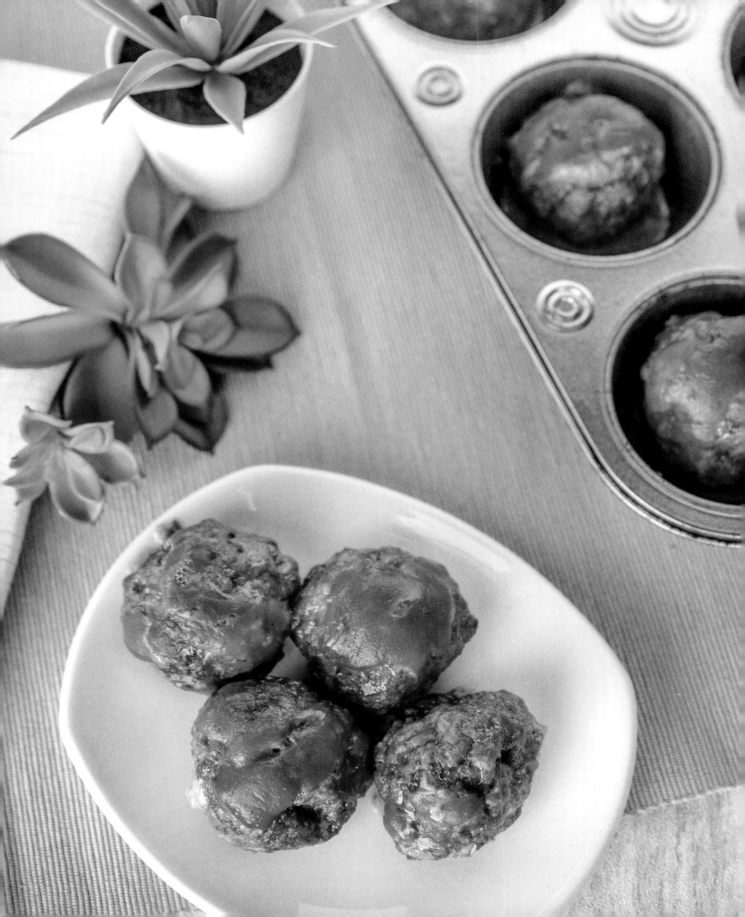

ONE-PAN COCONUT LIME CHICKEN

MAKES 4 servings   **PREP TIME: 10 minutes**   **COOK TIME: 30 minutes**

This dish is bursting with flavor! I always say that my favorite flavors are cilantro and lime. Add coconut cream, and it is basically my dream dinner. I also love that you don't have to dirty a bunch of dishes for this recipe—one pan and it's done! Serve over a bed of cauliflower rice, if desired.

INGREDIENTS

2 tablespoons coconut oil

4 boneless, skinless chicken breast halves (about 3 ounces each)

Salt and ground black pepper

¾ cup diced red onions

1 red bell pepper, diced

Juice of 1 lime, plus more for serving

½ cup finely chopped fresh cilantro, plus more for garnish

¼ teaspoon xanthan gum

¼ teaspoon red pepper flakes, or more if you like it spicy

1 cup chicken bone broth

1½ cups coconut cream

½ teaspoon turmeric powder

DIRECTIONS

1. Heat the coconut oil in a large skillet over medium-high heat.

2. While the oil is heating, place a chicken breast between two pieces of plastic wrap. Pound the chicken to an even thickness. (If you don't have a meat mallet, a rolling pin works like a charm!) Repeat with the remaining chicken breasts. This step isn't 100 percent necessary, but it will help the chicken cook more evenly.

3. Sprinkle both sides of the chicken with salt and pepper. Place the chicken in the hot skillet and cook for 5 to 7 minutes per side, until golden brown and crispy. It does not need to be cooked all the way through at this point. Remove the chicken from the pan and set aside.

4. Add the diced onions and bell pepper to the hot skillet and sprinkle with salt and pepper. Sauté until the onions are translucent and the bell pepper is soft.

5. Add the lime juice, cilantro, xanthan gum, and red pepper flakes to the skillet and cook, stirring, for 1 minute.

6. Stir in the broth, then bring the mixture to a boil. Once boiling, reduce the heat to low and simmer for 5 minutes to thicken the sauce.

7. Turn the heat to medium-high, add the coconut cream and turmeric, and bring to a boil again. Once the sauce is boiling, return the chicken to the pan.

8. Cover, reduce the heat to medium, and cook until the chicken is cooked all the way through, 5 to 7 minutes.

9. Add some more lime juice and garnish with cilantro before serving.

10. Store leftovers in the refrigerator for up to 5 days. Reheat in the microwave or a skillet.

Nutritional information (per serving)

Calories: 469	Total Carbs: 7g
Fat: 31g	Fiber: 1g
Protein: 44g	Net Carbs: 6g

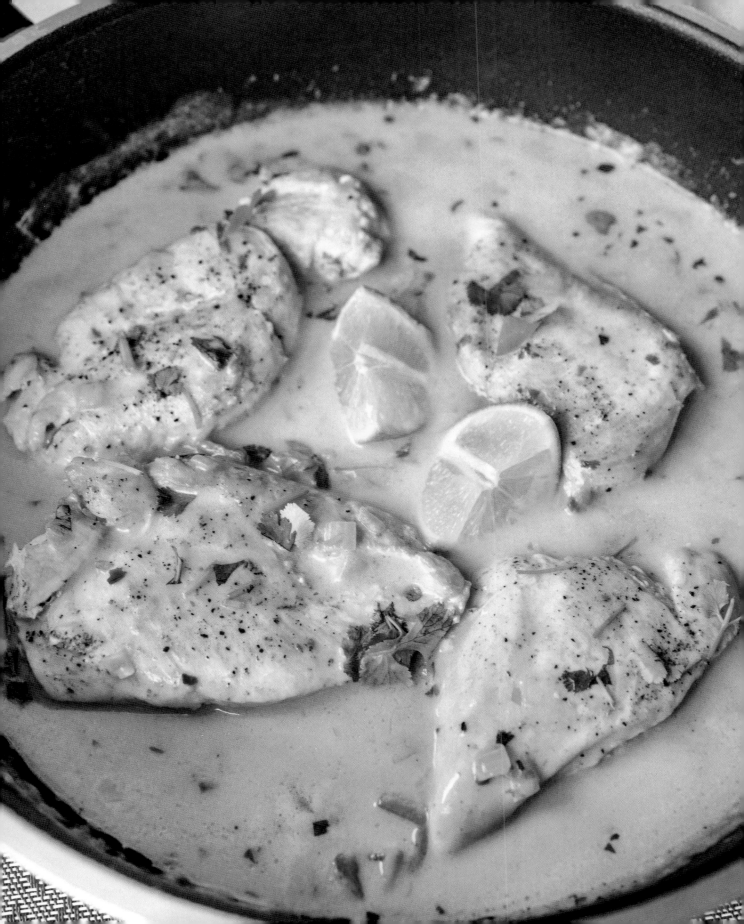

KOREAN BBQ BEEF

MAKES 4 servings   PREP TIME: 5 minutes   COOK TIME: 12 minutes

This recipe could not get much simpler! It takes less than fifteen minutes to make, and you'll scarf it down even quicker. Serve over a bed of cauliflower rice or in lettuce wraps!

INGREDIENTS

1 tablespoon unsalted butter or ghee

1 pound ground beef

2 cloves garlic, minced

¼ cup gluten-free soy sauce (tamari)

¼ cup brown sugar substitute

2 teaspoons toasted sesame oil

¼ teaspoon red pepper flakes

1 teaspoon freshly grated ginger (optional)

1 tablespoon sesame seeds (optional)

1 green onion, chopped (optional)

DIRECTIONS

1. In a medium-sized skillet, melt the butter over high heat. Add the ground beef and garlic and cook until the beef is browned, about 10 minutes. We like to cook it until the meat is a little crispy! There is no need to salt and pepper the meat because the sauce is salty enough.

2. In a small bowl, combine the soy sauce, sweetener, sesame oil, and red pepper flakes. Pour the sauce over the beef and stir until the meat is fully coated.

3. Top the beef mixture with the ginger, sesame seeds, and green onion, if desired, and serve.

4. Store leftovers in the refrigerator for up to 5 days. Reheat in a skillet with butter or ghee.

Nutritional information (per serving)

Calories: 265	Total Carbs: 2g
Fat: 17g	Fiber: 0g
Protein: 25g	Net Carbs: 2g

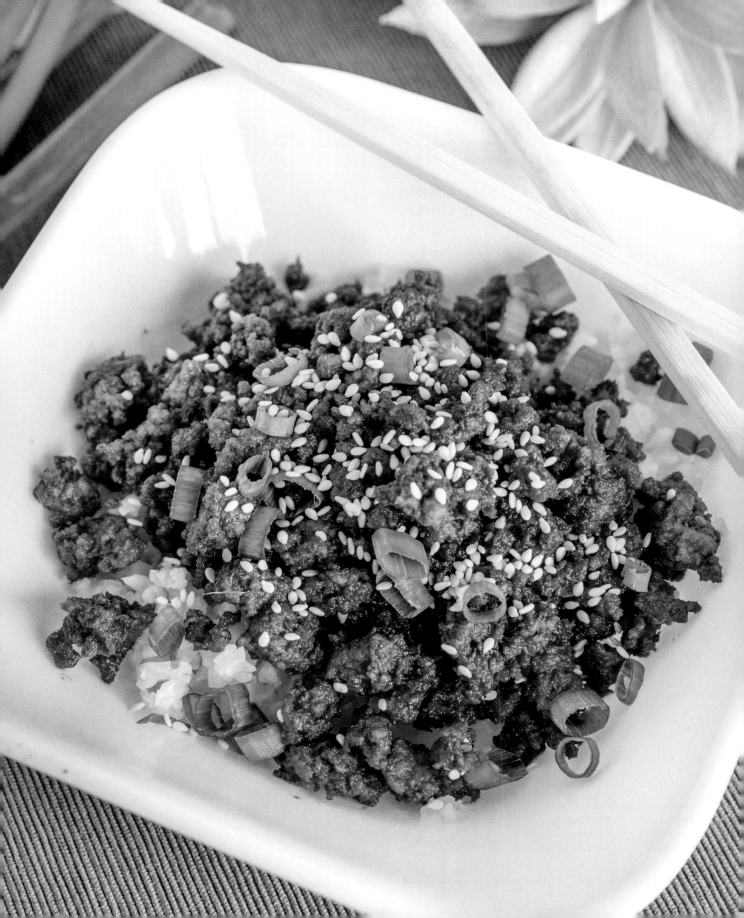

SHRIMP AND GRITS

MAKES 4 servings   PREP TIME: 10 minutes   COOK TIME: 30 minutes

Whenever I hear the word grits, I immediately think of the classic movie My Cousin Vinny. There's a scene where a man says, "No self-respecting Southerner uses instant grits. I take pride in my grits!" Well, I'm no Southerner, but I do take pride in my "grits"...even though they are made with cauliflower.

INGREDIENTS

1 cup chicken bone broth

½ cup heavy whipping cream

3 tablespoons unsalted butter

6 slices bacon

Florets from 1 small head cauliflower (about 1 pound), chopped and then grated into rice

1 pound large raw shrimp

1 teaspoon Old Bay seasoning

Salt and pepper

4 ounces cheddar cheese, shredded (about 1 cup)

¼ cup chopped green onions, for garnish

DIRECTIONS

1. In a medium saucepan, bring the broth, heavy cream, and butter to a boil over medium-high heat, whisking to combine.

2. Meanwhile, chop the bacon into tiny pieces. Place in a skillet over medium-high heat and cook for about 10 minutes, until the bacon is cooked all the way through. Remove the bacon from the pan and place on a plate lined with a paper towel. Drain most of the bacon fat from the skillet, leaving 2 tablespoons in the pan.

3. When the broth mixture reaches a boil, add the cauliflower and stir to combine. Reduce the heat to low, cover, and simmer for 20 minutes, stirring occasionally.

4. While the cauliflower grits are simmering, peel, devein, and rinse the shrimp. Pat dry with a paper towel to remove the excess water. Season the shrimp with the Old Bay seasoning and a generous sprinkling of salt and pepper. Place the shrimp in the skillet with the bacon grease, still over medium-high heat, and cook for 2 minutes on each side.

5. Add the cheddar cheese to the cauliflower grits mixture and whisk until the cheese is fully melted.

6. Place the grits on a plate and top with the shrimp, bacon, and green onions. Serve immediately! This dish is best served fresh, but you can store leftovers in the refrigerator for up to 4 days. Reheat in a skillet with butter or olive oil.

Nutritional information (per serving)

Calories: 474	Total Carbs: 7g
Fat: 32g	Fiber: 2g
Protein: 38g	Net Carbs: 5g

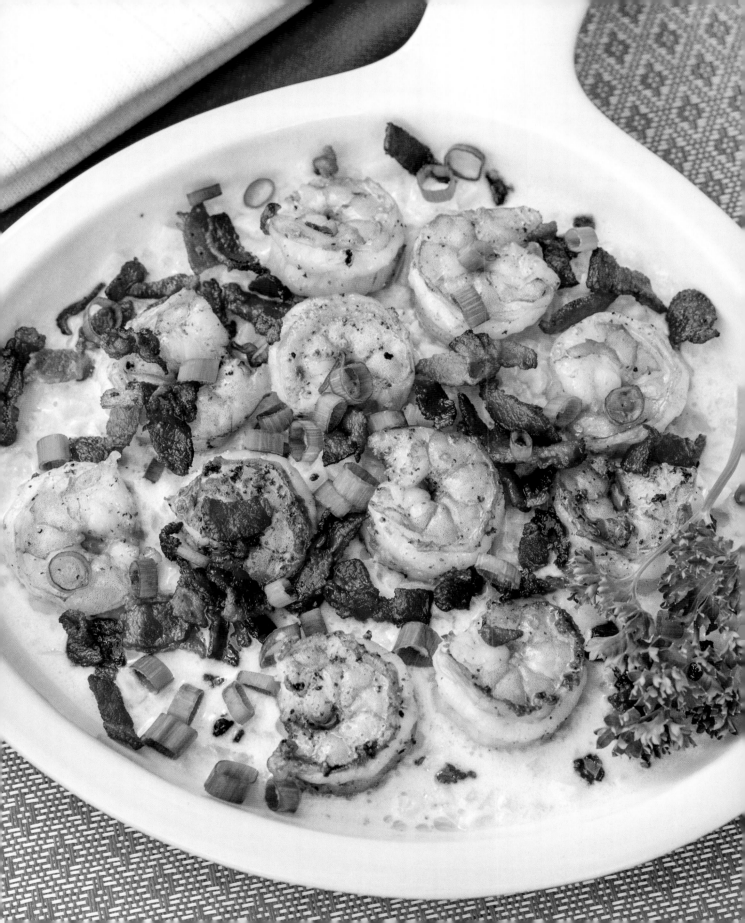

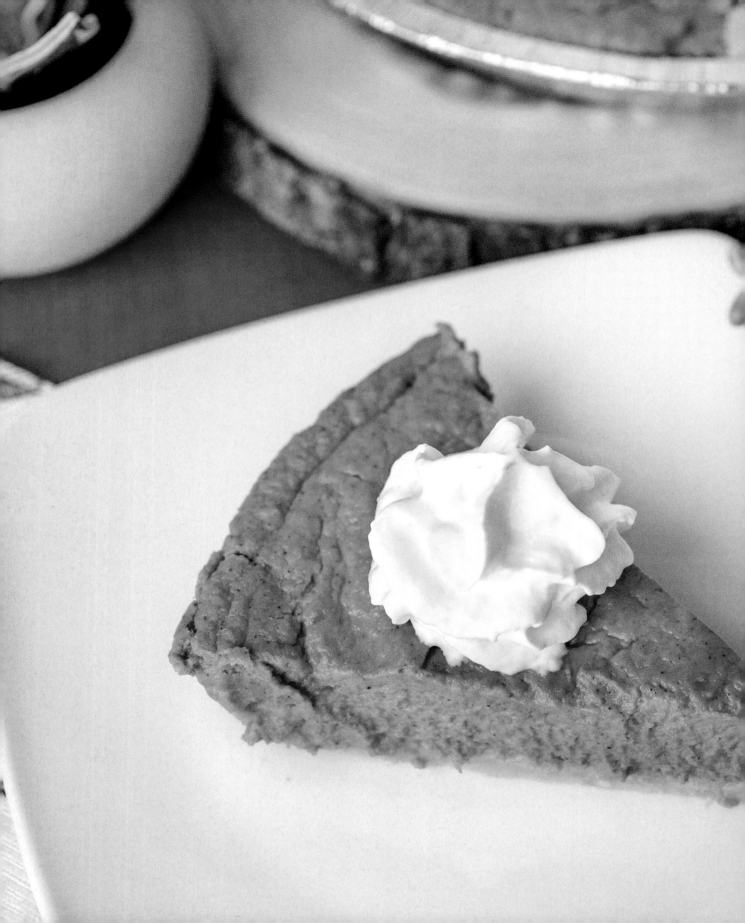

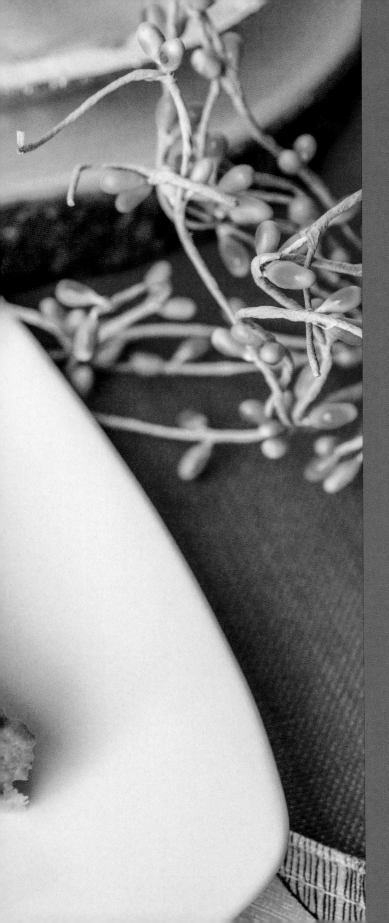

6 SWEET TOOTH

STRAWBERRY COCONUT SMOOTHIE

MAKES four 8-ounce servings   **PREP TIME:** 5 minutes   **COOK TIME:** —

It's funny how you start a new way of eating and all of a sudden, you crave things you never used to eat. For me, it's smoothies! I can't tell you how many times I've driven by a smoothie shop and been crushed that I couldn't have one. I was never a smoothie person before, but now, every once in a while, it's all I crave. Luckily, we can keto-fy just about anything. You can use this recipe as a base for whatever mix-ins you want. Blueberries, raspberries, spinach, avocado...the options are endless.

INGREDIENTS

1 (13½-ounce) can coconut cream

1 cup frozen strawberries

1 cup ice

¼ cup heavy whipping cream or unsweetened almond milk

1 teaspoon granulated sweetener

1 teaspoon vanilla extract

DIRECTIONS

Place all the ingredients in a blender and blend until the mixture has the consistency of a smoothie or milkshake. If it is too thick to blend, add a tablespoon of water at a time and try again. Enjoy!

Nutritional information (per serving)

Calories: 266   Total Carbs: 6g

Fat: 27g   Fiber: 1g

Protein: 1g   Net Carbs: 5g

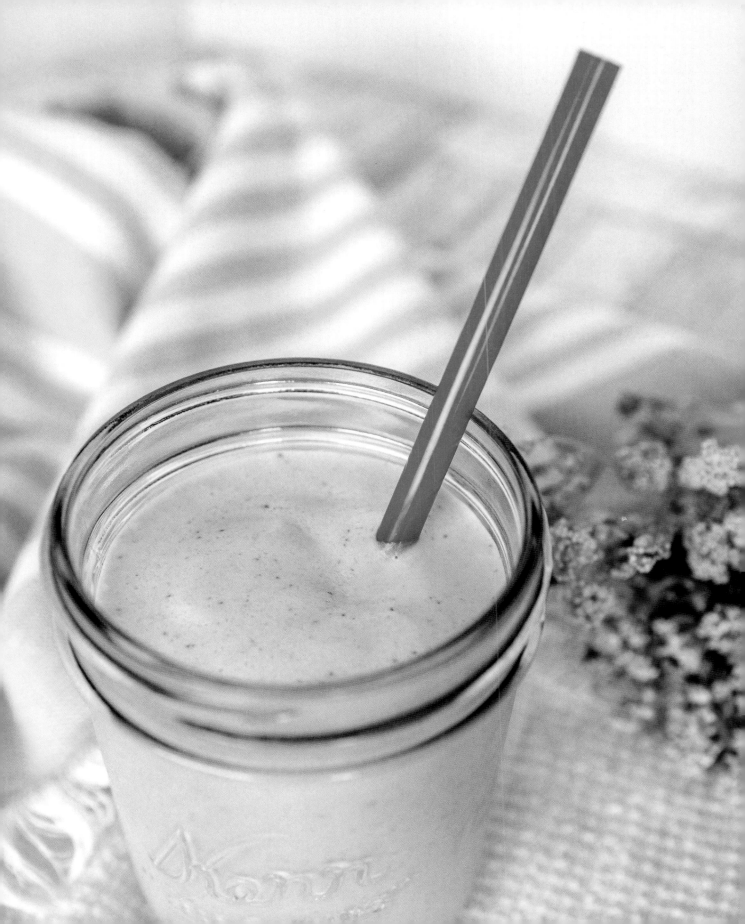

LEMON JULIUS

OPTION OPTION   OPTION

MAKES 2 servings   PREP TIME: 5 minutes   COOK TIME: —

My kids are weird and love to eat lemons like they are oranges. It gives me a bit of a panic attack to see them do it because it'll ruin the enamel on their teeth. This drink is the perfect tart, refreshing treat that I'm totally okay with them having instead. While it satisfies their taste for lemons, I don't need to worry about them ruining their beautiful (crooked) teeth. Win-win!

INGREDIENTS

⅔ cup unsweetened almond milk or coconut milk

½ cup heavy whipping cream or coconut cream

½ cup lemon juice (about 2 lemons)

¼ cup granulated sweetener

1 teaspoon vanilla extract

3 cups ice

FOR GARNISH (OPTIONAL):

Grated lemon zest

2 lemon slices

DIRECTIONS

1. Place all the ingredients, except the ice, in a blender. Blend on high until well combined.

2. Add the ice to the blender and blend on high until the drink reaches your desired consistency. Garnish each serving with lemon zest and/or a lemon slice, if desired. Yum!

Nutritional information (per serving)

Calories: 222	Total Carbs: 5g
Fat: 21g	Fiber: 0g
Protein: 1g	Net Carbs: 5g

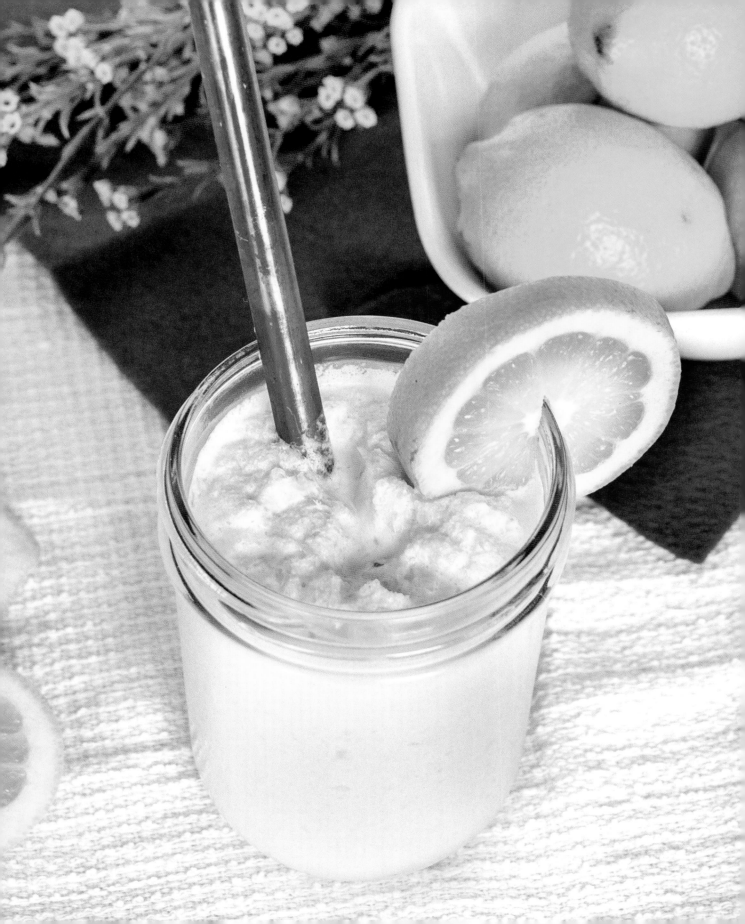

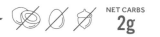

BUTTERBEER

MAKES eight 8-ounce servings   PREP TIME: 12 minutes   COOK TIME: —

My sister-in-law threw a Harry Potter–themed birthday party for her son and served homemade butterbeer. It was the cutest thing! I was determined to go home and create a keto version, and this is what I came up with—pretty dang good, if you ask me!

INGREDIENTS

1 (2-liter) bottle diet cream soda, chilled

2 tablespoons butter extract

1 cup heavy whipping cream

1 teaspoon rum extract

½ teaspoon granulated sweetener

3 ounces cream cheese (about ⅓ cup), softened

DIRECTIONS

1. Open the bottle of cream soda and pour the butter extract into the bottle. Seal the cap and gently roll the bottle so that the extract gets distributed without losing the carbonation. Set aside.

2. Make the whipped topping: Place the heavy cream, rum extract, and sweetener in a mixing bowl. Using a hand mixer, mix until soft peaks form, 8 to 10 minutes. Alternatively, you can use a stand mixer fitted with the whisk attachment.

3. Cut the cream cheese into small chunks so it's easier to blend. Add the cream cheese chunks to the cream mixture and mix until it has the consistency of whipped topping.

4. Pour the cream soda into chilled mugs, top with the whipped topping, and serve!

5. Store the whipped topping in the refrigerator for up to 1 week.

Nutritional information (per serving)

Calories: 183	Total Carbs: 2g
Fat: 18g	Fiber: 0g
Protein: 1g	Net Carbs: 2g

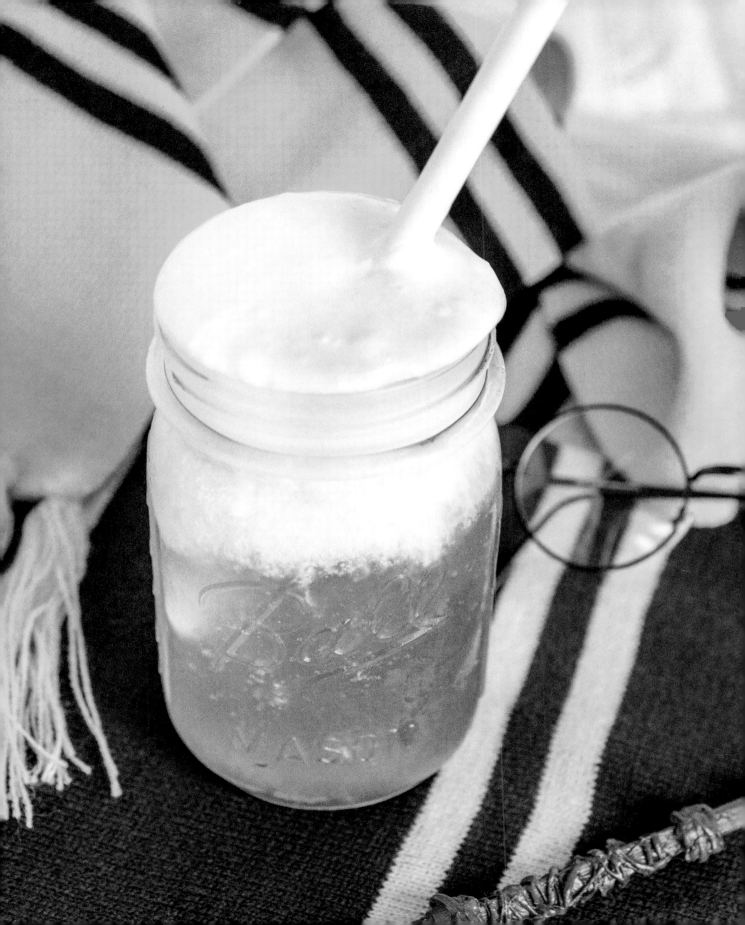

EGGNOG

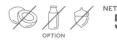

NET CARBS
5g

MAKES four 4-ounce servings   PREP TIME: 5 minutes, plus 3½ hours to chill   COOK TIME: 15 minutes

"Can I refill your eggnog for you? Get you something to eat? Drive you out to the middle of nowhere and leave you for dead?" —Clark W. Griswold, *National Lampoon's Christmas Vacation*

INGREDIENTS

6 large egg yolks

½ cup granulated sweetener

3 cups heavy whipping cream (or coconut cream for dairy-free)

1½ tablespoons freshly grated nutmeg, plus more for garnish

Pinch of salt

½ teaspoon vanilla extract

¼ teaspoon rum extract

DIRECTIONS

1. In a medium-sized bowl, whisk together the egg yolks and sweetener. Set aside.

2. In a medium-sized saucepan over medium-high heat, bring the heavy cream, nutmeg, and salt to a boil. Stir occasionally to prevent the mixture from sticking to the bottom of the pan.

3. Once the cream mixture reaches a boil, ladle it into the egg yolk mixture, about ½ cup at a time, whisking vigorously so the heat of the cream doesn't cook the eggs.

4. Pour the eggnog back into the saucepan over low heat, add the extracts, and simmer for about 5 minutes, whisking occasionally.

5. Remove from the heat and pour into a pitcher or medium-sized bowl. Let cool for 30 minutes, then cover the bowl and place in the fridge to chill for 3 hours.

6. Serve chilled, garnished with a sprinkle of nutmeg.

7. Store leftovers in the refrigerator for up to 5 days.

Nutritional information (per serving)

Calories: 688	Total Carbs: 5g
Fat: 67g	Fiber: 0g
Protein: 4g	Net Carbs: 5g

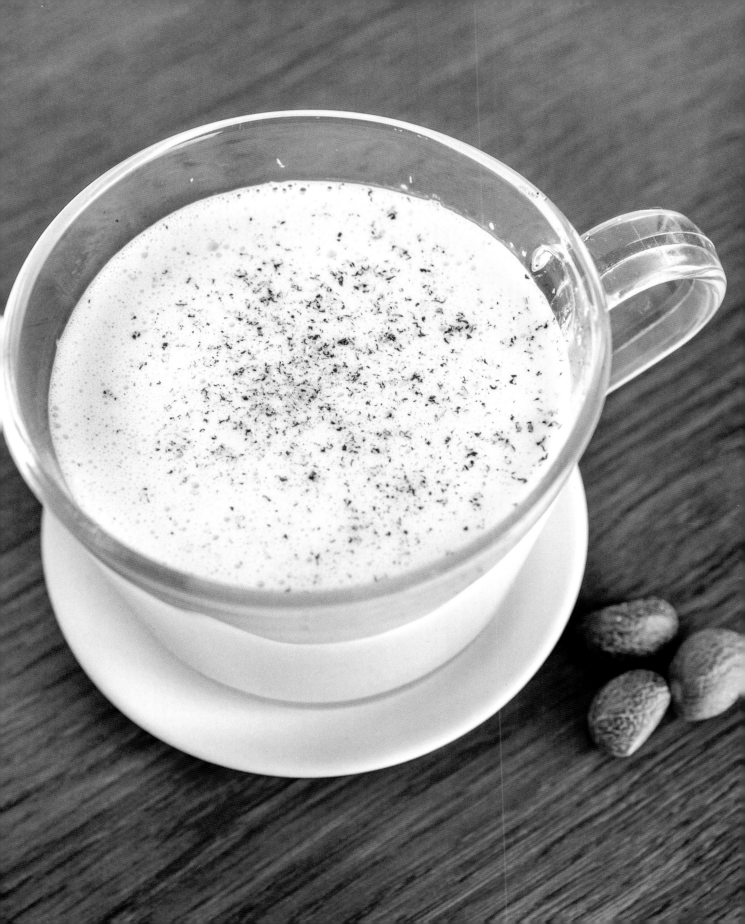

CINNAMON ICE CREAM

NET CARBS
1g

MAKES 3 quarts (½ cup per serving)   **PREP TIME: 20 minutes, plus 1 hour to chill**   **COOK TIME: —**

When I was in high school, I worked at Cold Stone Creamery in San Diego. I used to play around with the flavors and come up with random concoctions. One day, someone came in and ordered sweet cream ice cream with cinnamon and graham cracker pie crust, and I took note! I ended up trying it later, and it quickly became my favorite. Although I haven't eaten there in years, I still remember how amazing that cinnamon ice cream was. Here's my keto version. You don't even need an ice cream maker to make it! If you have yet to try butter extract, add it to your grocery list. It makes this ice cream so rich and creamy. Fun fact: You can make this recipe with any extract you can find and get a totally different flavor of ice cream.

INGREDIENTS

2 cups heavy whipping cream

1 (13½-ounce) can coconut cream

¾ cup granulated sweetener

1 teaspoon ground cinnamon

1 teaspoon butter extract

DIRECTIONS

1. Place the heavy cream in the bowl of a stand mixer and beat until it starts to thicken and form soft peaks, 6 to 7 minutes. (You can use a hand mixer, but a stand mixer saves a ton of time.)

2. Add the coconut cream, sweetener, cinnamon, and butter extract. Continue mixing until the mixture resembles whipped cream, about 2 minutes.

3. Transfer the whipped cream mixture to a 5 by 9-inch glass loaf pan and cover with plastic wrap. Put in the freezer to set for at least 1 hour.

4. Store in the freezer for up to 1 month.

Nutritional information (per serving)

Calories: 100	Total Carbs: 1g
Fat: 10g	Fiber: 0g
Protein: 0g	Net Carbs: 1g

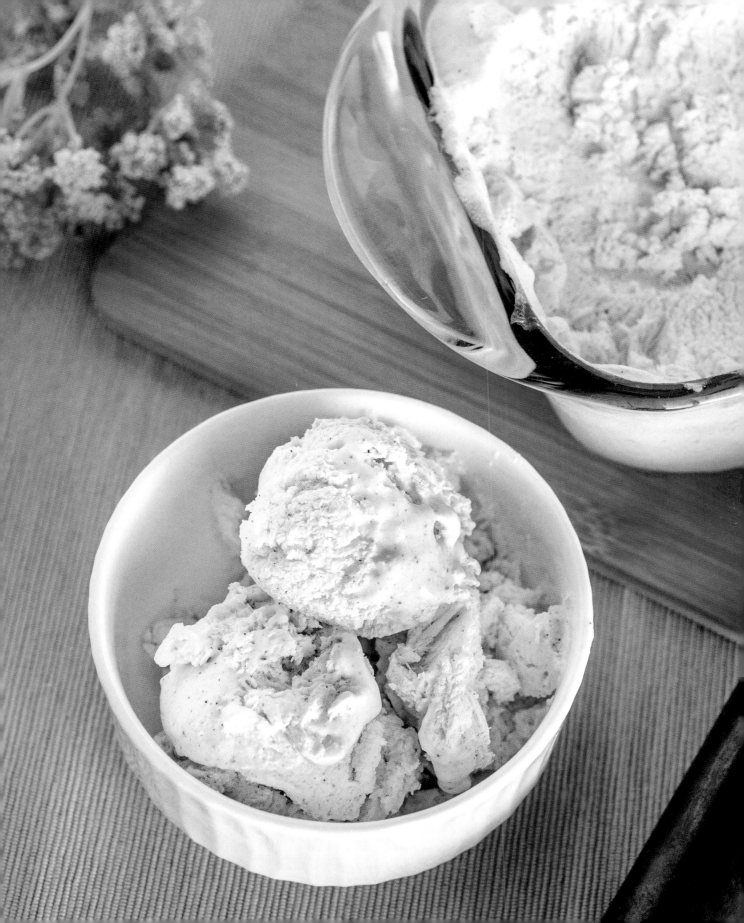

CARAMEL DIP

MAKES 10 servings (about 2 tablespoons per serving)   PREP TIME: 2 minutes   COOK TIME: —

Don't worry, there isn't any actual caramel in this dip. And I know what you're thinking...we can't have fruit on keto. Yes, we can! Small amounts of berries are perfectly fine; just be mindful of the carb count and try not to go overboard. This dip pairs extremely well with strawberries, but honestly, I'd eat it with a spoon. What can I say? I'm classy.

INGREDIENTS

1 (8-ounce) package cream cheese, softened

¾ cup brown sugar substitute

DIRECTIONS

Place the cream cheese and brown sugar substitute in a medium-sized bowl and mix with a hand mixer until smooth and creamy. This dip can get gritty, so make sure to mix well! Serve with your favorite berries. Store leftovers in the refrigerator for up to 1 week.

Nutritional information (per serving)

Calories: 79	Total Carbs: 1g
Fat: 8g	Fiber: 0g
Protein: 1g	Net Carbs: 1g

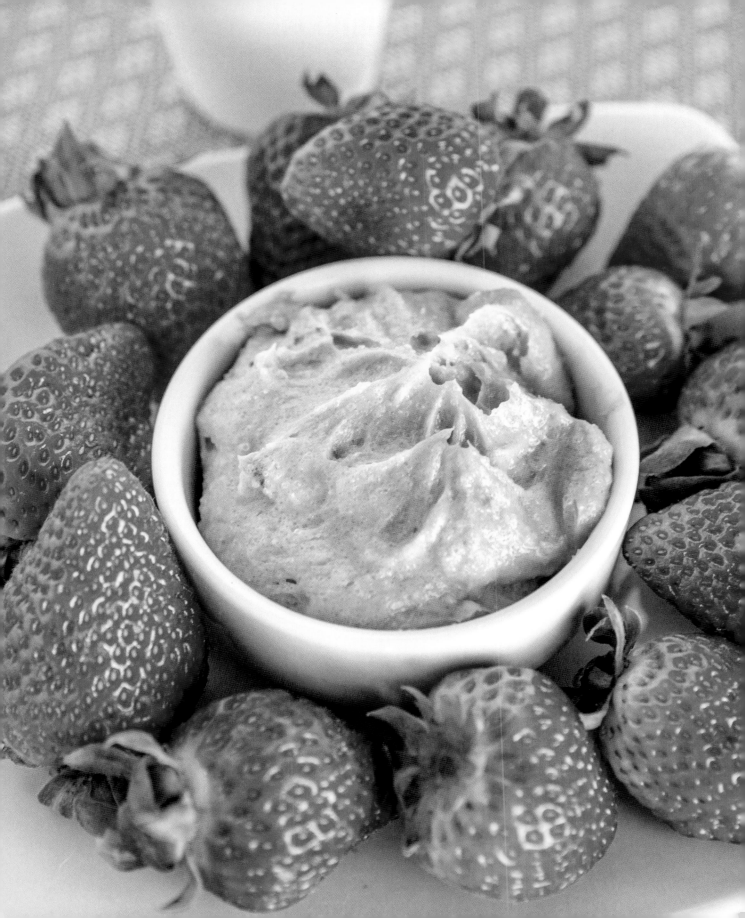

OOEY GOOEY MONKEY BREAD

MAKES one 8½ by 4½-inch loaf (6 servings)   **PREP TIME: 20 minutes**   **COOK TIME: 35 minutes**

You do not have to sacrifice flavor when you switch to a ketogenic lifestyle. Over the course of my journey, I've learned that you can keto-fy just about anything. This sweet bread is one of those dishes that translates to keto so beautifully! Keep it away from your kids, though, because they won't save any for you. Trust me, I know from experience.

INGREDIENTS

FOR THE DOUGH:

12 ounces mozzarella cheese, shredded (about 3 cups)

2 ounces cream cheese (¼ cup)

1½ cups blanched almond flour

2 large eggs

2 tablespoons granulated sweetener

1 tablespoon ground cinnamon

Cooking spray

FOR THE GLAZE:

⅓ cup unsalted butter or ghee, melted

2 tablespoons granulated sweetener

1 tablespoon ground cinnamon

¼ teaspoon maple extract

DIRECTIONS

1. Preheat the oven to 350°F. Generously spray an 8½ by 4½-inch loaf pan with cooking spray.

2. Make the dough: Place the mozzarella and cream cheese in a large microwave-safe bowl; there is no need to stir at this point. Microwave on high for 1 minute. Remove from the microwave and stir the cheeses with a fork. Microwave for an additional 30 seconds. Remove and stir again. Repeat until the cheeses are melted and easy to stir together.

3. Add the almond flour, eggs, sweetener, and cinnamon. Stir with a fork or spoon until the eggs are mixed in, then wet your hands and knead the dough until the cinnamon and sweetener are evenly distributed. You may need to wet your hands a few times to get everything fully mixed in. When the dough is combined, set it aside.

4. Wet your hands again. Pull off a small chunk of the dough and form it into a 1-inch ball. Repeat with the remaining dough, making a total of 20 to 25 balls. The dough will get sticky, so just re-wet your hands and continue.

5. Place the balls in the greased loaf pan, in no special arrangement. The pieces should look random.

6. Make the glaze: Put the melted butter, sweetener, cinnamon, and maple extract in a small bowl and stir until well incorporated. Pour the glaze evenly over the balls of dough in the loaf pan.

7. Bake for 30 to 35 minutes, until the glaze has browned. The bread will look very buttery when it comes out of the oven, but that's totally normal.

8. Remove from the oven and let cool in the pan for 5 minutes before diving in! There's no need for cutting here; simply break off pieces and enjoy. Store leftovers in the refrigerator for up to 5 days.

Nutritional information (per serving)

Calories: 438	Total Carbs: 7g
Fat: 39g	Fiber: 3g
Protein: 21g	Net Carbs: 4g

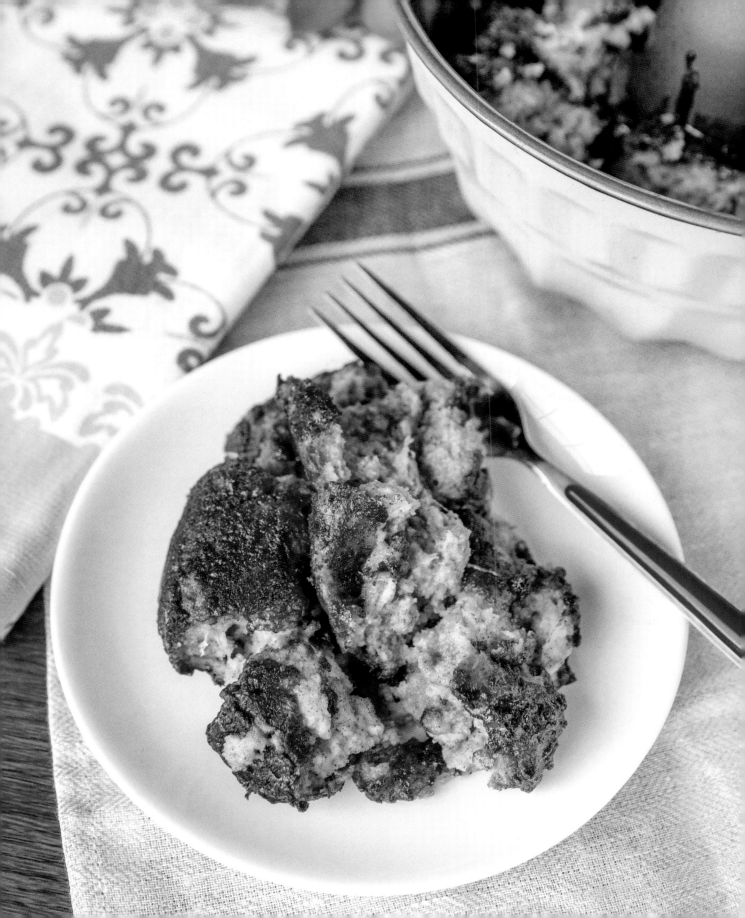

PUMPKIN FRY BREAD

NET CARBS
3g
OPTION

MAKES 6 breads (1 per serving)   PREP TIME: 30 minutes, plus 15 minutes to chill   COOK TIME: 20 minutes

This pumpkin fry bread was born on a rainy, fall, football-filled day. I was craving something with pumpkin spice and voilà! Along came this pumpkin fry bread. This one is a little more labor-intensive than most of my recipes, but it's so worth it!

INGREDIENTS

6 ounces shredded mozzarella cheese, shredded (about 1½ cups)

2 ounces cream cheese (¼ cup)

1 cup blanched almond flour

1 large egg

2 tablespoons pumpkin puree (not pumpkin pie filling)

½ teaspoon granulated sweetener, plus more for garnish

¼ teaspoon pumpkin pie spice

¼ teaspoon ground cinnamon, plus more for garnish

Avocado oil or coconut oil, for frying

DIRECTIONS

1. Preheat the oven to 425°F. Line a baking sheet with parchment paper or a silicone baking mat.

2. Place the mozzarella and cream cheese in a large microwave-safe bowl. Microwave on high for 30 seconds. Remove from the microwave and stir the cheeses with a fork, then microwave for another 30 seconds. Remove and stir again until the cheeses are melted. If it needs a little longer, microwave for another 30 seconds, then stir once more.

3. Add the almond flour, egg, pumpkin puree, sweetener, pumpkin pie spice, and cinnamon to the melted cheese mixture. Wet your hands and knead the dough until everything is well combined. This task may take some elbow grease, so don't rush. If the dough starts to stick to your hands, wet your hands again and continue working the dough.

4. Once the dough is well incorporated, place it in the refrigerator to chill for 15 minutes.

5. Take the dough out of the refrigerator and place on a piece of parchment paper. Put another piece of parchment on top of the dough and use a rolling pin to roll out the dough between the two sheets of parchment until it is about ½ inch thick. Then, using a 5-inch circular cookie cutter (or the rim of a small bowl, about 5 inches in diameter), cut out circles of dough. Repeat, gathering up the scraps and rerolling as needed, until all the dough has been used.

6. Place the circles on the lined baking sheet and use a fork to poke holes in the dough to prevent it from rising. Bake for 10 to 12 minutes, until the outsides are golden brown and a toothpick inserted in the center of a bread comes out clean.

7. Pour about ¼ inch of oil into a large skillet over high heat. Fry the circles, about three at a time, until they puff up and turn a nice golden-brown color on both sides, about 2 minutes on the first side and 1 minute on the other side.

8. Remove the fry bread from the oil and sprinkle with cinnamon and sweetener. Serve hot! Store leftovers in the refrigerator for up to 1 week. Reheat in the microwave or oven.

Nutritional information (per serving)

Calories: 221	Total Carbs: 5g
Fat: 19g	Fiber: 2g
Protein: 12g	Net Carbs: 3g

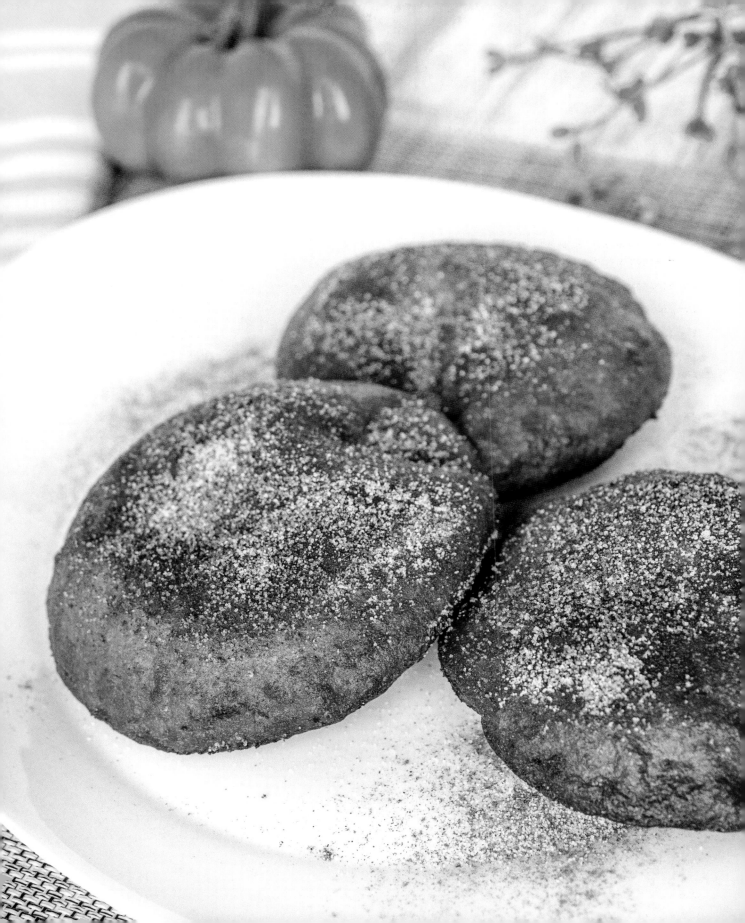

LOADED FAT BOMB

MAKES about 2 cups (2 tablespoons per serving)   PREP TIME: 5 minutes, plus 30 minutes to chill   COOK TIME: —

This is one thing I always tell my Instagram followers: If you're just starting out on keto, do not attempt to make any fat bombs that you find on Pinterest. Your taste buds haven't adjusted yet, and they simply won't taste good to you. I learned this the hard way! I tried every fat bomb there was, and it wasn't until I was fully fat-adapted that I actually started to enjoy them. With that said, this is my absolute favorite fat bomb that I've ever made. Try to find the peanut butter with the lowest amount of carbs/sugar, or grind your own.

INGREDIENTS

1 (8-ounce) package cream cheese, softened

¾ cup natural peanut butter

½ cup coconut cream

¼ cup sour cream

1 tablespoon granulated sweetener

½ cup sugar-free chocolate chips

Variation: To make individual fat bombs, portion the chilled mixture into 16 balls (2 tablespoons each), place on a baking sheet or tray, and freeze until firm. Transfer the balls to a freezer bag or, for taking on the go, wrap individually in plastic wrap and store in the freezer for up to 3 months.

DIRECTIONS

1. Place the cream cheese, peanut butter, coconut cream, sour cream, and sweetener in a large mixing bowl. Using a hand mixer, mix until well combined.

2. Add the chocolate chips and stir with a rubber spatula. Place the bowl in the refrigerator to chill for 30 minutes before enjoying. Simply grab a spoonful at a time!

3. Store in the refrigerator for up to 10 days or place in a resealable container and freeze for up to 3 months.

Nutritional information (per serving)

Calories: 171	Total Carbs: 4g
Fat: 15g	Fiber: 1g
Protein: 5g	Net Carbs: 3g

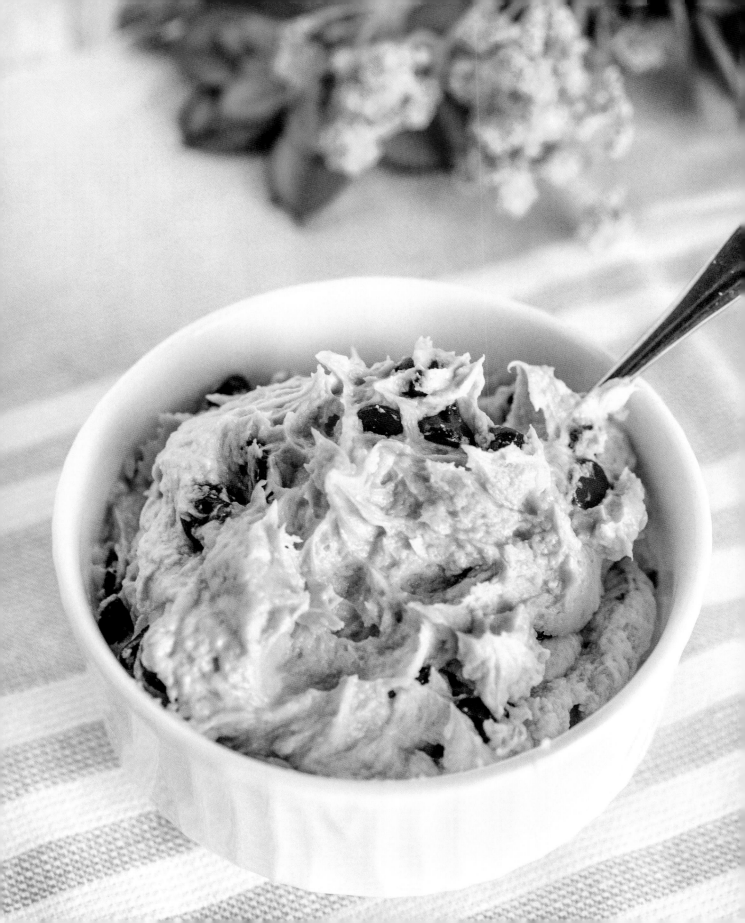

PUPPY CHOW

NET CARBS
3g

OPTION

MAKES 4 servings   PREP TIME: 10 minutes   COOK TIME: Up to 2 minutes

I know what you're thinking...I'm crazy for turning pork rinds into puppy chow. You're correct, I'm crazy, but that has nothing to do with the pork rinds. I think you'll be shocked at how yummy these are!

INGREDIENTS

½ cup sugar-free chocolate chips

¼ cup natural peanut butter

2 ½ tablespoons unsalted butter or ghee

2 tablespoons granulated sweetener

½ teaspoon vanilla extract

1 (3-ounce) bag plain pork rinds

¾ cup powdered sweetener

DIRECTIONS

1. Place the chocolate chips, peanut butter, and butter in a large microwave-safe bowl. Microwave on high for 30 seconds, then stir. Microwave for an additional 15 seconds and stir again. Repeat as needed until the mixture is fully melted and smooth.

2. Add the granulated sweetener and vanilla extract and stir until combined.

3. Break the pork rinds into ½-inch chunks. Be careful not to crush them completely; you don't want dust. Stir the pork rinds into the chocolate mixture until evenly coated.

4. Transfer the pork rind mixture to a gallon-sized resealable plastic bag. Pour in the powdered sweetener, seal the bag, and shake until evenly coated.

5. Pour into a bowl to serve. Store leftovers in the plastic bag at room temperature for up to 1 week.

Nutritional information (per serving)

Calories: 410	Total Carbs: 5g
Fat: 33g	Fiber: 2g
Protein: 20g	Net Carbs: 3g

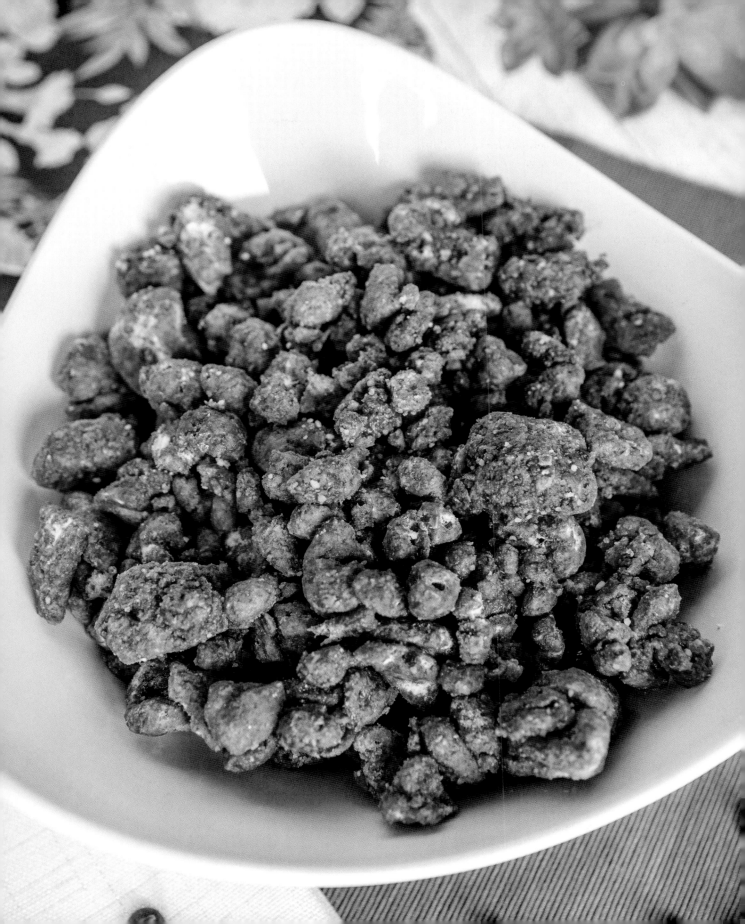

VANILLA SHORTBREAD CAKE FOR TWO

MAKES 2 servings   PREP TIME: 5 minutes   COOK TIME: 25 minutes

This is one of those recipes that just occurred to me one day out of nowhere. I intended to make something completely different and ended up with this cake instead. But, just like Bob Ross said, "There are no mistakes, just happy little accidents."

INGREDIENTS

¼ cup unsweetened vanilla-flavored macadamia nut milk, almond milk, or cashew milk

2 tablespoons unsalted butter or ghee, melted but not hot

1 large egg

½ teaspoon vanilla extract

½ cup blanched almond flour

2 tablespoons granulated sweetener

¼ teaspoon baking powder

Cooking spray

FOR SERVING:

Next-Level Whipped Cream (page 268)

1 large fresh strawberry, sliced

DIRECTIONS

1. Preheat the oven to 350°F.

2. In a medium-sized bowl, whisk together the nut milk, melted butter, egg, vanilla extract, almond flour, sweetener, and baking powder until smooth.

3. Spray two 6- to 8-ounce ramekins with cooking spray and pour an equal amount of the batter into each ramekin, making sure not to fill them more than three-quarters full. (Any more than that and the batter will spill over the edges during baking.)

4. Bake for 25 minutes, or until the edges have browned.

5. Serve warm, topped with whipped cream and a sliced strawberry.

Nutritional information (per serving)

Calories: 317	Total Carbs: 6g
Fat: 29g	Fiber: 3g
Protein: 11g	Net Carbs: 3g

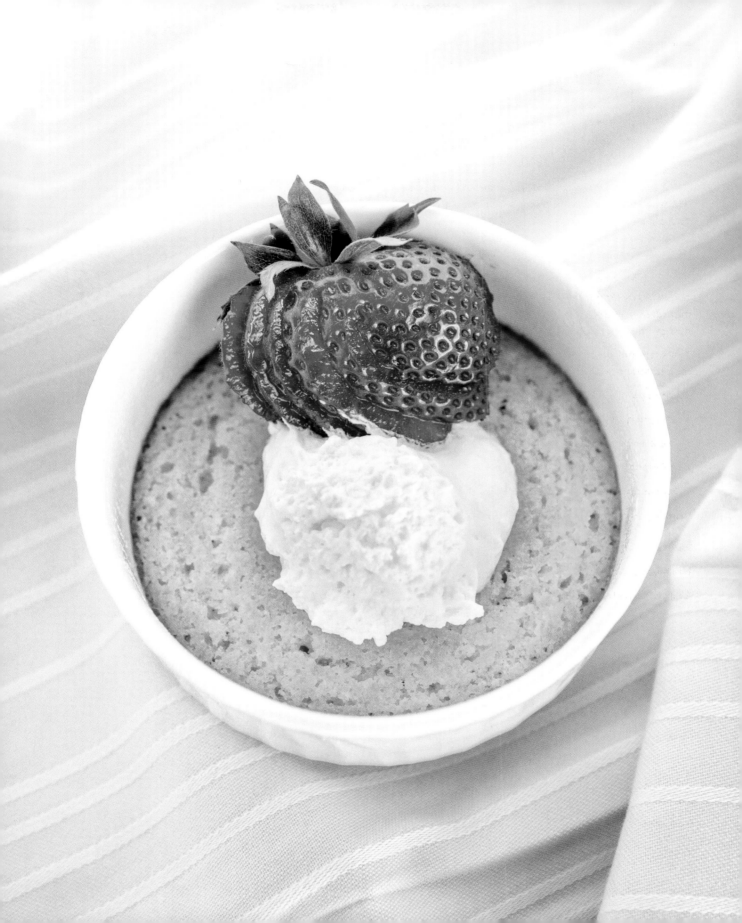

PUMPKIN PIE

MAKES one 9-inch pie (9 servings)   **PREP TIME:** 22 minutes, plus 4 hours to chill   **COOK TIME:** 52 minutes

Ahh...pumpkin pie. What a great gift to human beings, right? I think it was the only thing I looked forward to as a kid on Thanksgiving. Give me all the pie! This keto version will not disappoint.

INGREDIENTS

FOR THE CRUST:

1 cup blanched almond flour

4 to 6 tablespoons unsalted butter or ghee, softened

¼ cup granulated sweetener

FOR THE FILLING:

1 (15-ounce) can pumpkin puree (not pumpkin pie filling)

½ cup granulated sweetener

½ teaspoon ground cinnamon

½ teaspoon ginger powder

½ teaspoon pumpkin pie spice

½ teaspoon vanilla extract

3 large egg yolks

1 large egg

⅔ cup heavy whipping cream or coconut cream

Next-Level Whipped Cream (page 268), for topping

DIRECTIONS

1. Preheat the oven to 375°F.

2. Make the crust: Place all the ingredients in a medium-sized mixing bowl and use a fork to mix together. Begin with 4 tablespoons of butter; if the mixture is too dry, add up to 2 tablespoons more butter and continue to mix until the ingredients are fully incorporated. The crust will be very crumbly.

3. Transfer the crust to a 9-inch pie pan. Using your fingers, press the crust into an even layer. If you have enough crust, you can take it up the sides of the pan as well, but it is not necessary.

4. Par-bake for 12 minutes, or until golden. Remove from the oven and set aside.

5. Make the filling: Place the pumpkin puree, sweetener, spices, and vanilla extract in a large mixing bowl. Using a hand mixer, mix on low until everything is well combined.

6. Add the egg yolks one at a time and mix after each addition. Then add the whole egg and mix well. Add the heavy cream and stir until everything is well incorporated.

7. Pour the filling on top of the crust and smooth out the top.

8. Bake for 35 to 40 minutes, until the filling is firm.

9. Remove from the oven and place on a cooling rack to cool completely. Once cool, place the pie in the refrigerator to set for at least 4 hours; overnight is best.

10. Slice and serve topped with whipped cream. Store leftovers in the refrigerator for up to 1 week.

Nutritional information (per serving)

Calories: 234	Total Carbs: 5g
Fat: 22g	Fiber: 2g
Protein: 6g	Net Carbs: 3g

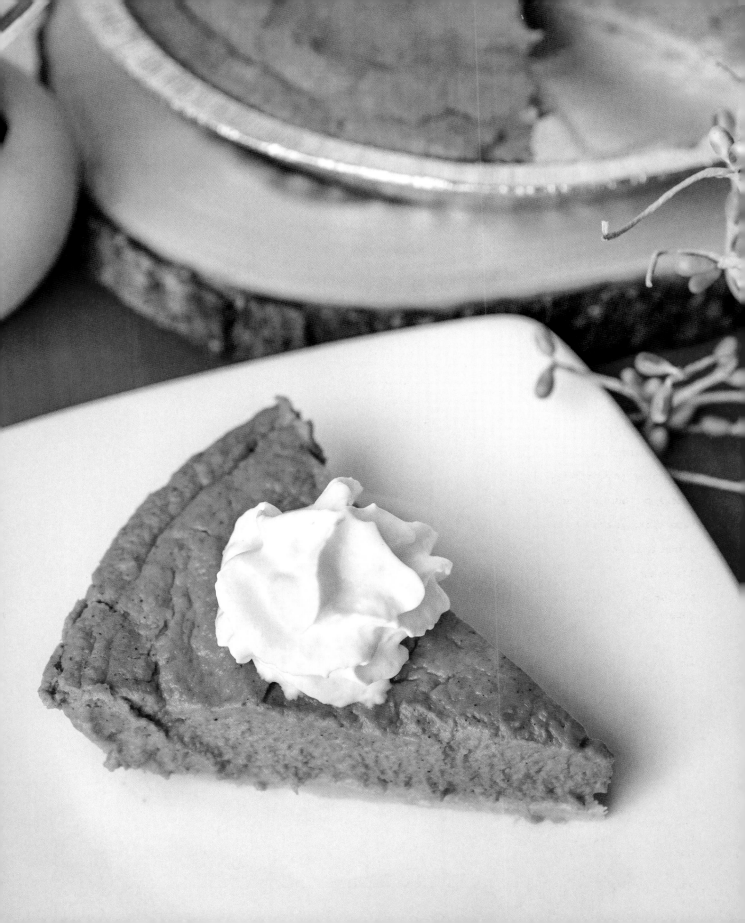

OLD-FASHIONED CHOCOLATE DONUTS

MAKES 8 to 10 donuts (1 per serving)   **PREP TIME: 12 minutes**   **COOK TIME: 20 minutes**

If you don't own a donut pan, I recommend getting one. They are fairly inexpensive, and there's something exciting about being able to eat a donut on keto. These donuts are so dang yummy and are such a great meal prep treat! You could make a batch at the beginning of the week and grab one for breakfast each morning when you're running out the door for work. The hardest part is not eating the entire batch all at once! My donut pan has six wells, so I bake the donuts in two batches. If your donut pan has at least eight wells, you can bake all the batter at one time.

INGREDIENTS

Cooking spray

3 tablespoons unsalted butter or ghee, softened

⅓ cup powdered sweetener, plus more for sprinkling

¼ cup heavy whipping cream or coconut cream

1 teaspoon vanilla extract

4 large eggs

1 cup blanched almond flour

3 tablespoons unsweetened cocoa powder or cacao powder

1 teaspoon baking powder

3 tablespoons sugar-free chocolate, melted

Special Equipment:
Two 6-cavity or one 12-cavity donut pan(s)

DIRECTIONS

1. Preheat the oven to 350°F. Spray 10 wells of one 12-cavity donut pan or two 6-cavity donut pans generously with cooking spray. Don't be shy with the cooking spray, even if you're using a silicone pan. This dough is sticky!

2. Put the butter, sweetener, and heavy cream in a large mixing bowl. Using a hand mixer or stand mixer, beat until well combined.

3. Add the vanilla extract and the eggs, one at a time, mixing well after each addition.

4. Add the almond flour, cocoa powder, baking powder, and melted chocolate. Mix until the ingredients are incorporated.

5. Pour the batter into the greased wells of the donut pan(s), filling each well about three-quarters full.

6. Bake for 18 to 20 minutes, until a toothpick inserted in the center of a donut comes out clean.

7. Remove from the oven and transfer the donuts to a wire cooling rack to cool for 5 minutes, then sprinkle the donuts with powdered sweetener. Store leftovers in the refrigerator for up to 1 week.

Nutritional information (per serving)

Calories: 163	Total Carbs: 8g
Fat: 14g	Fiber: 6g
Protein: 6g	Net Carbs: 2g

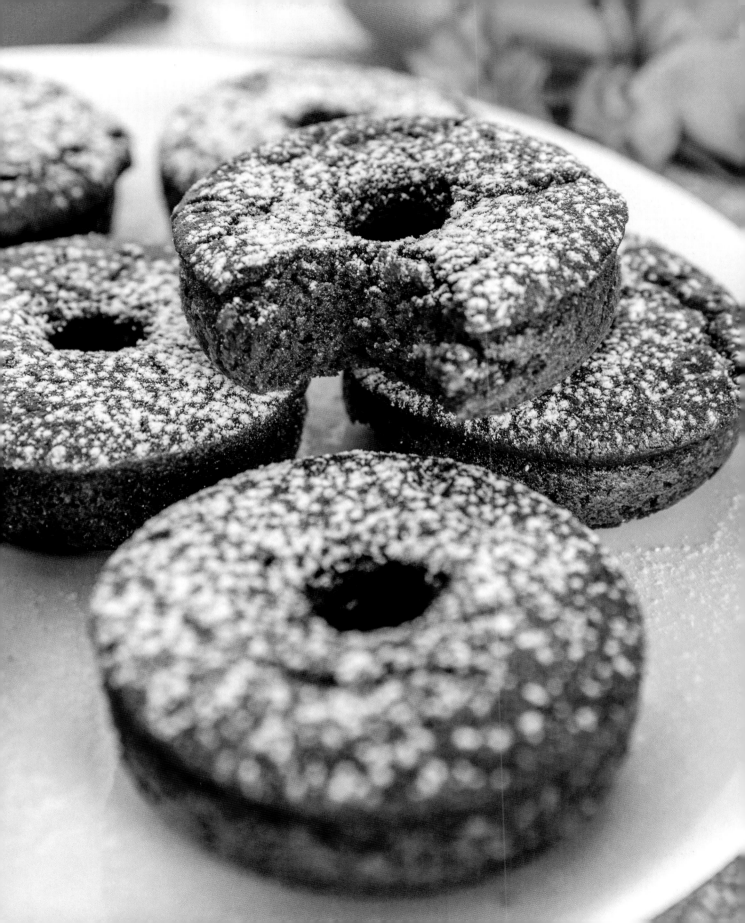

PEANUT BUTTER BALLS

MAKES 12 balls (1 per serving)   **PREP TIME: 15 minutes, plus 30 minutes to chill**

Peanut butter balls are my all-time favorite treat. My mom made these every year during the holidays, and we always looked forward to them. Serve them topped with Jam on the Fly (page 286), dip them in melted sugar-free chocolate, or eat them straight up for a delicious fat bomb!

INGREDIENTS

¾ cup natural peanut butter

½ cup (1 stick) unsalted butter or ghee, softened

1 teaspoon vanilla extract

1½ tablespoons granulated sweetener

DIRECTIONS

1. Place the peanut butter, butter, vanilla extract, and sweetener in a large mixing bowl. Mash with a fork until the ingredients are well incorporated. The mixture will be a bit liquid-y, but don't worry, it'll set up nicely.

2. Line a tray or baking sheet with parchment paper. Using an ice cream scoop or a large spoon, scoop up a portion of the peanut butter mixture and form into a 1-inch ball. Repeat with the remaining peanut butter mixture, forming a total of 12 balls. Place the balls on the lined tray and place in the freezer to set for 30 minutes. Let sit out at room temperature for about 5 minutes before enjoying.

3. Store in the freezer for up to 1 month.

Nutritional information (per serving)

Calories: 171	Total Carbs: 3g
Fat: 17g	Fiber: 2g
Protein: 4g	Net Carbs: 1g

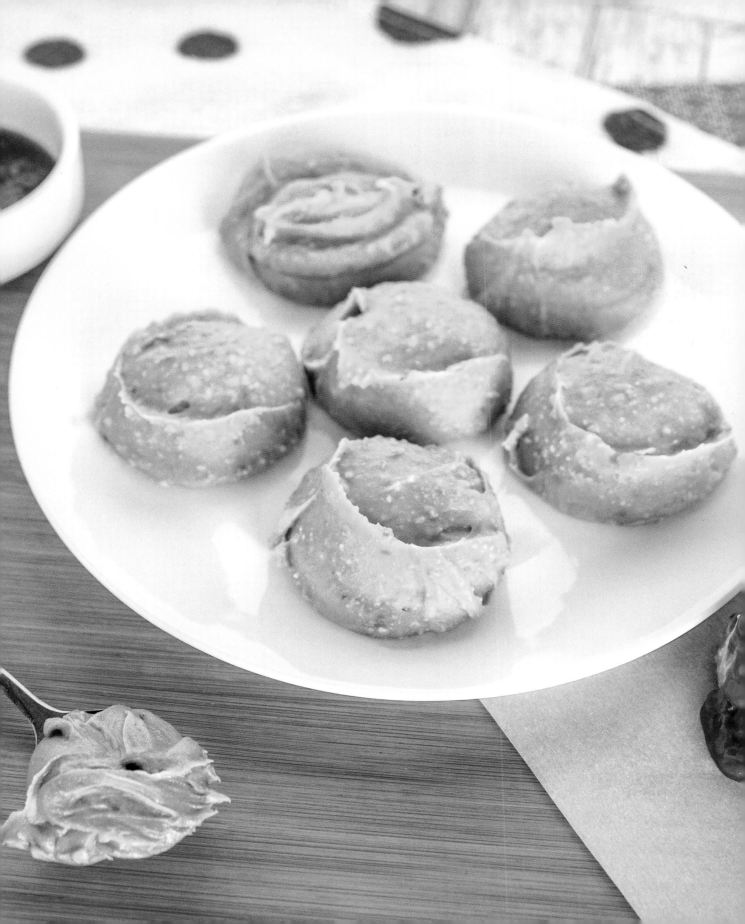

SNICKERDOODLE MUG CAKE

MAKES 1 serving   PREP TIME: 2 minutes   COOK TIME: 1½ minutes

This mug cake is so light and fluffy and really hits the spot when you need something sweet!

INGREDIENTS

Cooking spray

2 tablespoons coconut flour

1 tablespoon granulated sweetener

¼ teaspoon baking powder

¼ teaspoon ground cinnamon, plus more for garnish

3 tablespoons heavy whipping cream or coconut cream

1 large egg

½ teaspoon vanilla extract

DIRECTIONS

1. Spray a microwave-safe 8-ounce mug with cooking spray.

2. Place all the ingredients in a small mixing bowl and mix with a fork until well combined; the mixture should resemble cake batter.

3. Pour the batter into the greased mug. Microwave on high for 1 minute 20 seconds. Insert a toothpick in the center to test that the cake is cooked all the way through; it should come out clean. If it needs a little more time, microwave for 15 seconds more.

4. Sprinkle cinnamon on top and enjoy straight from the mug!

Nutritional information

Calories: 293	Total Carbs: 10g
Fat: 23g	Fiber: 5g
Protein: 9g	Net Carbs: 5g

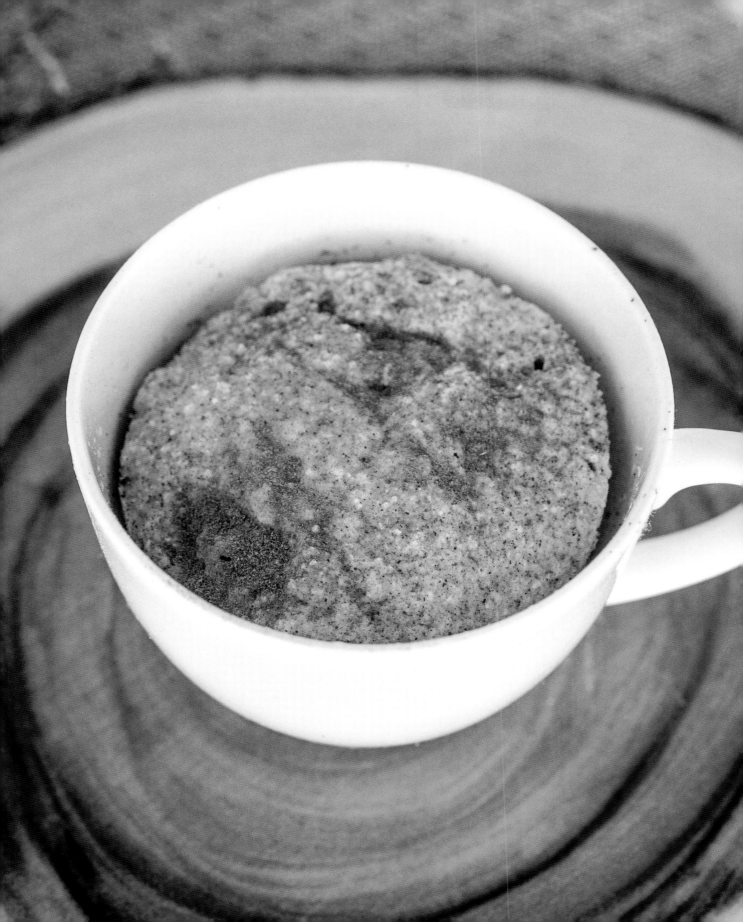

CAMERON'S PINK STUFF

MAKES 6 cups (¼ cup per serving)   PREP TIME: 3 minutes   COOK TIME: —

My husband, Cameron, has lived off of "Pink Stuff" since he was a little kid. This is his keto version of his family's favorite recipe, and it is to die for! I'm just throwing this out there as a disclaimer...this is dirty keto at its finest. Sugar-free whipped topping and Jell-O don't have the cleanest ingredients, so if that bothers you, try using fresh whipped cream or my Next-Level Whipped Cream (page 268) in place of the whipped topping and a powdered drink mix like Ultima or Go Everly, which are made with natural sweeteners, in place of the Jell-O.

INGREDIENTS

1 (24-ounce) container cottage cheese

1 (16-ounce) tub sugar-free whipped topping (such as Cool Whip)

1 (0.3-ounce) package sugar-free raspberry Jell-O

2 (8-ounce) packages cream cheese

DIRECTIONS

1. Put the cottage cheese, whipped topping, and Jell-O powder in a large bowl. Stir until well incorporated.

2. Cut the cream cheese into tiny chunks, about ¼ inch, and place the chunks in the bowl. Fold the mixture with a rubber spatula.

3. Serve cold! Store leftovers in the refrigerator for up to a week.

Nutritional information (per serving)

Calories: 70	Total Carbs: 3g
Fat: 5g	Fiber: 0g
Protein: 4g	Net Carbs: 3g

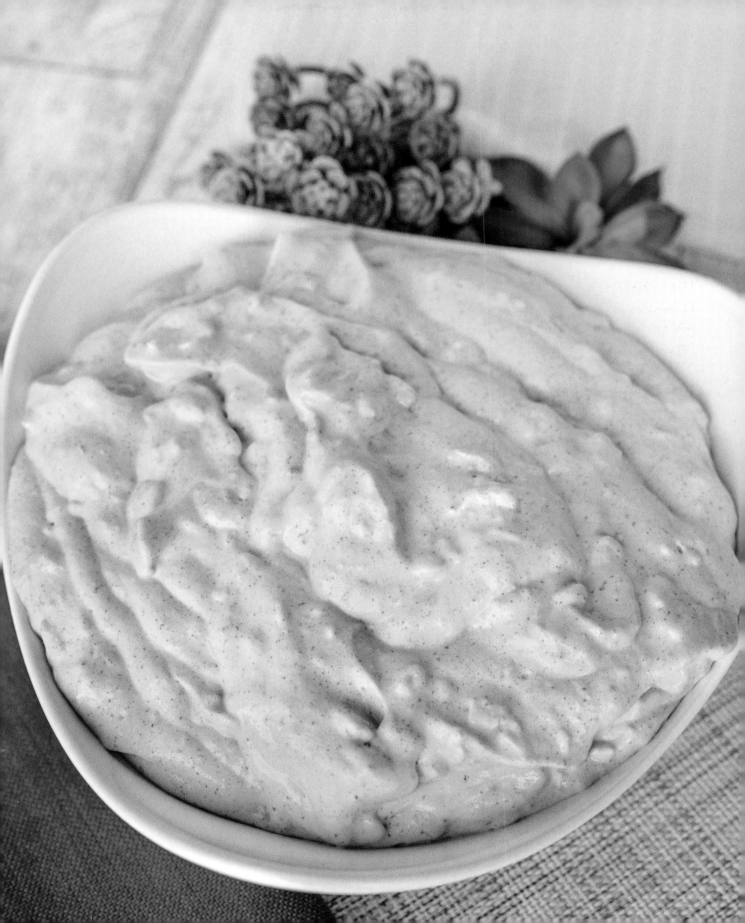

LEMON MUG CAKE

MAKES 1 serving   PREP TIME: 5 minutes   COOK TIME: 1½ minutes

Mug cake was my saving grace during my first few months on keto. It's the perfect quick-and-easy treat! This lemon version may be my favorite.

INGREDIENTS

Cooking spray

1 large egg

2½ tablespoons lemon juice

2 tablespoons heavy whipping cream or coconut cream

2 tablespoons coconut flour

1½ teaspoons granulated sweetener

¼ teaspoon baking powder

Pinch of salt

FOR TOPPING (OPTIONAL):

Next-Level Whipped Cream (page 268)

Grated lemon zest

DIRECTIONS

1. Spray a microwave-safe 8-ounce mug with cooking spray.

2. Place all the ingredients in a small mixing bowl and mix with a fork or whisk until the coconut flour is mixed well with the other ingredients and there are no chunks.

3. Pour the batter into the greased mug. Microwave on high for 1 minute 20 seconds. Insert a toothpick in the center to test that the cake is cooked all the way through; it should come out clean. If it needs a little more time, microwave for 15 seconds more.

4. Top with whipped cream and lemon zest, if desired, and serve right in the mug!

Nutritional information

Calories: 236	Total Carbs: 10g
Fat: 18g	Fiber: 5g
Protein: 9g	Net Carbs: 5g

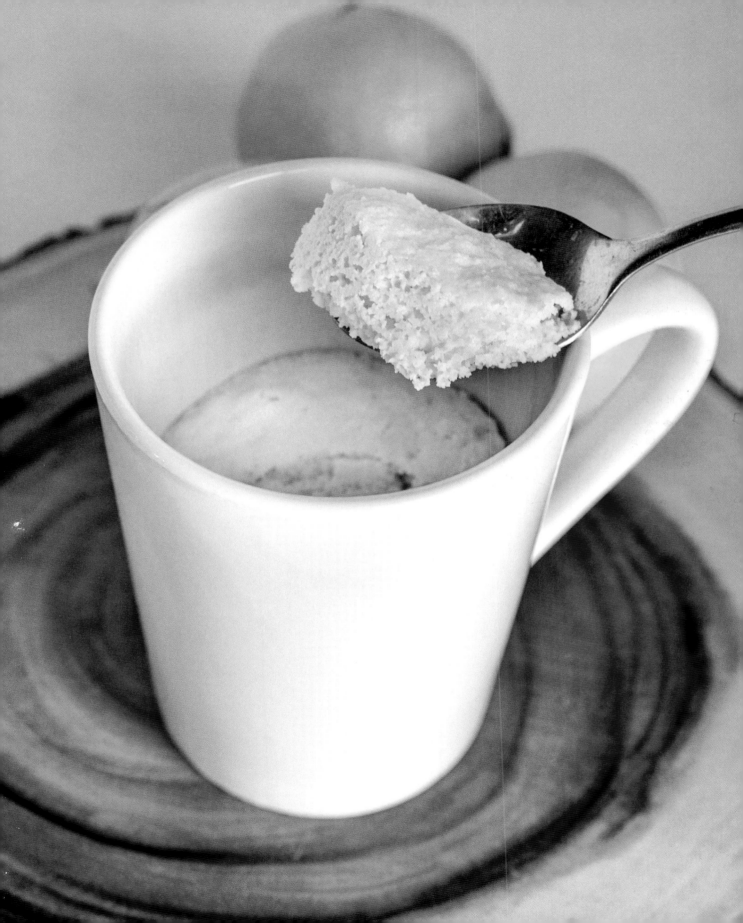

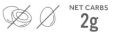

CHOCOLATE CHIP PEANUT BUTTER FAT BOMBS

MAKES 12 fat bombs (1 per serving)   **PREP TIME: 7 minutes, plus 1 hour to freeze**   **COOK TIME: —**

After doing keto for about seven months, I decided to allow myself a cheat day on my birthday. The first food on my list was chocolate chip cookie dough. I immediately regretted it. Although it was tasty, I quickly developed the biggest bellyache of all time. I learned my lesson. I decided that I needed to learn how to re-create those cheat foods to fit my keto lifestyle, saving myself the bellyache and the guilt. These fat bombs are perfect to keep on hand in the freezer. Just pop one in your mouth when the sweet tooth hits!

This recipe appears similar to the Loaded Fat Bomb recipe on page 218, but the butter used in these bites gives them a totally different flavor. They are denser and richer than the Loaded Fat Bomb, which is more like ice cream.

INGREDIENTS

1 (8-ounce) package cream cheese, softened

½ cup (1 stick) unsalted butter or ghee, softened

½ cup natural peanut butter or unsweetened almond butter

2 teaspoons vanilla extract

2 teaspoons granulated sweetener

¾ cup sugar-free chocolate chips

DIRECTIONS

1. Line a baking sheet or tray with parchment paper or a silicone baking mat and set aside.

2. Place the cream cheese, butter, peanut butter, vanilla extract, and sweetener in a large bowl. Using a hand mixer, mix until well incorporated.

3. Add the chocolate chips and mix in with a rubber spatula.

4. Use a cookie scoop or large spoon to form twelve 1½-inch balls, placing each ball on the lined baking sheet.

5. Place the baking sheet in the freezer for 1 hour to harden the fat bombs.

6. Put the frozen fat bombs in a gallon-sized resealable plastic bag and store in the refrigerator for up to 1 week or in the freezer for up to 4 weeks. Enjoy straight from the fridge or freezer, or, if frozen, let them sit out at room temperature for a couple of minutes to soften before eating.

Nutritional information (per serving)

Calories: 269	Total Carbs: 3g
Fat: 25g	Fiber: 1g
Protein: 5g	Net Carbs: 2g

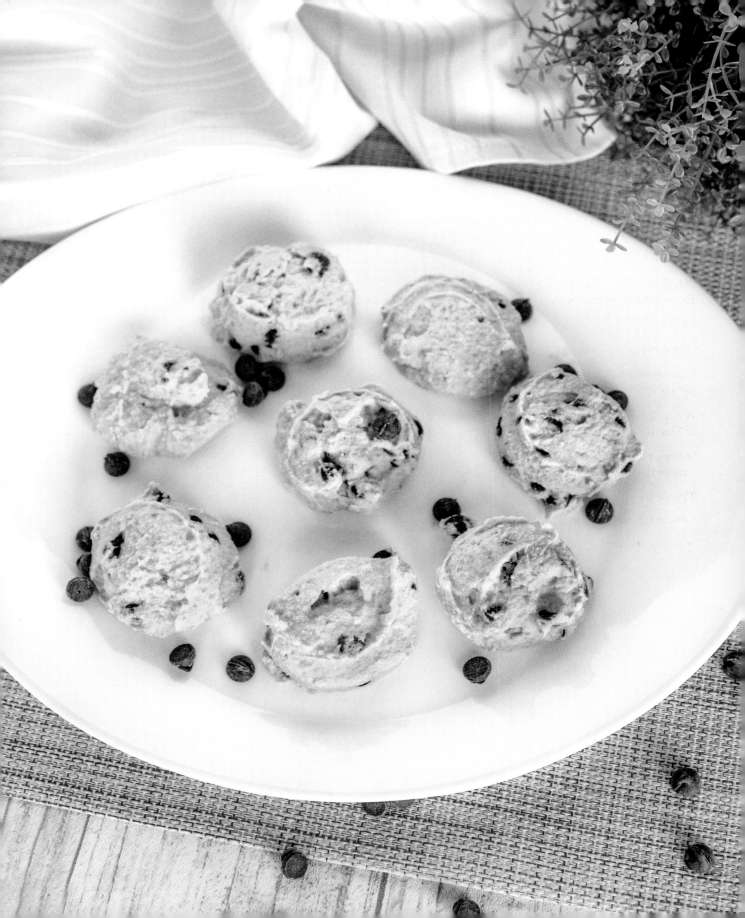

CINNAMON SPICE BREAD

MAKES one 8½ by 4½-inch loaf (9 servings)   **PREP TIME:** 10 minutes   **COOK TIME:** 32 minutes

Do you miss bread? Probably. I'm at a point now where I just don't crave it anymore, thankfully. But every once in a while, I want it. This is my favorite bread. It tastes like Christmas to me.

INGREDIENTS

Cooking spray

½ cup heavy whipping cream

¼ cup (½ stick) unsalted butter or ghee, melted but not hot

3 large eggs

½ teaspoon vanilla extract

¼ cup granulated sweetener

1 cup blanched almond flour

1 tablespoon coconut flour

2 teaspoons baking powder

1 teaspoon ground cinnamon

Pinch of salt

Cream Cheese Frosting (page 302), for topping (optional)

DIRECTIONS

1. Preheat the oven to 350°F. Spray a 8½ by 4½-inch loaf pan with cooking spray.

2. In a large mixing bowl, whisk together the heavy cream, melted butter, eggs, vanilla extract, and sweetener until well combined.

3. Add the almond flour, coconut flour, baking powder, cinnamon, and salt to the wet mixture. Whisk again until the ingredients are well incorporated.

4. Pour the batter into the greased loaf pan and bake for 28 to 32 minutes, until a toothpick inserted in the center of the loaf comes out clean.

5. Serve warm with butter or let cool completely and then top with cream cheese frosting, if desired. Store leftovers in the refrigerator or simply cover and keep on the counter for up to 4 days. We love ours reheated in the microwave and topped with butter.

Nutritional information (per serving)

Calories: 193	**Total Carbs:** 3g
Fat: 18g	**Fiber:** 2g
Protein: 6g	**Net Carbs:** 1g

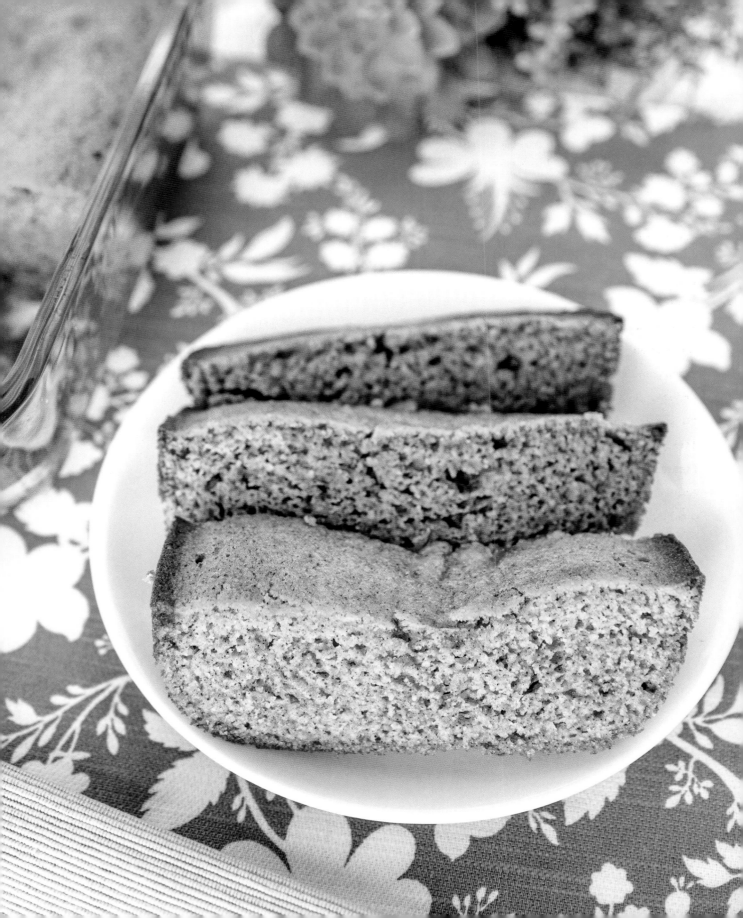

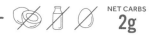

CANDIED PECANS

MAKES 6 servings   **PREP TIME:** 2 minutes   **COOK TIME:** 8 minutes

You know those candied nut places in the mall that smell like heaven when you walk by? That's what these are. I remember passing one of those shops when I first started keto, and I almost cried. Little did I know that I could make a keto-friendly version at home, and for a fraction of the cost! These nuts are perfect for holiday parties, neighbor gifts, or even just to keep on hand when you need something sweet. Feel free to switch out the pecans for another nut. This recipe would be amazing with almonds!

INGREDIENTS

¼ cup water

¾ cup granulated sweetener

1 teaspoon vanilla extract

½ teaspoon ground cinnamon

Pinch of salt

3 cups raw pecan halves

DIRECTIONS

1. Put the water and sweetener in a medium-sized saucepan and bring to a boil over medium-high heat.

2. Reduce the heat to low and add the vanilla extract, cinnamon, and salt. Stir until well combined.

3. Remove from the heat, add the pecans, and stir to coat. Let sit for 1 to 2 minutes. Meanwhile, line a rimmed baking sheet with parchment paper or a silicone baking mat.

4. Spread the candied pecans on the lined baking sheet and let cool completely. Break them up, if necessary, and serve! Store leftovers in the pantry for up to a week or in the refrigerator for up to 2 weeks.

Nutritional information (per serving)

Calories: 385   **Total Carbs:** 8g
Fat: 42g   **Fiber:** 6g
Protein: 6g   **Net Carbs:** 2g

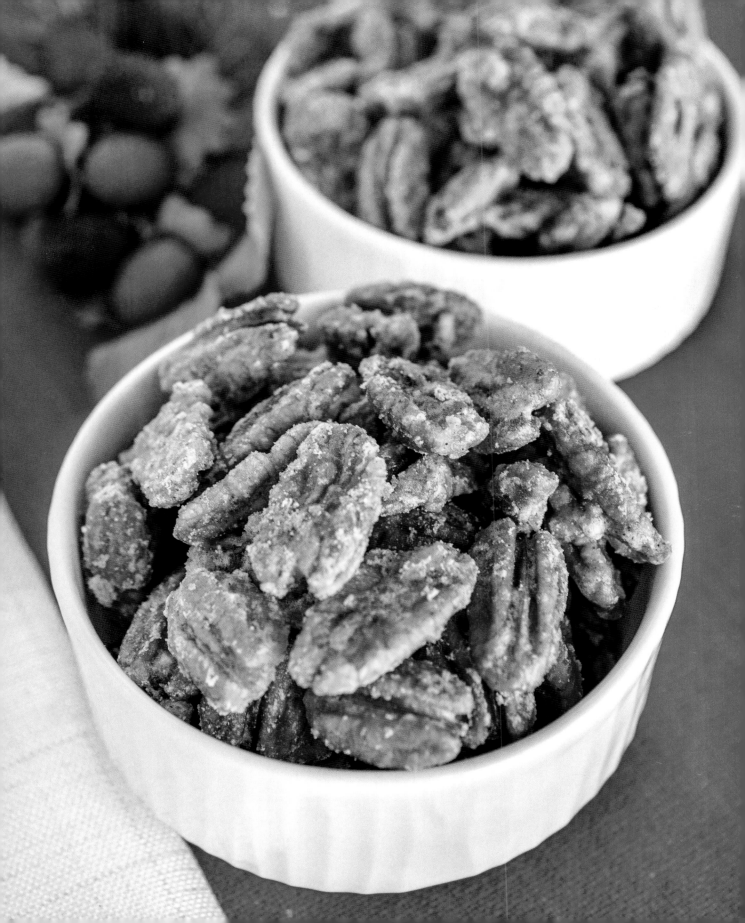

BLUEBERRY COBBLER

MAKES 6 servings   **PREP TIME: 5 minutes**   **COOK TIME: 30 minutes**

This is one of my favorite treats. Lucky for me, my husband doesn't like blueberries, so I usually get this cobbler all to myself, and that's something I'll always cherish. No, but seriously, sometimes I don't like to share my food, and this dessert falls into that category.

INGREDIENTS

3 cups blueberries (fresh or frozen)

3½ tablespoons granulated sweetener, divided

1 teaspoon xanthan gum

1½ teaspoons lemon juice

1 cup blanched almond flour

3 tablespoons unsalted butter or ghee, softened

DIRECTIONS

1. Preheat the oven to 350°F.

2. Place the blueberries, 2 tablespoons of the sweetener, the xanthan gum, and lemon juice in a medium-sized bowl. Stir with a spoon to coat the blueberries evenly.

3. Put the almond flour and the remaining 1½ tablespoons of sweetener in a separate bowl and stir.

4. Transfer the blueberry mixture to a 9-inch square baking dish or divide it evenly among six 4-ounce ramekins. Sprinkle the almond flour mixture on top of the blueberries.

5. Cut the butter into small pieces and scatter them over the almond flour topping. It doesn't have to look pretty; just make sure to distribute the butter evenly.

6. Bake until the top is golden brown, 18 to 20 minutes if using fresh blueberries or 25 to 30 minutes if using frozen blueberries.

7. Let cool for about 2 minutes, then serve! Store in the refrigerator for up to 5 days. Reheat in the oven or microwave.

Nutritional information (per serving)

Calories: 206	**Total Carbs:** 14g
Fat: 16g	**Fiber:** 4g
Protein: 6g	**Net Carbs:** 10g

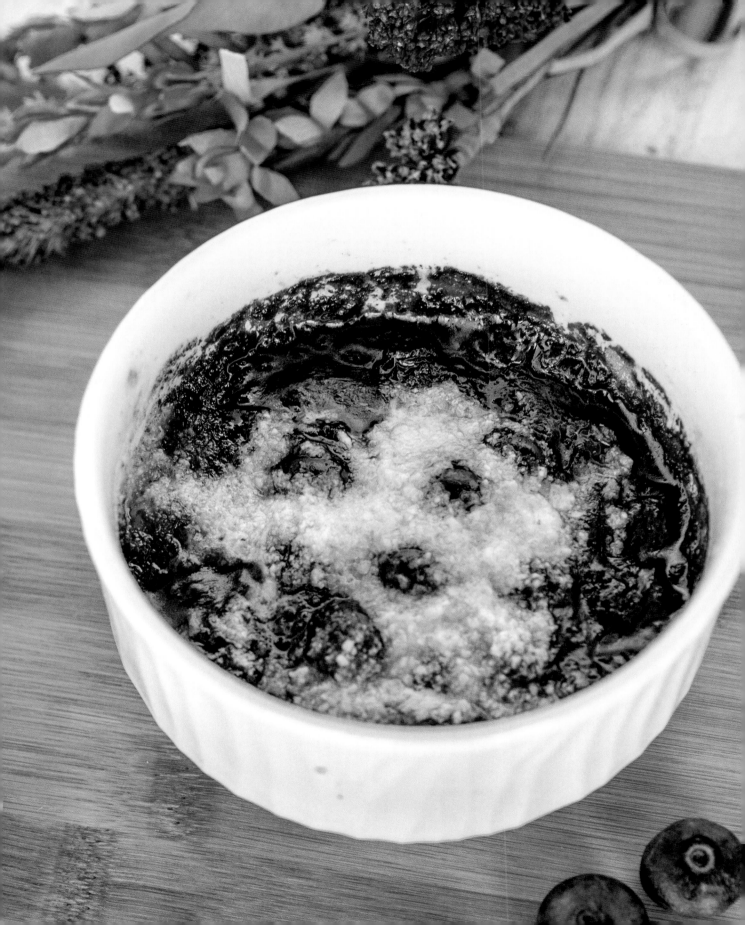

SALTED CHOCOLATE MACADAMIA NUT CLUSTERS

MAKES 12 clusters (1 per serving)   PREP TIME: 10 minutes, plus 30 minutes to chill   COOK TIME: —

This treat is a crowd-pleaser for sure—even for the non-keto peeps in your life. I love to make these for parties or just to keep a few stored in the refrigerator for when my sweet tooth is calling.

INGREDIENTS

1½ cups sugar-free chocolate chips

3 ounces raw macadamia nuts (about ½ cup)

Pink Himalayan salt, for topping

DIRECTIONS

1. Line a baking sheet with parchment paper or a silicone baking mat.

2. Place the chocolate chips in a microwave-safe bowl and microwave on high for 1 minute. Stir, then microwave for another 30 seconds. Repeat as needed in 30-second increments until the chocolate is fully melted.

3. Put a cluster of 3 or 4 macadamia nuts on the lined baking sheet. Repeat until you have 12 nut clusters.

4. Pour the melted chocolate over the nut clusters, using about 1½ tablespoons for each cluster. Then top each cluster with a dash of salt.

5. Place the clusters in the fridge to chill for 30 minutes before enjoying. Store in the refrigerator for up to 2 weeks.

Nutritional information (per serving)

Calories: 175	Total Carbs: 3g
Fat: 14g	Fiber: 1g
Protein: 3g	Net Carbs: 2g

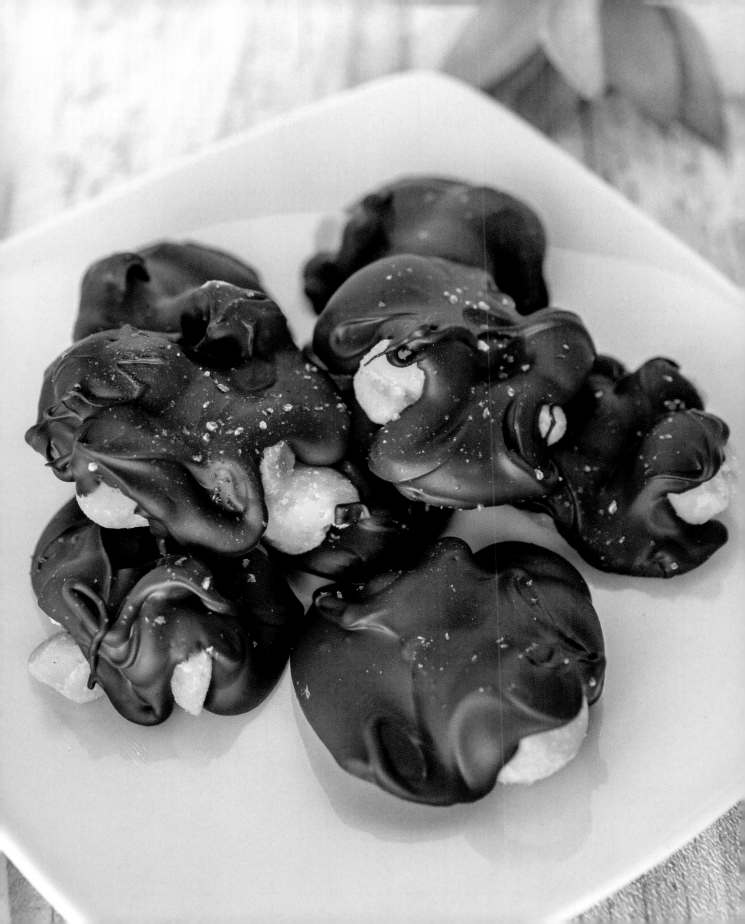

PUMPKIN PIE DONUT MUFFINS

MAKES 14 mini muffins (2 per serving)   **PREP TIME: 25 minutes**   **COOK TIME: 20 minutes**

Have you ever had a muffin so confoundingly good that you don't really know how to identify it? Well, you're about to experience that with this recipe, hence the funky name. These taste just like pumpkin pie, but also donuts, and also muffins. Try them and you'll get it.

INGREDIENTS

Cooking spray

2½ cups blanched almond flour

¼ cup plus 2 tablespoons granulated sweetener, divided

1 tablespoon pumpkin pie spice

1 teaspoon baking powder

½ teaspoon salt

2 large eggs

½ cup pumpkin puree (not pumpkin pie filling)

⅓ cup sugar-free maple syrup, store-bought or homemade (page 269)

¼ cup coconut oil, melted but not hot

1 teaspoon vanilla extract

¾ cup sugar-free chocolate chips (optional)

1 tablespoon ground cinnamon

Special Equipment:
Mini muffin pan

DIRECTIONS

1. Preheat the oven to 325°F. Spray 14 wells of a mini muffin pan with cooking spray and set aside. (If your mini muffin pan has fewer than 16 wells, you'll need to bake the muffins in batches.)

2. In a large bowl, combine the almond flour, ¼ cup of the sweetener, the pumpkin pie spice, and salt.

3. Put the eggs, pumpkin puree, maple syrup, melted coconut oil, and vanilla extract in a medium-sized bowl. Using a stand mixer or hand mixer, mix until well incorporated.

4. Pour the wet mixture into the dry ingredients and mix on high until thoroughly combined. The mixture should look like cookie dough. Fold in the chocolate chips, if using.

5. Using a spoon or 1¼-ounce cookie scoop, place a small scoop of the dough in each of the greased wells of the mini muffin pan. Bake for 18 to 20 minutes, until golden.

6. While the muffins are baking, place the cinnamon and remaining 2 tablespoons of sweetener in a small bowl and stir with a fork.

7. Remove the muffins from the oven. While they are hot, use a spoon to sprinkle the cinnamon mixture on top of the muffins.

8. Serve warm. Store leftovers in the refrigerator for up to 1 week.

Nutritional information (per serving)

Calories: 317	Total Carbs: 16g
Fat: 27g	Fiber: 11g
Protein: 12g	Net Carbs: 5g

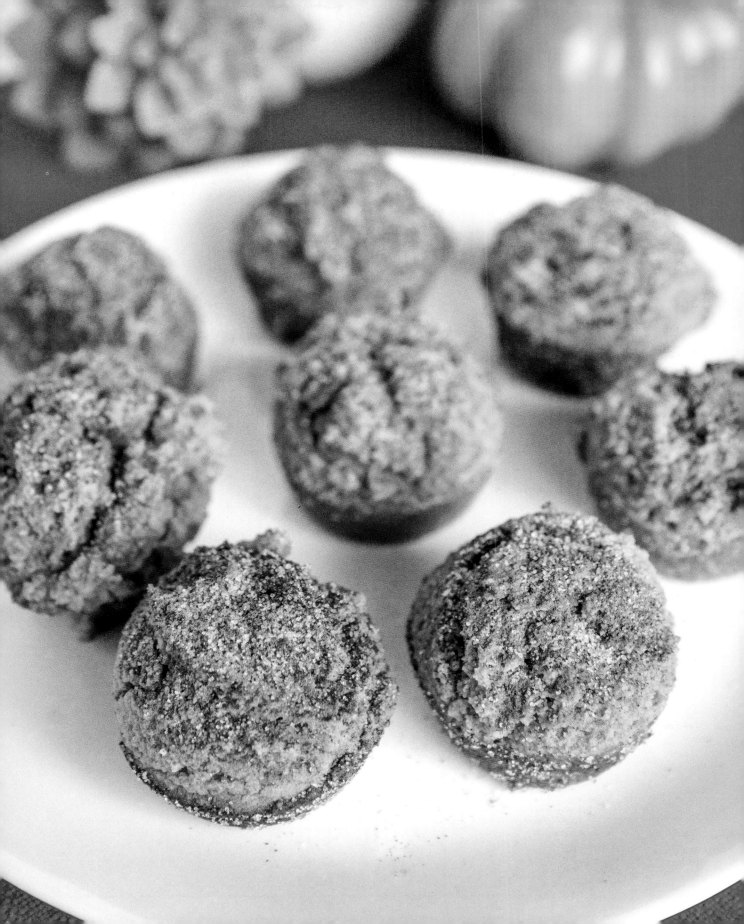

STRAWBERRY BANANA MUG CAKE

MAKES 1 serving   **PREP TIME:** 2 minutes   **COOK TIME:** 1½ minutes

Oh, how I miss bananas. Anytime I can add banana extract to something, you better believe I'm on it! If you're not a banana fan, you can simply omit the banana extract or substitute the extract of your choice: orange, lemon, coconut...

INGREDIENTS

Cooking spray

3 fresh strawberries, cut into small pieces

2 tablespoons coconut flour

1 tablespoon granulated sweetener

½ teaspoon baking powder

2 tablespoons heavy whipping cream or coconut cream

1½ teaspoons coconut oil

1 large egg

1 teaspoon banana extract

DIRECTIONS

1. Spray a microwave-safe 8-ounce mug with cooking spray.

2. Place all the ingredients in a small mixing bowl and mix with a fork until well incorporated.

3. Pour the batter into the greased mug. Microwave on high for 1 minute 20 seconds. Insert a toothpick in the center to test that the cake is cooked all the way through; it should come out clean. If it needs a little more time, microwave for 15 seconds more.

4. Remove from the microwave and enjoy straight from the mug!

Nutritional information

Calories: 302   Total Carbs: 11g
Fat: 25g   Fiber: 5g
Protein: 9g   Net Carbs: 6g

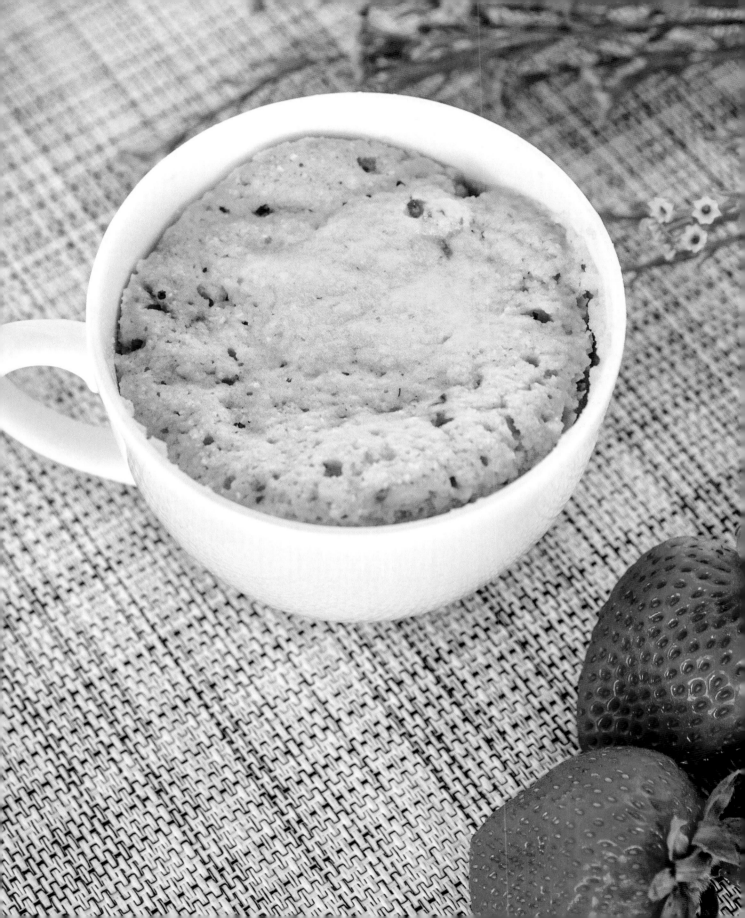

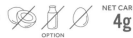
ROMAN'S CHOCOLATE-COVERED PEANUT BUTTER BARS

MAKES 9 bars (1 per serving)   **PREP TIME: 10 minutes, plus 1 hour to chill**   **COOK TIME: 1 minute**

This yummy treat is named after our second child, Roman. He's our peanut butter kid. Now that I think of it, he's also our chocolate kid. Roman is obsessed with these bars and always has to tell me, "These don't even taste keto!" Coming from a child, that's a super good indicator of how tasty these are!

INGREDIENTS

¾ cup blanched almond flour

½ cup natural peanut butter

¼ cup (½ stick) unsalted butter or ghee, softened

2 tablespoons granulated sweetener

½ teaspoon vanilla extract

Cooking spray

1 cup sugar-free chocolate chips

DIRECTIONS

1. Place the almond flour, peanut butter, butter, sweetener, and vanilla extract in a large bowl. Use a hand mixer to blend until combined.

2. Spray an 8-inch square glass baking dish with cooking spray. Press the peanut butter mixture into the pan in an even layer and smooth out the top.

3. Place the chocolate chips in a small microwave-safe bowl. Microwave on high for 30 seconds, then stir. If necessary, microwave for another 30 seconds, or until the chocolate is fully melted.

4. Pour the melted chocolate on top of the peanut butter mixture and smooth it into an even layer.

5. Place the dish in the refrigerator for at least 1 hour to allow the flavors to blend and the chocolate to harden. Cut into bars and enjoy.

6. Store in the refrigerator for up to 6 days or freeze for up to 3 months. If frozen, let the bar sit out at room temperature for about 5 minutes before eating.

Nutritional information (per serving)

Calories: 296	Total Carbs: 6g
Fat: 26g	Fiber: 2g
Protein: 8g	Net Carbs: 4g

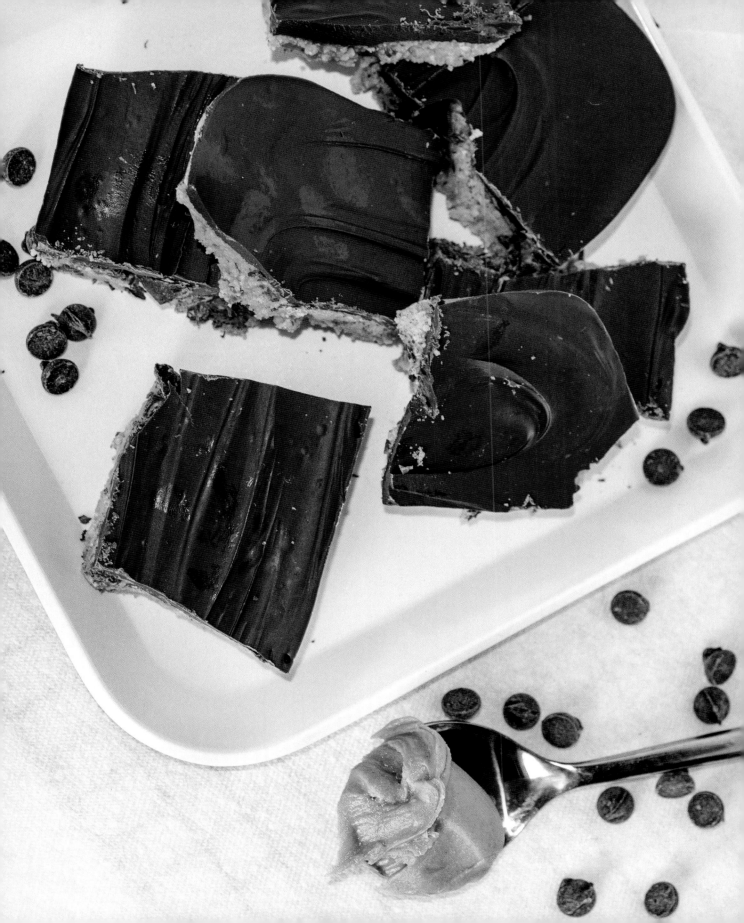

FLOURLESS CHOCOLATE MUG CAKE

MAKES 1 serving   **PREP TIME: 2 minutes**   **COOK TIME: 1½ minutes**

This mug cake has been a huge hit with my Instagram followers. I will give a brief disclaimer, though. If you haven't been doing keto for very long, desserts like these probably will not taste great to you. Give your taste buds some time to adjust before giving this recipe a try. If you are fat-adapted, make this cake ASAP! Your sweet tooth will thank you. I like to top this cake with a few sugar-free chocolate chips and whipped cream.

INGREDIENTS

Cooking spray

2 tablespoons unsweetened cocoa powder or cacao powder

2 tablespoons granulated sweetener

1 large egg

1 tablespoon heavy whipping cream or coconut cream

½ teaspoon vanilla extract

¼ teaspoon baking powder

Pinch of salt

DIRECTIONS

1. Spray a microwave-safe 8-ounce mug with cooking spray.

2. Place all the ingredients in a small mixing bowl and mix with a fork until well incorporated.

3. Pour the batter into the greased mug. Microwave on high for 1 minute 20 seconds. Insert a toothpick in the center to test that the cake is cooked all the way through; it should come out clean. If it needs a little more time, microwave for 15 seconds more.

4. Remove from the microwave and serve right in the mug!

Nutritional information

Calories: 153   **Total Carbs:** 7g
Fat: 11g   **Fiber:** 4g
Protein: 8g   **Net Carbs:** 3g

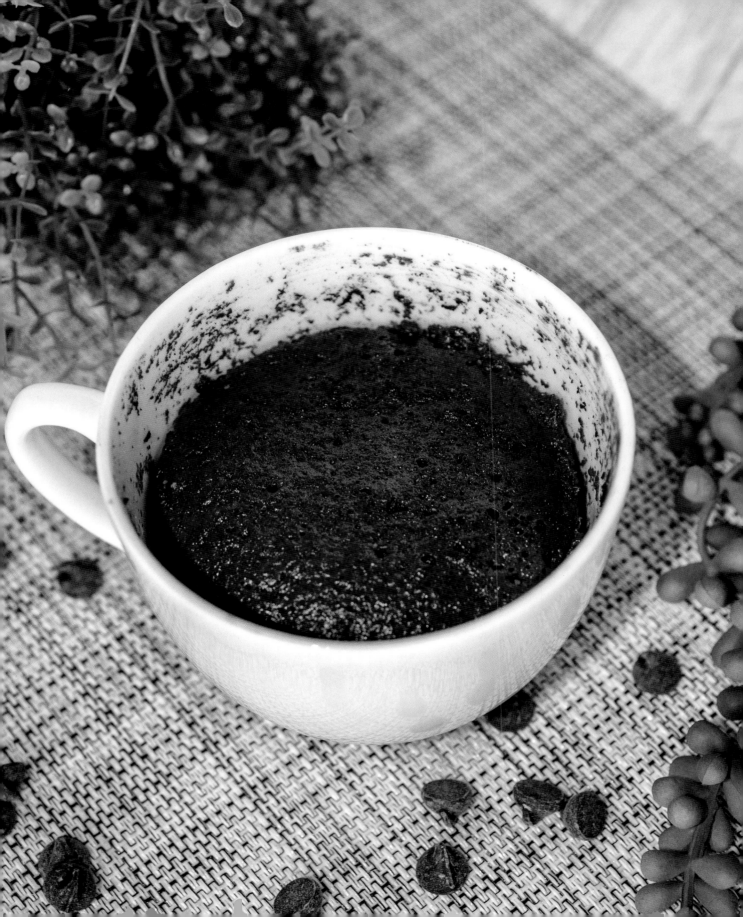

CHEESECAKE

MAKES one 9-inch cake (12 servings)   PREP TIME: 18 minutes, plus time to chill overnight   COOK TIME: 55 minutes

Did someone say cheesecake? Seriously, I'll do any diet for life if I can still have cheesecake. Am I right? This is an excellent low-carb dessert. Just try to not eat the whole thing in one sitting.

INGREDIENTS

FOR THE CRUST:

1½ cups blanched almond flour

3 tablespoons granulated sweetener

¼ cup (½ stick) unsalted butter or ghee, softened

Cooking spray

FOR THE FILLING:

3 (8-ounce) packages cream cheese, softened

¼ cup heavy whipping cream

3 large eggs

⅓ cup granulated sweetener

1 teaspoon vanilla extract

DIRECTIONS

1. Preheat the oven to 300°F.

2. Make the crust: Place the almond flour, sweetener, and butter in a medium-sized mixing bowl. Stir with a fork until the crust mixture has a crumbly consistency.

3. Spray a 9-inch springform pan generously with cooking spray. Then press the crust mixture into the bottom of the prepared pan, smoothing it out in an even layer. Set aside.

4. Make the filling: Place the cream cheese and heavy cream in another mixing bowl. Using a hand mixer, mix until a whipped texture develops.

5. Add the eggs one at a time, mixing well after each addition. Add the sweetener and vanilla extract and mix until well incorporated.

6. Pour the filling over the crust and smooth into an even layer.

7. Bake for 45 to 55 minutes, until the cheesecake is slightly golden brown on the edges but still a little jiggly in the middle. Allow to cool completely in the pan, then cover and place in the refrigerator to chill and set overnight.

8. Remove the outer ring of the springform pan, then slice and serve cold!

Nutritional information (per serving)

Calories: 353   Total Carbs: 5g
Fat: 32g   Fiber: 2g
Protein: 10g   Net Carbs: 3g

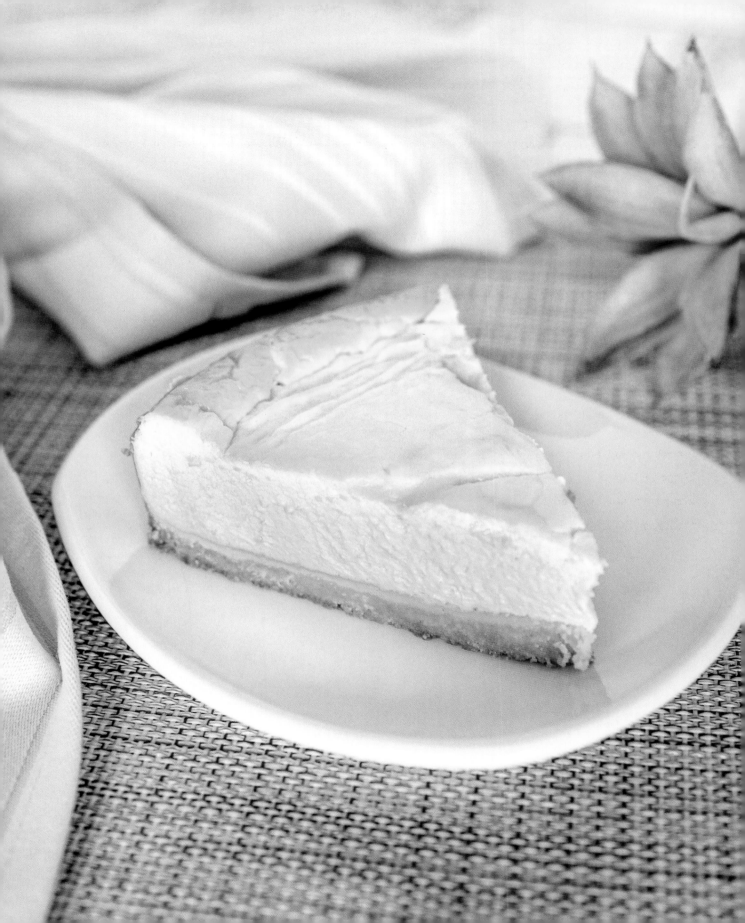

CRÈME BRÛLÉE

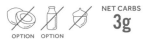

NET CARBS
3g

MAKES 4 servings   PREP TIME: 5 minutes, plus 1 hour to chill   COOK TIME: 40 minutes

Crème brûlée is such a decadent treat—rich, creamy, and perfectly sweet. I think everyone would agree that the best part is cracking that beautiful caramelized sweetener on top to find the creamy inside. There is really nothing better.

INGREDIENTS

4 large egg yolks

1 teaspoon vanilla extract

2 cups heavy whipping cream or coconut cream

5 tablespoons granulated sweetener, divided

DIRECTIONS

1. Preheat the oven to 325°F.

2. In a small bowl, whisk together the egg yolks and vanilla extract.

3. Place the heavy cream and 1 tablespoon of the sweetener in a saucepan over medium heat. Whisk constantly until the mixture starts to boil. Remove from the heat and slowly add the egg yolk mixture while whisking. Continue whisking until well combined.

4. Divide the mixture evenly among four 6-ounce ramekins. Place the ramekins in a glass baking dish and pour hot water into the dish so that it comes halfway up the sides of the ramekins.

5. Bake for 30 minutes, or until the edges are set but the center is slightly jiggly.

6. Remove the ramekins from the baking dish and place on a cooling rack to cool for 10 minutes. Then place the ramekins in the refrigerator for 1 hour to chill and fully set.

7. Once the crème brûlée has set, preheat the oven to the broil setting.

8. Top each ramekin with a tablespoon of the remaining sweetener and place under the broiler for 3 to 5 minutes, just until the sweetener caramelizes and hardens. (Alternatively, you can use a kitchen torch to caramelize the sweetener.) Serve immediately. Store leftovers in the refrigerator for up to 2 days.

Nutritional information (per serving)

Calories: 455	Total Carbs: 3g
Fat: 45g	Fiber: 0g
Protein: 3g	Net Carbs: 3g

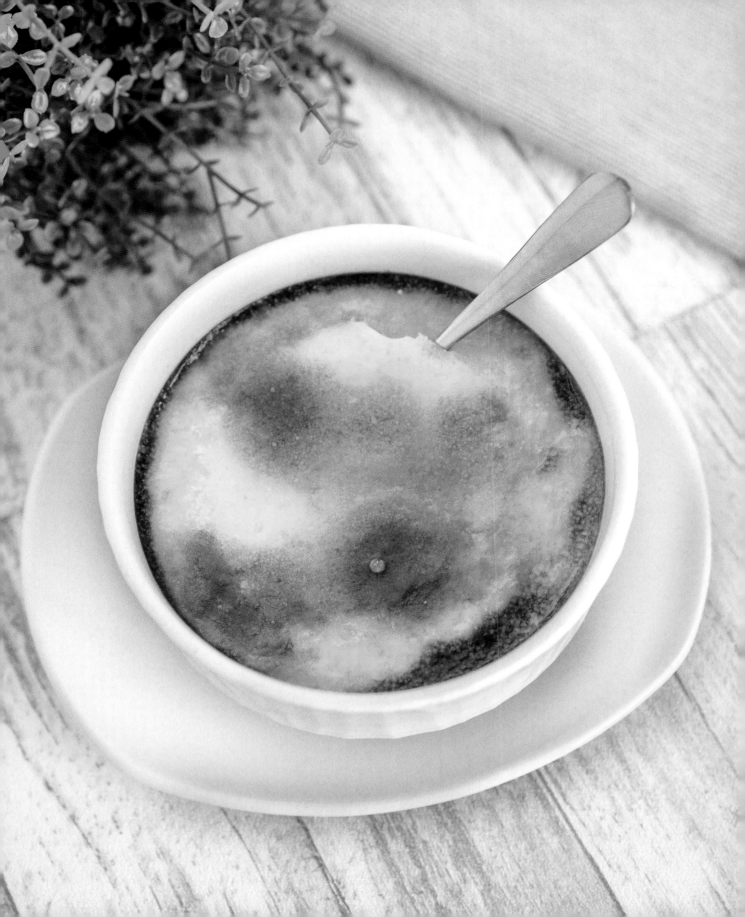

CHOCOLATE CHIP COOKIES

MAKES 12 cookies (1 per serving)   PREP TIME: 10 minutes   COOK TIME: 15 minutes

One of my favorite traditions is making chocolate chip cookies every Sunday. When I first started keto, I gave up that tradition for a while because I couldn't resist the temptation. I've since come up with this chocolate chip cookie recipe, which is the perfect mix of fluffy and sweet—almost like a sweet chocolate biscuit consistency. It has taken over my Sunday chocolate chip cookie baking sessions!

INGREDIENTS

2 cups blanched almond flour

¼ cup granulated sweetener

2 teaspoons baking powder

2 large eggs, beaten

⅓ cup unsalted butter or ghee, melted but not hot

1 teaspoon vanilla extract

1 cup sugar-free chocolate chips

DIRECTIONS

1. Preheat the oven to 350°F. Line a baking sheet with parchment paper or a silicone baking mat.

2. Place the almond flour, sweetener, and baking powder in a large bowl and combine with a whisk. Stir in the remaining ingredients and mix until everything is well incorporated.

3. Use a cookie scoop or spoon to form the dough into twelve 1-inch balls and place on the lined baking sheet, spacing them about 2 inches apart.

4. Bake for 12 to 15 minutes, until slightly browned.

5. Remove the cookies to a cooking rack and allow to cool completely before serving. Store leftovers in the refrigerator for up to 2 weeks.

Nutritional information (per serving)

Calories: 253   Total Carbs: 5g
Fat: 22g   Fiber: 2g
Protein: 8g   Net Carbs: 3g

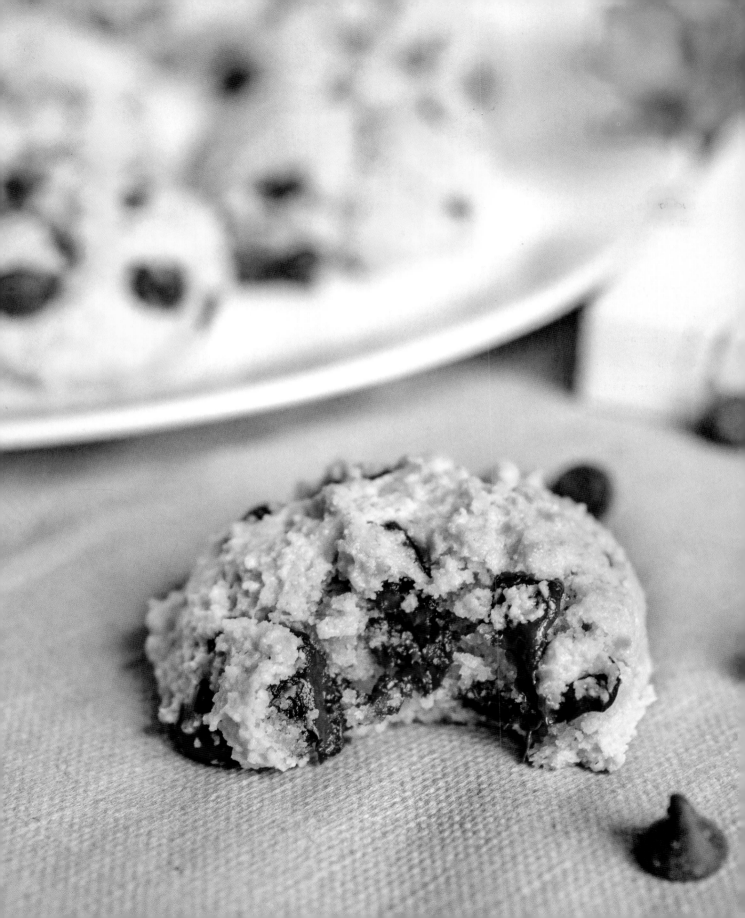

EGG-FREE PEANUT BUTTER MUG CAKE

MAKES 1 serving   **PREP TIME:** 2 minutes   **COOK TIME:** 1½ minutes

Mug cakes are some of the best creations in existence—perfect portion size and endless possibilities. Swap out the peanut butter in this recipe for any nut butter, and you'll get a totally different flavor!

INGREDIENTS

Cooking spray

3 tablespoons natural peanut butter

2 tablespoons blanched almond flour

2 teaspoons granulated sweetener

¼ teaspoon baking powder

¼ cup heavy whipping cream or coconut cream

DIRECTIONS

1. Spray a microwave-safe 8-ounce mug with cooking spray.

2. Place all the ingredients in a small mixing bowl and mix with a fork until well combined.

3. Scoop the batter into the greased mug. Microwave on high for 1 minute 20 seconds. Insert a toothpick in the center to test that the cake is cooked all the way through; it should come out clean. If it needs a little more time, microwave for 15 seconds more.

4. Remove from the microwave and enjoy straight from the mug!

Nutritional information

Calories: 555	**Total Carbs:** 11g
Fat: 52g	**Fiber:** 6g
Protein: 16g	**Net Carbs:** 5g

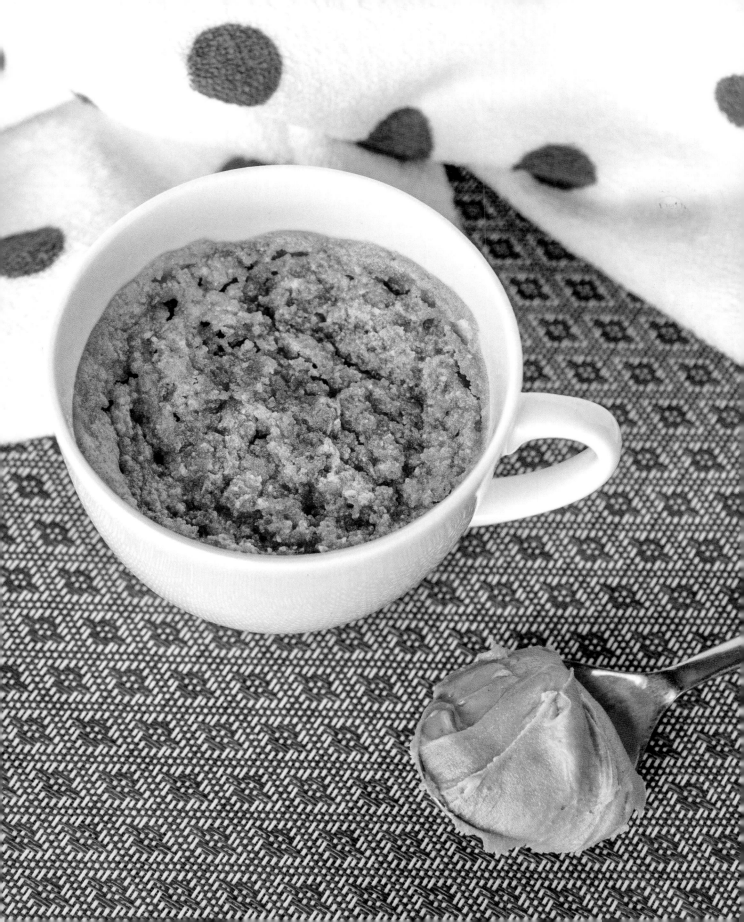

CINNAMON CRISPS

MAKES 4 servings   PREP TIME: 5 minutes   COOK TIME: —

I know what you're thinking...pork rinds turned into cinnamon crisps? Gross! Well, I'm here to tell you that these taste so much like the cinnamon twists from Taco Bell, it's shocking!

INGREDIENTS

3 cups plain pork rinds

¼ cup (½ stick) unsalted butter or ghee, melted but not hot

2 tablespoons granulated sweetener

1 tablespoon ground cinnamon

DIRECTIONS

Place the pork rinds in a gallon-sized resealable plastic bag. Pour the melted butter, sweetener, and cinnamon into the bag and shake until the pork rinds are evenly coated. These are best served immediately so the pork rinds don't get soggy.

Nutritional information (per serving)

Calories: 282	Total Carbs: 0g
Fat: 23g	Fiber: 0g
Protein: 20g	Net Carbs: 0g

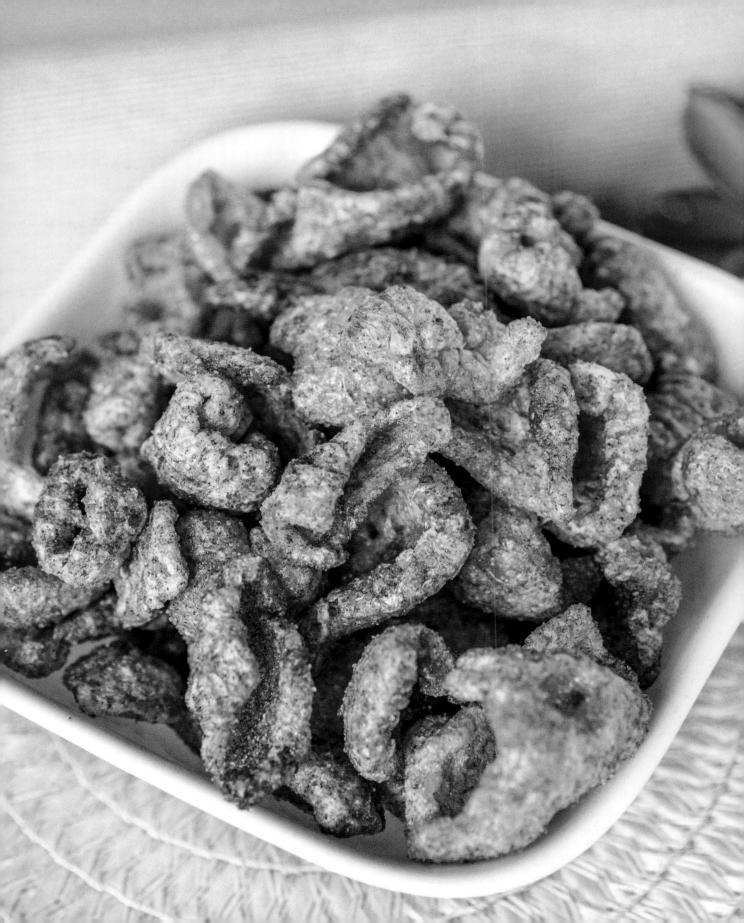

PUMPKIN CHOCOLATE CHIP COOKIES

MAKES 12 cookies (1 per serving)   PREP TIME: 10 minutes   COOK TIME: 15 minutes

The thing I love about keto is that you can turn just about anything into a keto-friendly treat. These cookies prove that you don't need to sacrifice flavor on a ketogenic diet. My whole family gobbles them up as soon as they come out of the oven. We love to dip ours in unsweetened almond milk. Yum!

INGREDIENTS

½ cup pumpkin puree (not pumpkin pie filling)

⅓ cup granulated sweetener

¼ cup (½ stick) unsalted butter or ghee, softened

1 large egg

½ teaspoon vanilla extract

1 cup blanched almond flour

1 teaspoon baking powder

1 teaspoon ground cinnamon

1 teaspoon pumpkin pie spice

½ teaspoon xanthan gum

Pinch of salt

¾ cup sugar-free chocolate chips

DIRECTIONS

1. Preheat the oven to 350°F. Line a baking sheet with parchment paper or a silicone baking mat.

2. Place the pumpkin puree, sweetener, butter, egg, and vanilla extract in a large mixing bowl. Using a hand mixer or stand mixer, mix on high until everything is well incorporated.

3. Add the almond flour, baking powder, cinnamon, pumpkin pie spice, xanthan gum, and salt to the bowl with the pumpkin mixture. Continue to mix until everything is thoroughly combined.

4. Fold in the chocolate chips with a rubber spatula.

5. Use a cookie scoop or spoon to form the dough into twelve 1½-inch balls and place on the lined baking sheet, spacing them about 2 inches apart.

6. Bake for 12 to 15 minutes, until the tops are golden brown.

7. Remove the cookies to a cooling rack and let cool completely before serving. Store leftovers in the refrigerator for up to 2 weeks.

Nutritional information (per serving)

Calories: 163	Total Carbs: 4g
Fat: 14g	Fiber: 1g
Protein: 4g	Net Carbs: 3g

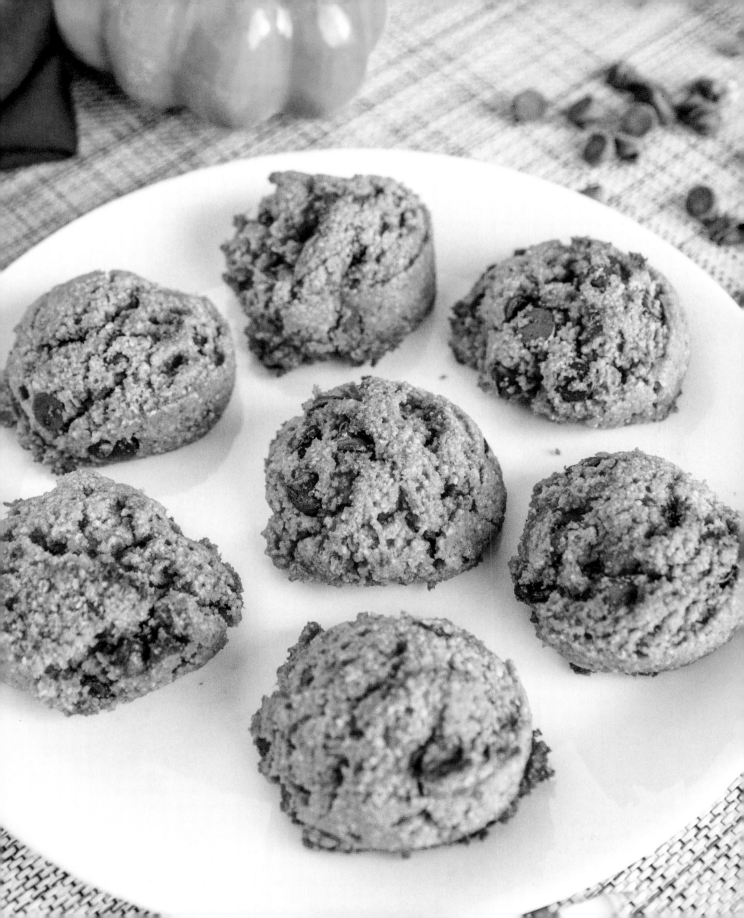

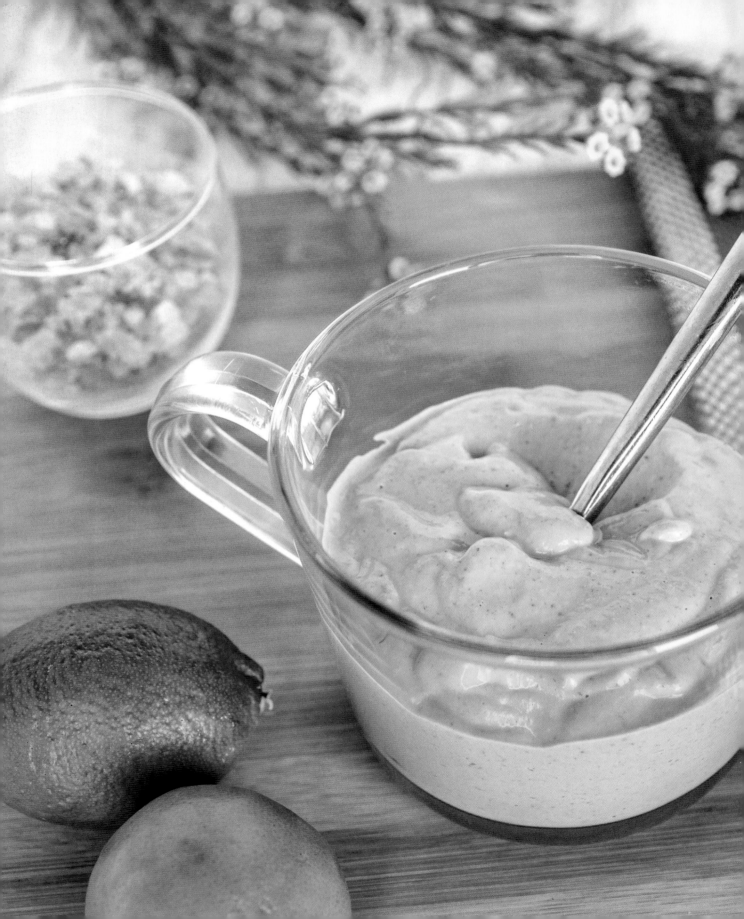

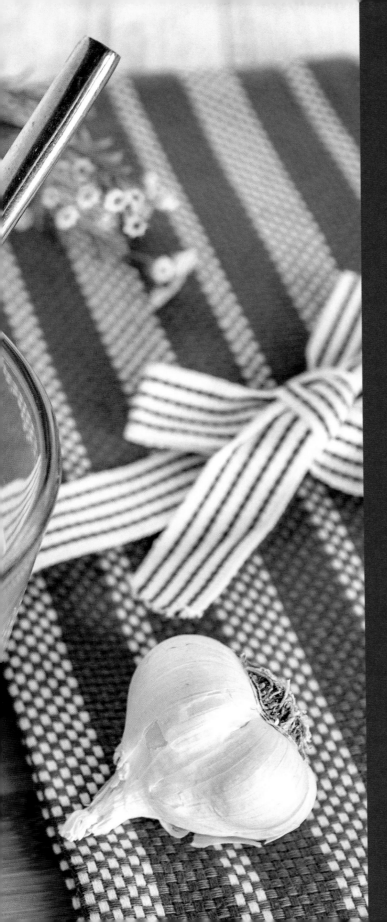

7 GET SAUCY

NEXT-LEVEL WHIPPED CREAM

MAKES 4 cups (2 tablespoons per serving)   PREP TIME: 5 minutes   COOK TIME: —

Sure, whipped cream is amazing, but have you ever tried it with cream cheese in it? Let the name speak for itself. Be careful with this recipe. Every time I sneak a spoonful, I end up eating more like ten spoonfuls.

INGREDIENTS

1 (8-ounce) package cream cheese, softened

2 cups heavy whipping cream

2 tablespoons granulated or powdered sweetener

DIRECTIONS

1. Place the cream cheese in a high-powered blender and blend on high for 1 to 2 minutes, until it is fluffy and about doubled in volume. Alternatively, beat it using a hand mixer or stand mixer.

2. Add the heavy cream and blend on high until the mixture has increased in volume, about 2 minutes.

3. Add the sweetener and continue to blend until the sweetener is thoroughly mixed in, about 1 minute.

4. Store in the refrigerator for up to 5 days.

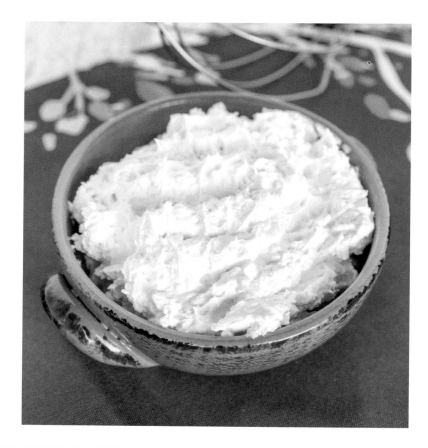

Nutritional information (per serving)

Calories: 75	Total Carbs: 1g
Fat: 7g	Fiber: 0g
Protein: 1g	Net Carbs: 1g

MAPLE SYRUP

MAKES 2 cups (2 tablespoons per serving)   **COOK TIME: 15 minutes**

Maple syrup is a staple in our home. Most days, we live on waffles and pancakes. This sugar-free syrup is great when you're in a pinch, and it is made with better-quality ingredients than the store-bought sugar-free stuff!

INGREDIENTS

2 cups water

½ cup granulated sweetener

½ teaspoon xanthan gum

2 teaspoons maple extract

DIRECTIONS

1. In a medium-sized saucepan, whisk together the water, sweetener, and xanthan gum. Bring to a boil, whisking occasionally.

2. When it starts to boil, add the maple extract and whisk. Reduce the heat to low and let the syrup simmer for about 8 minutes so that it thickens.

3. Serve warm. Store in the refrigerator for up to 2 weeks.

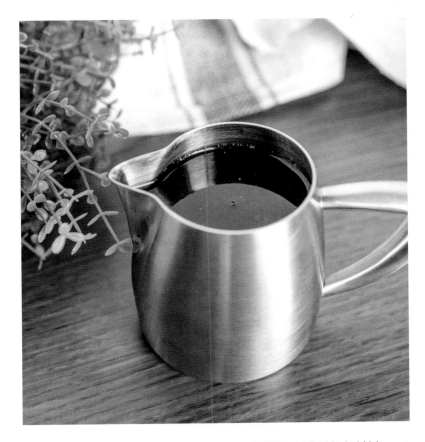

Nutritional information (per serving)

Calories: 0

Fat: 0g

Protein: 0g

Total Carbs: 0g

Fiber: 0g

Net Carbs: 0g

SWEETENED CONDENSED MILK

MAKES 1¼ cups (2 tablespoons per serving) **PREP TIME: 2 minutes** **COOK TIME: 50 minutes**

This sweetened condensed milk is liquid gold! Plan on doubling or even tripling this recipe so you always have some on hand. It keeps for up to two weeks in the fridge, or you can freeze it and thaw as needed. Add it to your favorite desserts or drinks; it is amazing in coffee or drizzled over mug cake. You can even pour it over cauliflower rice to make a sweet coconut rice.

INGREDIENTS

2 cups half-and-half

½ cup granulated sweetener

1 heaping tablespoon coconut oil

½ teaspoon vanilla extract

DIRECTIONS

1. In a medium-sized saucepan, combine the half-and-half, sweetener, and coconut oil. Bring to a boil, then reduce the heat to medium. Continue to cook until it is reduced by about half, stirring occasionally to prevent burning, about 40 minutes.

2. Stir in the vanilla and reduce the heat to low. Simmer, uncovered, for about 5 minutes, allowing it to thicken further. Remove from the heat and let cool completely before using.

3. Store in a sealed jar in the refrigerator for up to 2 weeks.

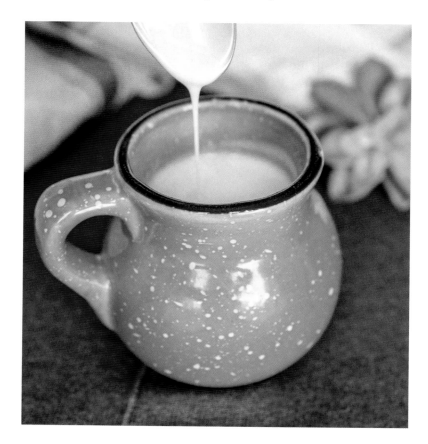

Nutritional information (per serving)

Calories: 69	Total Carbs: 2g
Fat: 6g	Fiber: 0g
Protein: 2g	Net Carbs: 2g

AIOLI

MAKES 1 cup (2 tablespoons per serving)   **PREP TIME: 5 minutes**   **COOK TIME: —**

Garlic is the best flavor in the entire world. Argue this with me, I dare you. I'm kidding, but garlic really is just so delicious. My family slathers this aioli on just about everything. It is a great way to add extra fats while packing a ton of flavor into your dishes. Go with eight cloves of garlic if you like things super garlicky!

INGREDIENTS

1 cup mayonnaise

6 to 8 cloves garlic, minced

1 tablespoon lemon juice

DIRECTIONS

1. Place all the ingredients in a medium-sized bowl and stir until well combined.

2. Serve immediately. Store in the refrigerator for up to 2 weeks.

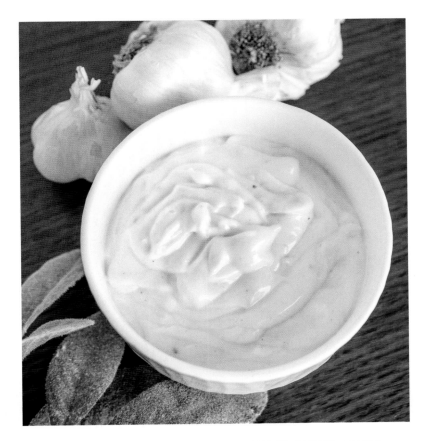

Nutritional information (per serving)

Calories: 181	Total Carbs: 0g
Fat: 20g	Fiber: 0g
Protein: 0g	Net Carbs: 0g

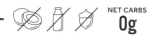

CHIPOTLE MAYO

MAKES 1 cup (2 tablespoons per serving)   **PREP TIME: 5 minutes**   **COOK TIME: —**

This is one of my favorite sauces to add to tacos and salads. It's rich and creamy, and the chipotle in adobo sauce gives it just the right amount of heat.

INGREDIENTS

1 cup mayonnaise

1 teaspoon lime juice

1 to 2 peppers from a small can of chipotle peppers in adobo sauce

DIRECTIONS

1. Place the mayonnaise and lime juice in a medium-sized bowl and stir to combine.

2. Open the can of chipotles and, using a fork, take out one or two peppers: one if you like it mild or two if you like it with a little kick! Mince the peppers and add them to the mayo mixture. Mix well. Feel free to add some of the sauce from the can to give the mayo even more heat.

3. Store in the refrigerator for up to 2 weeks.

> *TIP: Don't throw away the rest of the can of chipotles in adobo sauce! Transfer the contents to a resealable plastic bag and store in the freezer. The peppers will keep in the freezer for up to a year.*

Nutritional information (per serving)

Calories: 183	Total Carbs: 0g
Fat: 20g	Fiber: 0g
Protein: 0g	Net Carbs: 0g

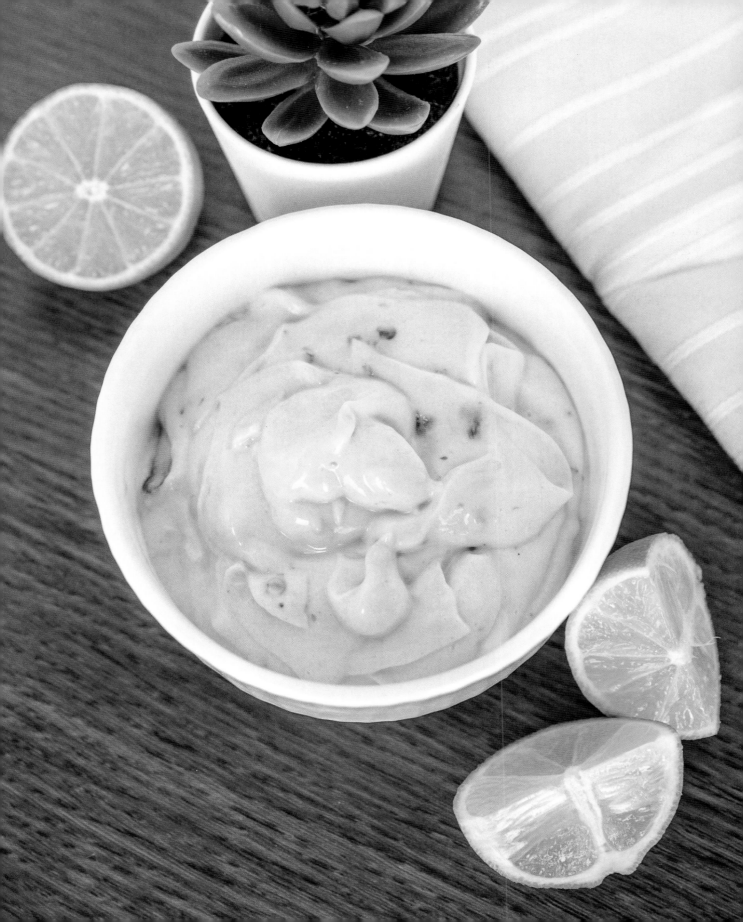

BLUE CHEESE DRESSING

NET CARBS
0g

MAKES 1½ cups (2 tablespoons per serving) PREP TIME: 10 minutes COOK TIME: —

Blue cheese is one of those funny foods that people don't really start to like until they're in their thirties. At least that's how it was for me. So the bad news is, if you're over thirty and you still don't like blue cheese, there's probably no hope for you; you're stuck with ranch for life. On the bright side, if you were born loving blue cheese, you are going to love this dressing! Spoon it over salads, serve it alongside chicken wings, or simply dip your celery and occasional carrot sticks in it.

INGREDIENTS

1 cup mayonnaise

2 tablespoons red wine vinegar

2 cloves garlic, minced

½ teaspoon salt

¼ teaspoon ground black pepper

Splash of heavy whipping cream, if needed

3 ounces blue cheese, crumbled (about ½ cup)

DIRECTIONS

1. In a medium-sized bowl, whisk together the mayonnaise, vinegar, garlic, salt, and pepper. If the dressing is too thick, add a splash of heavy cream to thin it out a bit.

2. Stir in the blue cheese crumbles and serve. Store in the refrigerator for up to 2 weeks.

Nutritional information (per serving)

Calories: 147   Total Carbs: 0g

Fat: 15g   Fiber: 0g

Protein: 2g   Net Carbs: 0g

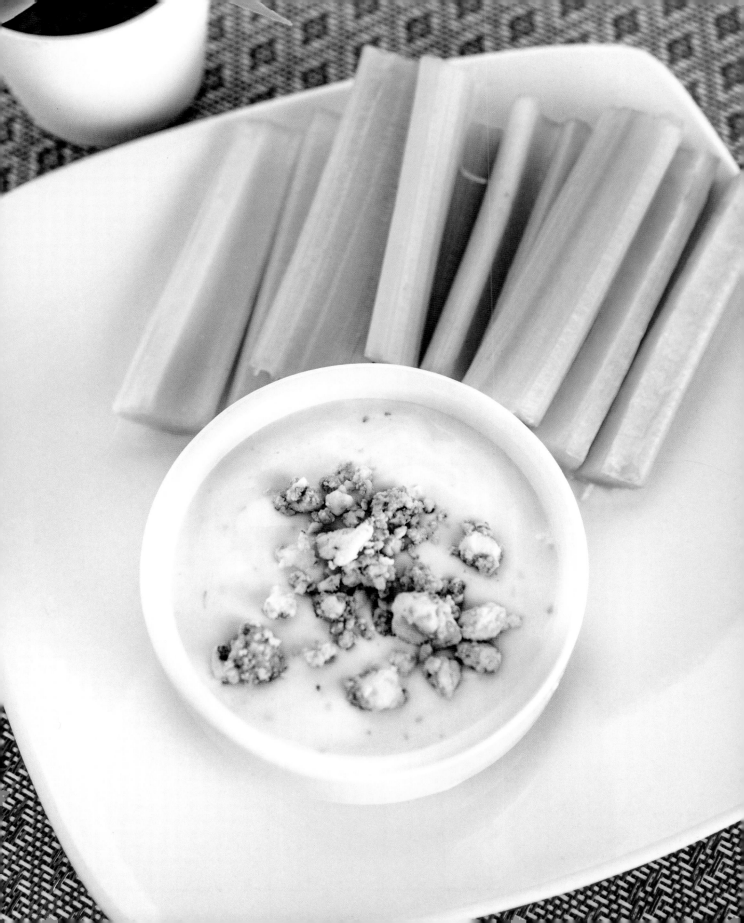

CHEESE SHELLS

MAKES 4 shells (2 per serving)   PREP TIME: 1 minute   COOK TIME: 6 minutes

Okay, so cheese shells aren't exactly "saucy," but like many of the basics in this chapter, these little guys are so versatile. You can use whatever cheese you like, make them whatever shape you like, and make them however big or small you want. We love them for tacos and tostadas and even as a crunchy topping for bunless burgers. The possibilities are endless, and I'm excited to see what you do with them! Although it's certainly not necessary, you could season the cheese with chili powder and cumin to give the shells an extra kick. These should be used when freshly made; they don't keep well.

INGREDIENTS

12 ounces cheddar cheese, shredded (3 cups)

DIRECTIONS

1. Preheat a griddle or a large nonstick skillet over medium-high heat (about 350°F if using an electric griddle).

2. Place ¾ cup of cheese on the griddle or skillet and form into a circle 4 to 5 inches in diameter. Repeat three more times until you have four piles of cheese cooking on the griddle or skillet. (If you don't have a griddle or large skillet, cook the shells in batches in a smaller nonstick skillet.)

3. Let the cheese melt and start to bubble, about 3 minutes. When it begins to crisp up on the edges, use a spatula to flip it over. If your cheese is too flimsy to work with, let it cook a little longer, until it's stable enough to flip. Cook the other side for about 2 minutes, or until golden.

4. Remove the cheese from the griddle and center each shell over the handle of a wooden spoon balanced on two glasses or cups. Let the cheese hang over the handle so that it forms a curved taco shell shape.

5. Serve immediately with your favorite taco ingredients!

Nutritional information (per serving)

Calories: 687	Total Carbs: 5g
Fat: 57g	Fiber: 0g
Protein: 39g	Net Carbs: 5g

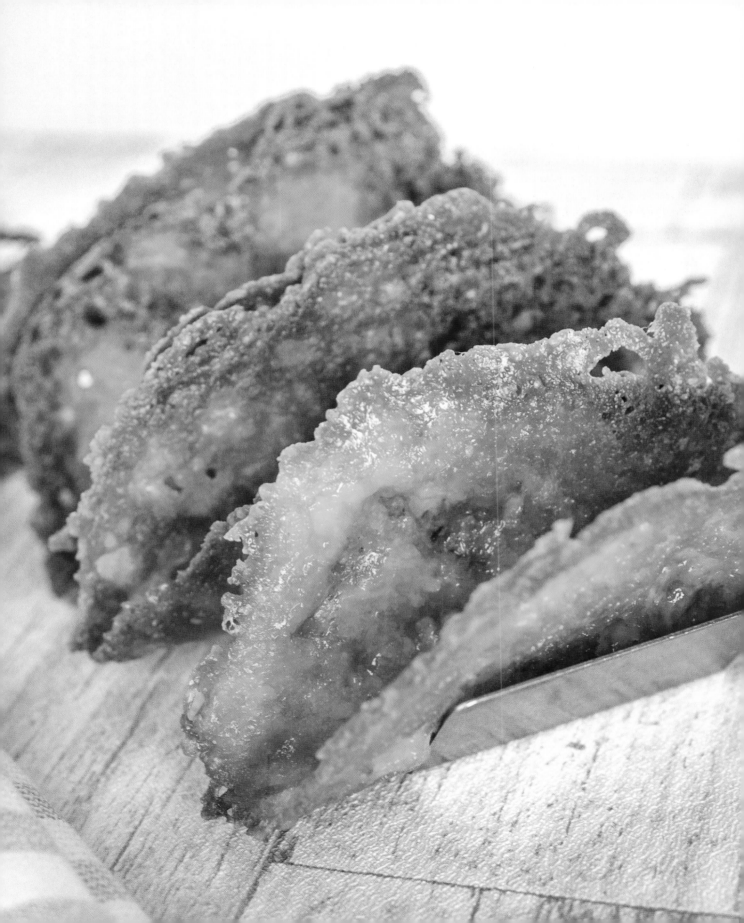

AVOCADO CILANTRO LIME DRESSING

MAKES 1½ cups (2 tablespoons per serving)   **PREP TIME: 10 minutes**   **COOK TIME: —**

This is the perfect dressing for any type of salad. It's creamy, tangy, and delicious! It's also vibrant in color, and we all know that pretty food tastes better.

INGREDIENTS

1 medium-sized ripe avocado

½ cup fresh cilantro leaves

¼ cup avocado oil

¼ cup sour cream (or mayonnaise for dairy-free)

3 tablespoons water

Juice of 1 lime

1 clove garlic, peeled

¼ teaspoon onion powder

Salt and ground black pepper, to taste

DIRECTIONS

1. Cut the avocado in half lengthwise. Remove the pit and discard. Scoop the flesh into a blender or food processor. Add the remaining ingredients and blend until smooth.

2. Store in the refrigerator for up to 10 days.

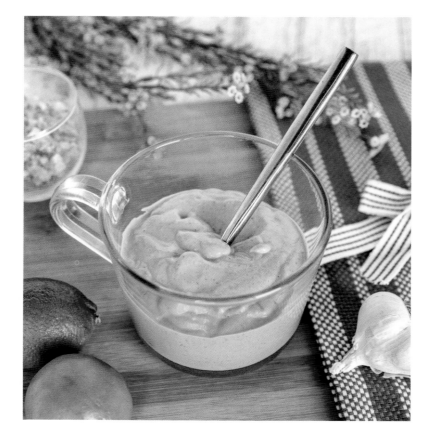

Nutritional information (per serving)

Calories: 73	Total Carbs: 2g
Fat: 8g	Fiber: 1g
Protein: 0g	Net Carbs: 1g

COCKTAIL SAUCE

MAKES 1 cup (2 tablespoons per serving)   PREP TIME: 2 minutes   COOK TIME: —

Back in the day, I was a server at Texas Roadhouse. When people would order the shrimp, they often asked for cocktail sauce. The only problem was that we didn't have cocktail sauce. Instead of upsetting people by telling them no, I'd run into the kitchen and whip up a version of this simple concoction for the perfect cocktail sauce! A total crowd-pleaser, and you can't get much easier. Serve it with your favorite shrimp.

INGREDIENTS

1 cup sugar-free ketchup

2 tablespoons prepared horseradish

1½ tablespoons lemon juice

1½ tablespoons Worcestershire sauce

DIRECTIONS

Place all the ingredients in a medium-sized bowl and stir to combine. Store in the refrigerator for up to 3 weeks.

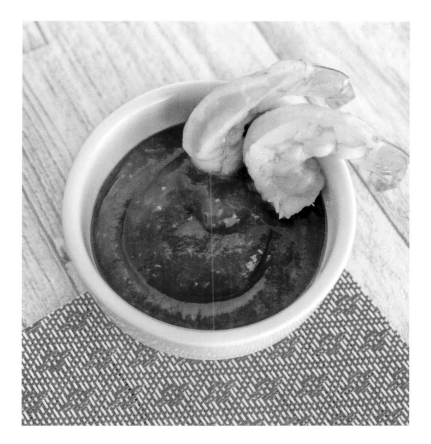

Nutritional information (per serving)

Calories: 13	Total Carbs: 3g
Fat: 0g	Fiber: 0g
Protein: 0g	Net Carbs: 3g

EASIEST ALFREDO SAUCE EVER

MAKES 3 cups (¼ cup per serving)   PREP TIME: 2 minutes   COOK TIME: 10 minutes

Alfredo is the ultimate comfort food. This sauce is great on zoodles or, my personal favorite, as a dip for my low-carb Dinner Rolls (page 134).

INGREDIENTS

½ cup (1 stick) unsalted butter

4 ounces cream cheese (½ cup)

2 cups heavy whipping cream

4 ounces Parmesan cheese, shredded (about 1 cup)

2 cloves garlic, minced, or 1 teaspoon garlic powder

Salt and ground black pepper

DIRECTIONS

1. Place the butter, cream cheese, and heavy cream in a medium-sized saucepan over medium-high heat. Bring to a boil, whisking constantly as the butter and cream cheese melt.

2. Add the Parmesan cheese (if desired, reserve a little for garnish) and garlic and season with salt and pepper. Whisk to combine and reduce the heat to low. Simmer, stirring occasionally, for 5 minutes to allow the flavors to meld.

3. Remove from the heat and serve! Store in the refrigerator for up to 5 days. Reheat in the microwave or on the stovetop.

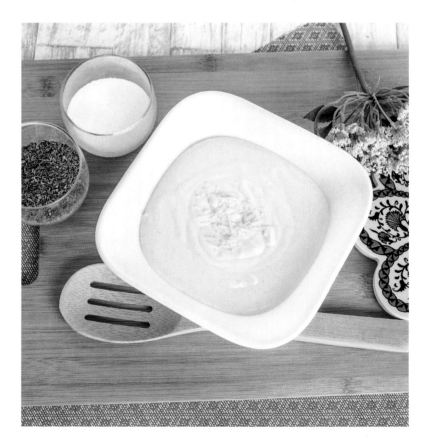

Nutritional information (per serving)

Calories: 263	Total Carbs: 2g
Fat: 26g	Fiber: 0g
Protein: 3g	Net Carbs: 2g

SWEET CREAM SAUCE

MAKES ¾ cup (2 tablespoons per serving)   PREP TIME: 1 minute   COOK TIME: 5 minutes

I think I lived off this cream sauce when I first discovered cream cheese pancakes. I craved it every day. It's buttery and sweet and tastes sinfully good. Use it to top Flourless Waffles (page 48) or pancakes, or simply eat it with a spoon when you want something sweet.

INGREDIENTS

1 tablespoon unsalted butter

1 cup heavy whipping cream

1 teaspoon granulated sweetener

1 teaspoon vanilla extract

DIRECTIONS

1. Melt the butter in a small skillet over medium-high heat. Once melted, add the heavy cream and let the mixture bubble for 1 minute.

2. Whisk in the sweetener and vanilla extract and cook for about 3 minutes, whisking occasionally. The sauce will continue to bubble and reduce.

3. Remove from the heat and serve! Store in the refrigerator for up to 1 week. Reheat on the stovetop.

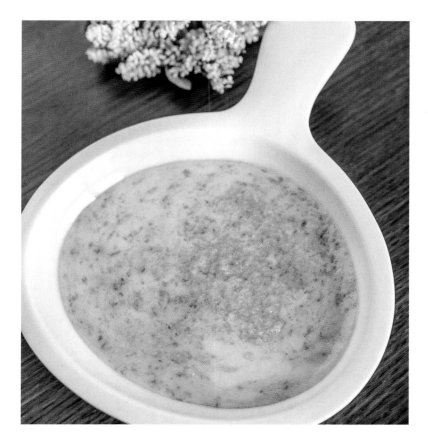

Nutritional information (per serving)

Calories: 151	Total Carbs: 1g
Fat: 15g	Fiber: 0g
Protein: 0g	Net Carbs: 1g

SAVORY TORTILLAS

MAKES 8 tortillas (2 per serving) **PREP TIME: 10 minutes** **COOK TIME: 10 minutes**

I love these tortillas for pretty much everything! They are perfect for tacos, enchiladas, and, my personal favorite, breakfast tacos filled with scrambled eggs and cheese. Getting them just right may take you some practice, but do not give up. I butchered these probably half a dozen times before I got the hang of it. The effort is totally worth it! Make a big batch and freeze them so you always have some on hand.

INGREDIENTS

6 large eggs

4 ounces cream cheese (½ cup), softened

½ teaspoon garlic powder

½ teaspoon onion powder

¼ teaspoon ground cumin

¼ teaspoon paprika

Salt and ground black pepper, to taste

DIRECTIONS

1. Preheat a griddle or a large nonstick skillet over medium-high heat (about 350°F if using an electric griddle).

2. Place all the ingredients in a blender and blend on high until the batter is smooth. It should be very runny at this point, with no chunks of cream cheese.

3. Pour roughly ¾ cup of the batter onto the griddle so it makes a thin 6-inch circle. (The size is mostly personal preference; just be sure to make them all the same size.) I can easily fit four 6-inch circles on my griddle at one time.

4. Cook until the edges of the tortillas are not sticking to the griddle, 3 to 4 minutes. Then gently flip and cook for another minute so the other side is cooked all the way through. Repeat with the remaining batter.

5. Serve immediately. Store leftovers in the refrigerator for up to 1 week or in the freezer for up to 1 month. Reheat in the microwave.

> *TIP:* *If you have a high-powered blender, it is not necessary to soften the cream cheese before adding it to the blender.*

Nutritional information (per serving)

Calories: 208	Total Carbs: 2g
Fat: 17g	Fiber: 0g
Protein: 11g	Net Carbs: 2g

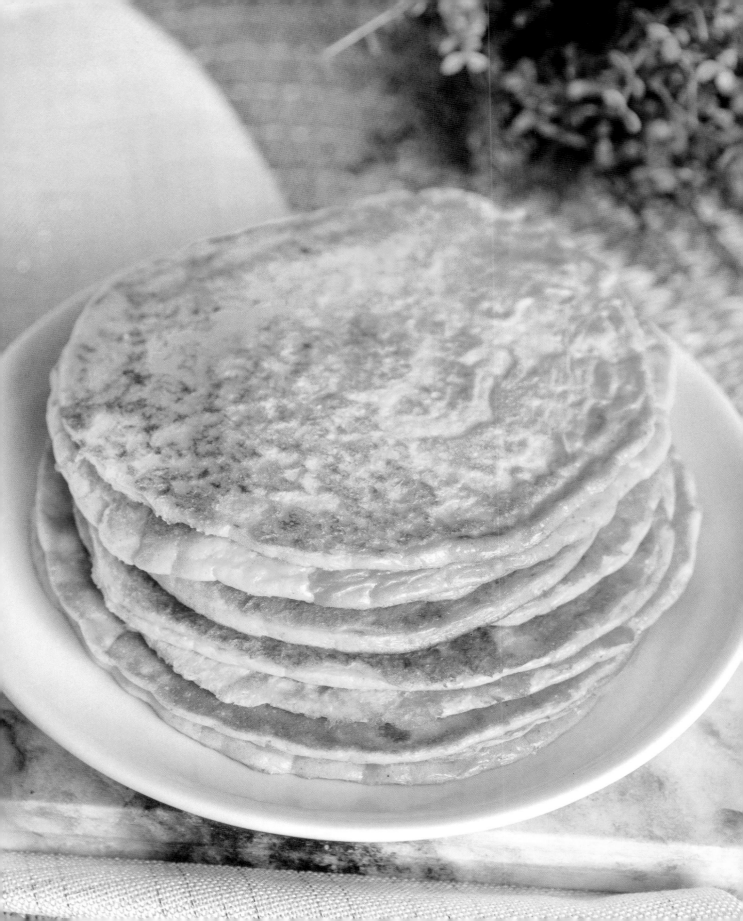

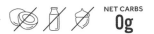

THOUSAND ISLAND DRESSING

MAKES 1½ cups (2 tablespoons per serving)   PREP TIME: 5 minutes   COOK TIME: —

When I first moved to Utah, I quickly learned that every restaurant carries "fry sauce." It's a Utah thing, for sure. Each rendition is slightly different, but it's basically just Thousand Island dressing. This super simple keto version reminds me of In-n-Out Burger's sauce. Smother it on bunless burgers, salads, or my Reuben in a Bowl (page 104).

INGREDIENTS

1 cup mayonnaise

¼ cup sugar-free ketchup

1 tablespoon dill pickle juice

1 to 2 baby dill pickles, finely chopped

Salt and ground black pepper, to taste

DIRECTIONS

Place all the ingredients in a small bowl and stir until well combined. Store in the refrigerator for up to 2 weeks.

Nutritional information (per serving)

Calories: 123   Total Carbs: 0g

Fat: 13g   Fiber: 0g

Protein: 0g   Net Carbs: 0g

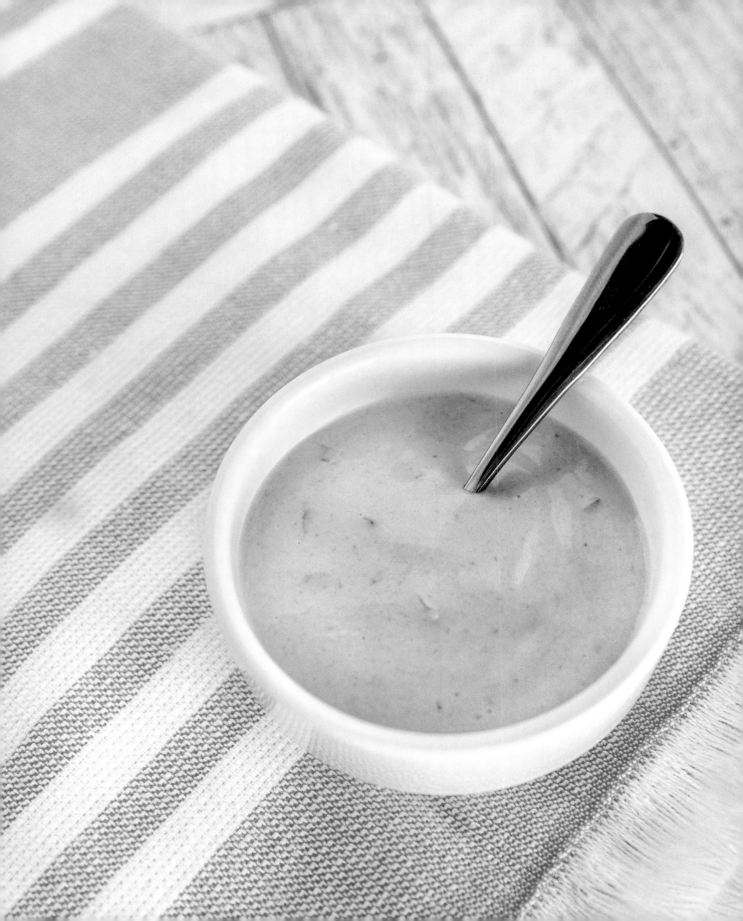

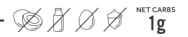

JAM ON THE FLY

MAKES 1 cup (2 tablespoons per serving)   PREP TIME: 8 minutes   COOK TIME: 5 minutes

This is the perfect jam to make when you're in a pinch. Actually, it's the perfect jam in general. It's quick, easy, and yummy, and you can add it to just about anything! Top mug cakes with it, spread it on pancakes, or eat it by the spoonful with some peanut butter.

INGREDIENTS

1 cup fresh berries of choice (we like strawberries)

1 teaspoon lemon juice

1 teaspoon granulated sweetener

1 teaspoon unflavored gelatin

DIRECTIONS

1. Place the berries and lemon juice in a medium-sized saucepan over medium-high heat. Mash with a potato masher to your desired texture. (I like a few chunks in mine, so I don't overmash.) Bring to a boil, stirring constantly so the mixture doesn't stick to the bottom of the pan.

2. Once boiling, remove from the heat and stir in the sweetener and gelatin until fully incorporated.

3. Let the jam sit for about 5 minutes to thicken, then serve! Store in the refrigerator for up to 2 weeks (although I'm sure you'll eat it up faster than that!).

Nutritional information (per serving)

Calories: 9	Total Carbs: 1g
Fat: 0g	Fiber: 0g
Protein: 1g	Net Carbs: 1g

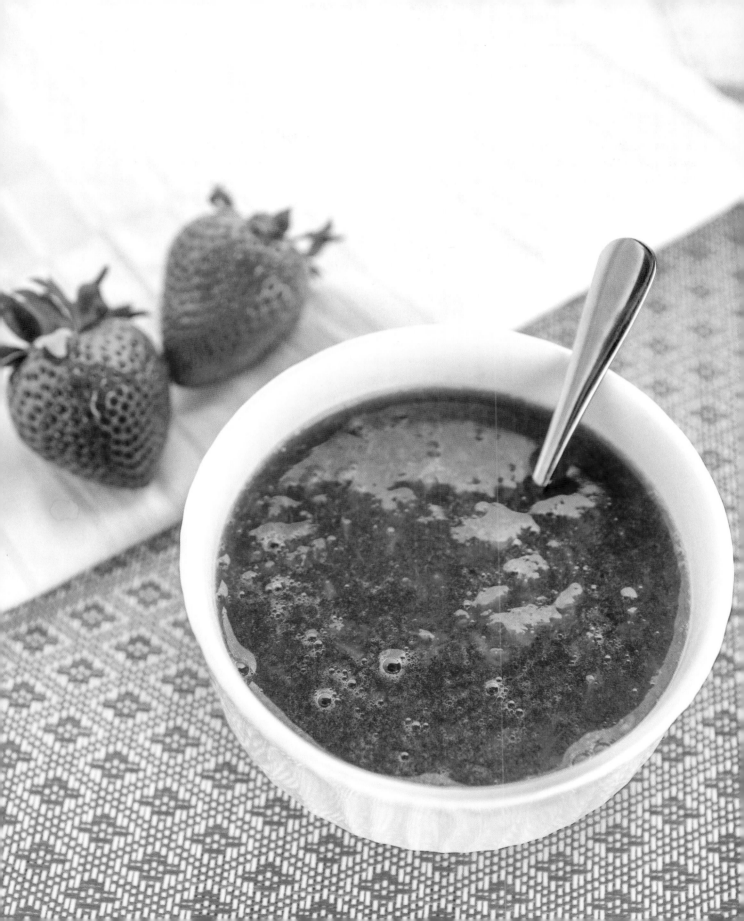

FATHEAD PIZZA CRUST

MAKES one 14-inch crust (8 servings)   **PREP TIME: 18 minutes**   **COOK TIME: 12 minutes**

The first time I made fathead dough, I was in heaven! Pizza is one of those things that I didn't eat a ton of before I started keto, yet after I started keto, I craved it like crazy. I'm so amazed at how many creative ways there are to use this crust. I make a variation of this recipe at least once a week, whether it's for pizza crust, rolls, or buns. To make rolls or buns from this fathead dough, simply adjust the shape and bake for 18 to 20 minutes, until golden brown.

INGREDIENTS

12 ounces mozzarella cheese, shredded (about 3 cups)

4 ounces cream cheese (½ cup)

1½ cups blanched almond flour

1 teaspoon garlic powder

1 teaspoon onion powder

1 teaspoon Italian seasoning

1 teaspoon garlic salt, plus more for topping

2 large eggs

DIRECTIONS

1. Preheat the oven to 425°F. Line a baking sheet with parchment paper or a silicone baking mat.

2. Place the mozzarella and cream cheese in a large microwave-safe bowl; there's no need to stir at this point. Microwave on high for 1 minute. Remove from the microwave and stir the cheeses with a fork, then microwave for another minute. At this point, you want the cheeses to be smooth. If necessary, microwave for another 30 seconds.

3. Add the remaining ingredients and combine the dough with your hands. If it gets too sticky, simply wet your hands and continue working the dough until it is well combined.

4. Place the dough on the lined baking sheet. Place a sheet of parchment paper on top of the dough and roll the dough between the two sheets with a rolling pin. Spread the dough evenly to a thickness of ½ to ⅓ inch; make it whatever shape you like.

5. Roll the edge of the dough toward the center to form a thick edge; that way, all the toppings will remain inside the crust, and it will look like a real pizza.

6. Use a fork to poke holes in the dough to prevent bubbling. Sprinkle some garlic salt on top and par-bake for 10 to 12 minutes, until golden brown on the edges.

7. Store in the refrigerator for up to 5 days.

> *TIP: To make a pizza using this crust, top the par-baked crust with your favorite toppings and bake for 10 to 12 minutes, until the toppings are heated through and the crust is browned on the edges.*

Nutritional information (per serving)

Calories: 287	Total Carbs: 6g
Fat: 24g	Fiber: 2g
Protein: 16g	Net Carbs: 4g

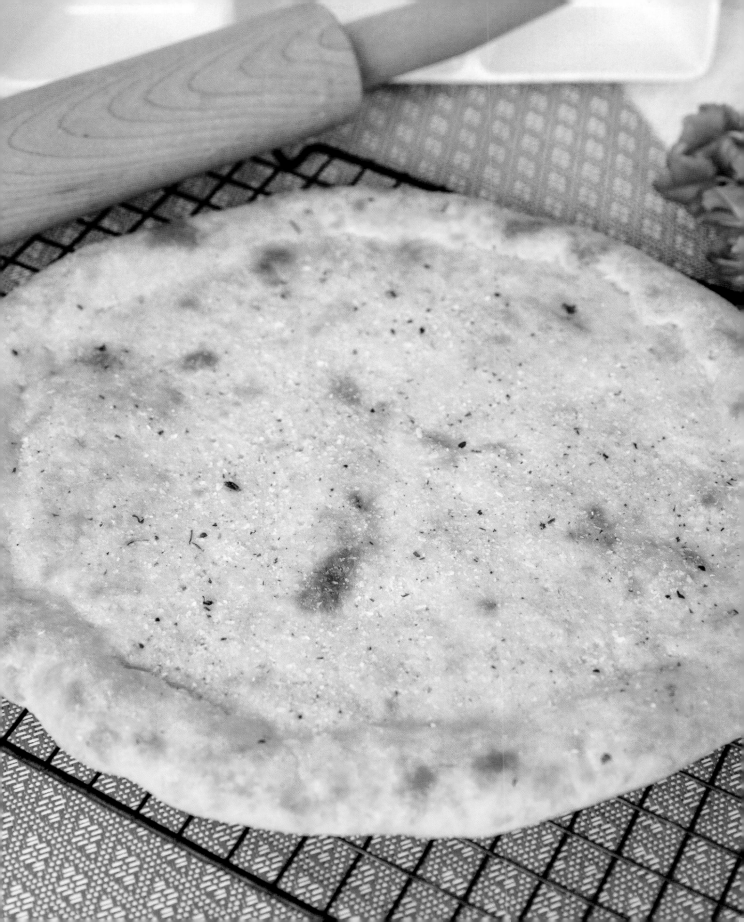

COPYCAT CHICK-FIL-A SAUCE

MAKES ¾ cup (2 tablespoons per serving) **PREP TIME: 5 minutes, plus 30 minutes to chill** **COOK TIME: —**

Pair this sauce with my Chicken Nuggets (page 174) and you have a delicious replica of a Chick-fil-A meal. Or, as my kids would say, "Holy cow, this tastes just like the real thing!" It's honestly the nicest thing they have ever said to me.

INGREDIENTS

½ cup mayonnaise

2 tablespoons Dijon mustard

1 tablespoon sugar-free BBQ sauce

1 teaspoon lemon juice

1 teaspoon prepared yellow mustard

DIRECTIONS

Place all the ingredients in a small bowl and stir until well combined. Place the sauce in the refrigerator to chill for 30 minutes so all the flavors can blend together. Store in the refrigerator for up to 10 days.

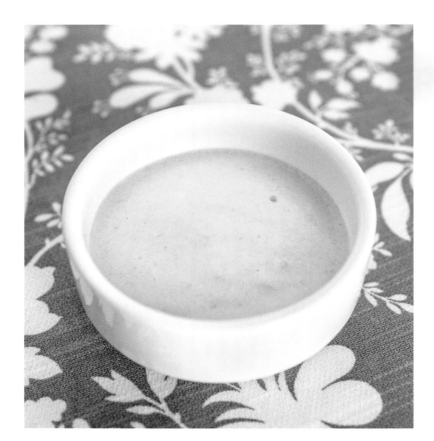

Nutritional information (per serving)

Calories: 126	Total Carbs: 0g
Fat: 13g	Fiber: 0g
Protein: 0g	Net Carbs: 0g

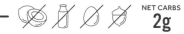

NET CARBS
2g

THANKSGIVING CRANBERRY SAUCE

MAKES 4 cups (2 tablespoons per serving)   **PREP TIME: 1 minute**   **COOK TIME: 40 minutes**

Cranberry sauce has always been one of my favorite parts of Thanksgiving. The tart cranberries and citrus pair so beautifully in this low-carb version. Serve this sauce hot or cold with your turkey dinner, or spread a little cream cheese on my Cheese Crackers (page 82) and then top them with this sauce. Yum!

INGREDIENTS

1 (32-ounce) bag fresh cranberries

2 cups water

⅓ cup brown sugar substitute

⅓ cup granulated sweetener

1 tablespoon orange extract

1 teaspoon ground cinnamon

DIRECTIONS

1. Bring the cranberries and water to a boil in a large, deep-sided skillet over medium-high heat.

2. Reduce the heat to low, add the remaining ingredients, and stir until well combined. Let the sauce simmer, covered, for 30 minutes, stirring occasionally and mashing the berries to help them burst. When all the berries have burst and the sauce has thickened, it is done. Serve immediately, or chill in the refrigerator until cold and then serve.

3. Store in the refrigerator for up to 10 days, or freeze for up to 1 year.

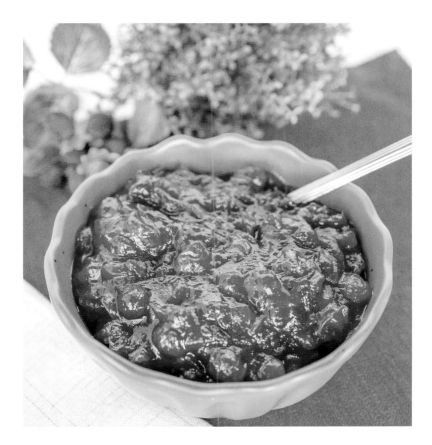

Nutritional information (per serving)

Calories: 13	Total Carbs: 3g
Fat: 0g	Fiber: 1g
Protein: 0g	Net Carbs: 2g

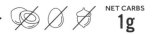

CREAMY HORSERADISH SAUCE

MAKES 1 cup (2 tablespoons per serving)   PREP TIME: 5 minutes   COOK TIME: —

Funny story about horseradish: When my oldest child was about eight years old, he asked me to make him a sandwich. I happily did, as usual. Except that time, I accidentally used horseradish sauce instead of mayo! In my defense, the squeezable bottles looked identical. He took one bite of the sandwich and started bawling and screaming about how much it burned. We laugh about it now, but to this day, Gavin will not touch horseradish. Oops!

If you ask me, one of the most delicious meals on the planet is prime rib with creamy horsey sauce. The other members of my family also love this sauce on steak, in chicken salad, and especially on leftover brisket sandwiches made with my Best 90-Second Bread Ever (page 70).

INGREDIENTS

1 cup sour cream

¼ cup prepared horseradish

1 tablespoon Dijon mustard

Pink Himalayan salt, to taste

DIRECTIONS

Place all the ingredients in a small bowl and mix until well combined. Store in the refrigerator until ready to use; it will keep for up to 3 weeks.

Nutritional information (per serving)

Calories: 63	Total Carbs: 1g
Fat: 6g	Fiber: 0g
Protein: 1g	Net Carbs: 1g

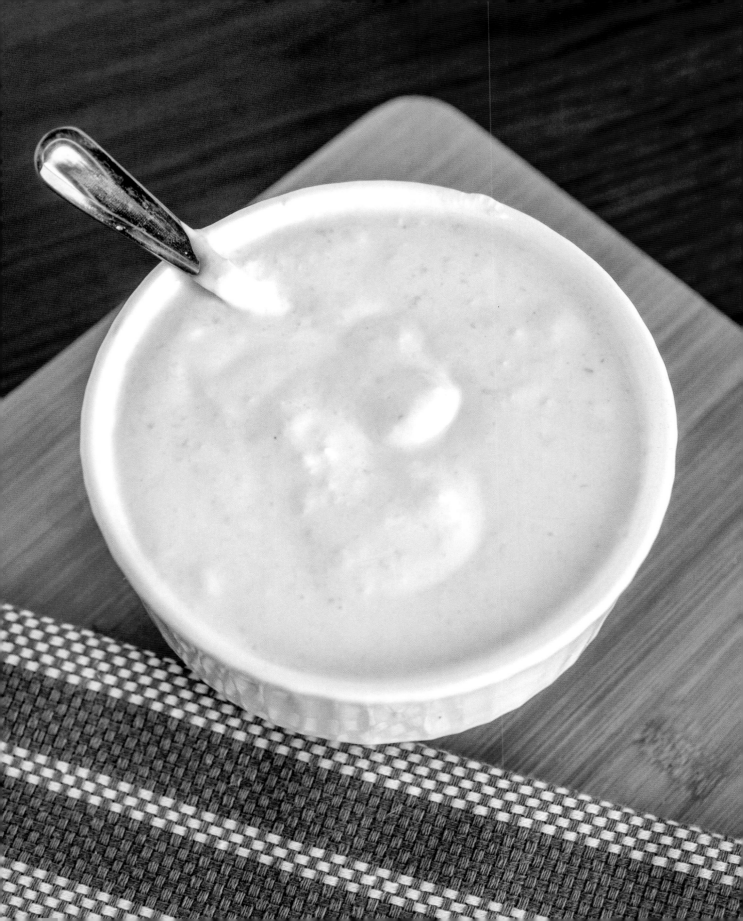

CHICKEN PIZZA CRUST

MAKES 1 crust (2 servings)   **PREP TIME: 10 minutes**   **COOK TIME: 18 minutes**

This is the perfect pizza crust for those who have a nut allergy and cannot have my Fathead Pizza Crust (page 288), which is made with almond flour. It's practically zero-carb, too! Serve with your favorite pizza toppings.

INGREDIENTS

1 (12½-ounce) can chunk chicken breast (see Notes)

1 ounce Parmesan cheese, grated (about ¼ cup)

1 large egg

¼ teaspoon garlic powder

¼ teaspoon onion powder

DIRECTIONS

1. Preheat the oven to 425°F. Line a baking sheet with parchment paper or a silicone baking mat.

2. Drain as much of the liquid from the can of chicken as possible. Place the chicken in a medium-sized mixing bowl. Add the remaining ingredients and stir with a fork until well combined.

3. Pour the chicken mixture onto the lined baking sheet. Using your hands, shape the "dough" into a circle about ⅓ inch thick. If you like a thin crust, form a larger, thinner circle. A smaller circle will result in a thicker crust.

4. Bake for 16 to 18 minutes, until golden brown.

5. Store in the refrigerator for up to 4 days. Reheat in the oven or in a skillet for a super crispy crust.

> *NOTES: I like Costco brand canned chicken.*
>
> *To make a pizza using this crust, simply top the baked crust with cheese and your favorite toppings and bake in a preheated 400°F oven for an additional 12 to 15 minutes, until the cheese is melted.*

Nutritional information (per serving)

Calories: 234	Total Carbs: 1g
Fat: 9g	Fiber: 0g
Protein: 36g	Net Carbs: 1g

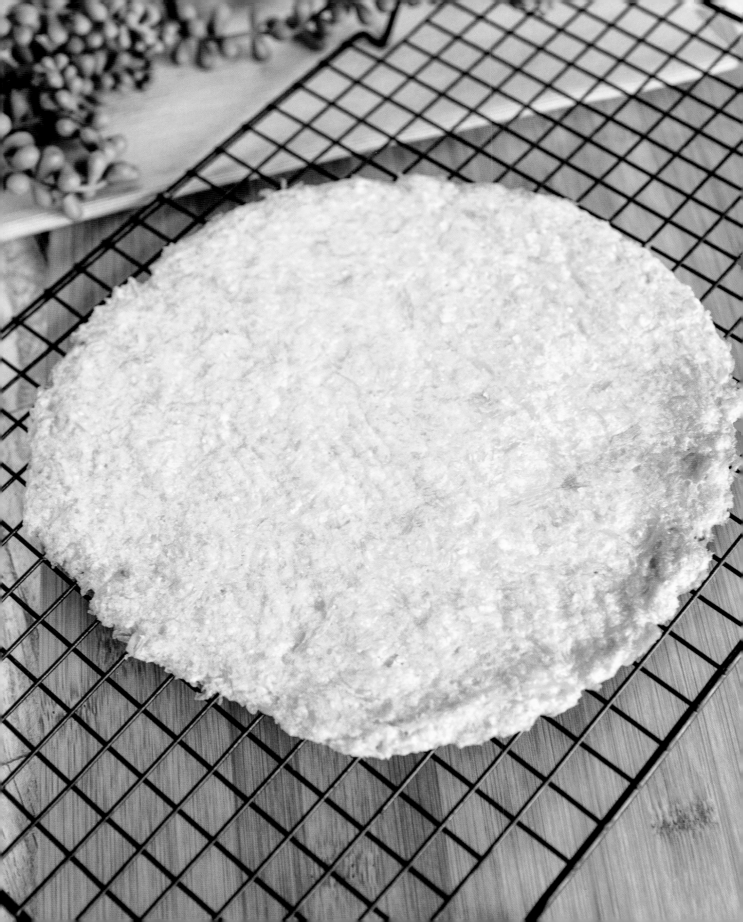

ROASTED GARLIC

NET CARBS
7g

MAKES 8 servings   PREP TIME: 5 minutes   COOK TIME: 40 minutes

"Let food be thy medicine and medicine be thy food."—Hippocrates

Did you know that throughout history, garlic has been used for health and medicinal purposes? Garlic can combat sickness and boost immune function. It can also reduce blood pressure, lower cholesterol, and improve athletic performance. Pretty amazing, right? I shared this photo on my Instagram and had people freaking out because it triggered their trypophobia. For that, I am genuinely sorry. (If you don't know what trypophobia is, I suggest not Googling it if you're hungry. It's gross!) But you cannot deny the health benefits or the deliciousness of roasted garlic.

INGREDIENTS

6 heads garlic

2 tablespoons extra-virgin olive oil

DIRECTIONS

1. Preheat the oven to 350°F.

2. Peel off the papery outer layers of the heads of garlic. Try to get as much off as possible.

3. Cut the tops off the heads of garlic, about ¼ inch from the top, so the tops of the cloves are exposed. Place in a small glass or ceramic baking dish, cut sides up.

4. Drizzle a teaspoon of olive oil over each head of garlic so that it soaks into the cloves.

5. Bake for 40 minutes, or until the garlic is soft. Do not overcook, as burned garlic can taste very bitter.

6. Simply squeeze the cloves out of the skin and add them to your favorite dishes or, if you're a true garlic lover, eat them plain! Store in the refrigerator for up to 2 weeks or in the freezer for up to 1 year.

Nutritional information (per serving)

Calories: 64	Total Carbs: 7g
Fat: 4g	Fiber: 0g
Protein: 1g	Net Carbs: 7g

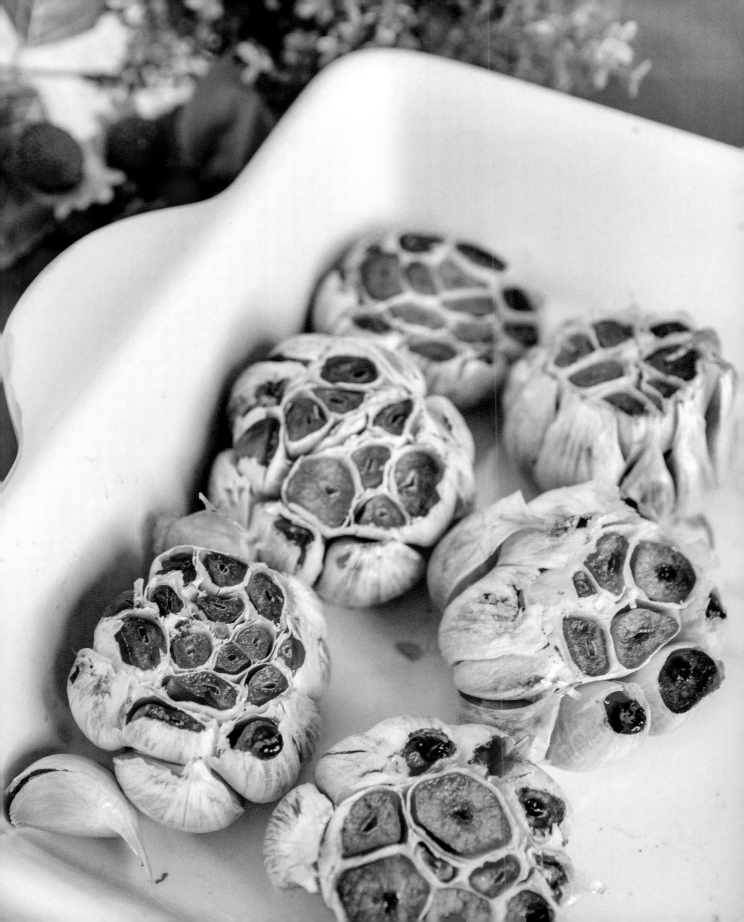

CARAMELIZED ONIONS

MAKES about 2 cups (½ cup per serving)   PREP TIME: 10 minutes   COOK TIME: 50 minutes

There's something magical about caramelizing onions; it really pulls out the sweetness. And caramelized onions make just about any dish taste like you've been slaving over it all day. These onions are so good on top of green beans or bunless burgers or, my favorite, in a Caramelized Onion Tart (page 166).

INGREDIENTS

2 tablespoons unsalted butter or ghee

2 tablespoons extra-virgin olive oil or avocado oil

3 to 4 large yellow onions, thinly sliced

Salt and ground black pepper

1 to 2 tablespoons balsamic vinegar

DIRECTIONS

1. Place the butter and oil in a large skillet over medium-high heat.

2. Add the sliced onions and stir to coat. Sprinkle with salt and pepper. Cook, stirring occasionally, for 20 minutes.

3. Reduce the heat to low. Add the balsamic vinegar and cook for another 20 to 30 minutes, stirring occasionally, until the onions have reduced in size. The key is to let them cook long enough that they become caramelized but not so long that they burn.

4. Serve as a side dish or on top of veggies or meat. Store in the refrigerator for up to 5 days. Reheat in the oven.

Nutritional information (per serving)

Calories: 124	Total Carbs: 3g
Fat: 13g	Fiber: 1g
Protein: 1g	Net Carbs: 2g

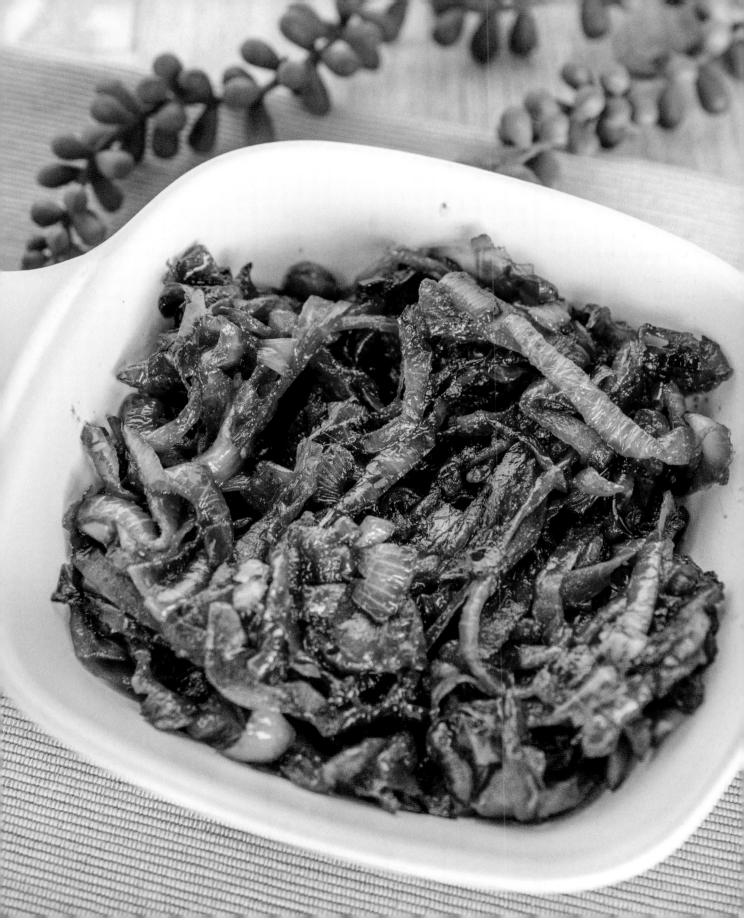

TZATZIKI SAUCE

MAKES 1½ cups (2 tablespoons per serving)   **PREP TIME: 10 minutes**   **COOK TIME: —**

I'm not sure there is a better combination than gyro meat and tzatziki sauce. The cucumber and lemon in this sauce are so fresh-tasting, and the dill adds a wonderful flavor. Add tzatziki to Greek salads, use it as a veggie dip, or serve it with my Greek Chicken (page 180).

INGREDIENTS

1 cucumber

1½ cups plain Greek yogurt

3 cloves garlic, minced

2 tablespoons chopped fresh dill, plus extra for garnish if desired

2 tablespoons extra-virgin olive oil, plus extra for drizzling if desired

1 tablespoon lemon juice

½ teaspoon pink Himalayan salt

¼ teaspoon ground black pepper

DIRECTIONS

1. Use a vegetable peeler to peel the cucumber. Discard the skin.

2. Use a cheese grater to grate the cucumber over a paper towel. When the entire cucumber has been grated, wrap the grated cucumber in the paper towel and squeeze out all the excess liquid.

3. Place the cucumber and the remaining ingredients in a medium-sized mixing bowl. Stir until everything is well incorporated. Drizzle with olive oil and garnish with more fresh dill, if desired.

4. Serve immediately, or store in the refrigerator for up to 1 week.

Nutritional information (per serving)

Calories: 36	Total Carbs: 2g
Fat: 3g	Fiber: 0g
Protein: 2g	Net Carbs: 2g

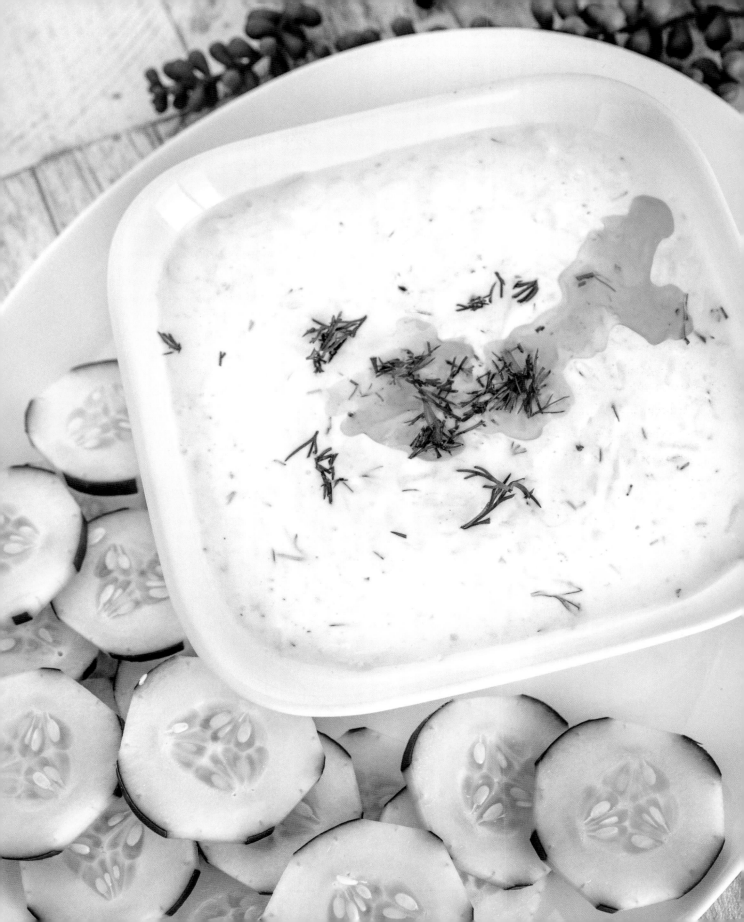

CREAM CHEESE FROSTING

MAKES about 1½ cups (2 tablespoons per serving)   **PREP TIME: 5 minutes**   **COOK TIME: —**

This frosting is an awesome topping for muffins, cookies, mug cakes, and so on. It tastes just like the sugar-filled version! You can jazz it up with any flavored extract you like—orange, coconut, strawberry...you name it.

INGREDIENTS

1 (8-ounce) package cream cheese, softened

¼ to ½ cup powdered sweetener

¼ cup (½ stick) unsalted butter or ghee, softened

1 tablespoon heavy whipping cream

1½ teaspoons vanilla extract

DIRECTIONS

Place all the ingredients in a medium-sized bowl, starting with ¼ cup of sweetener, and thoroughly combine with a hand mixer until smooth. Taste and add up to ¼ cup more sweetener, as desired, and mix again to combine. Store leftovers in the refrigerator for up to 6 days. Stir before using.

Nutritional information (per serving)

Calories: 106   Total Carbs: 1g

Fat: 10g   Fiber: 0g

Protein: 1g   Net Carbs: 1g

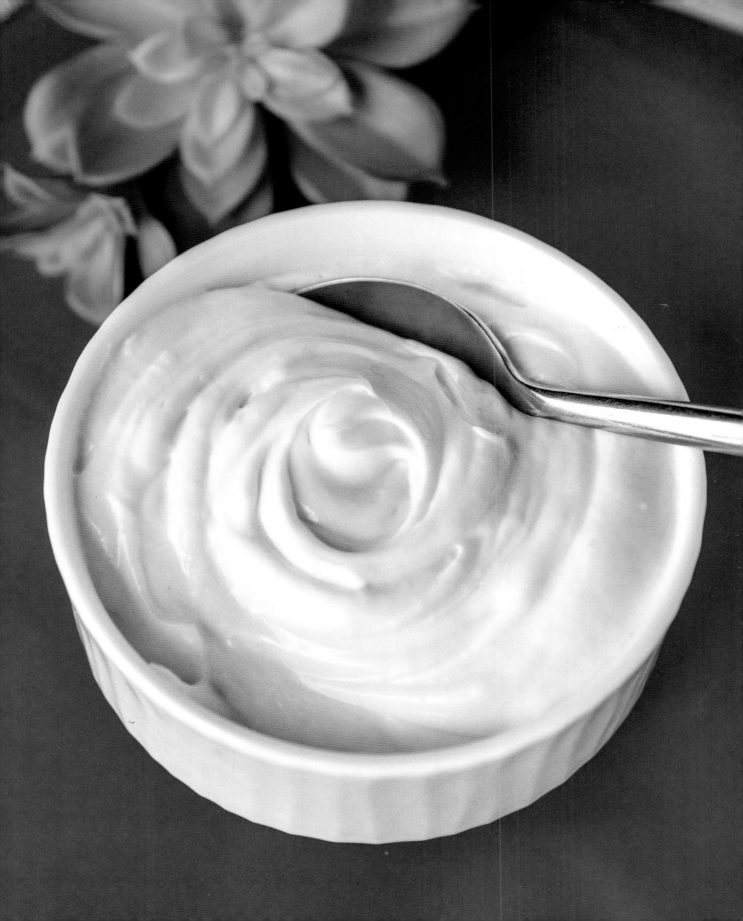

SAVORY BREADCRUMBS

MAKES 2 cups (2 tablespoons per serving)   **PREP TIME: 4 minutes**   **COOK TIME: —**

Not a pork rind fan? That's okay; neither am I. They are just too...porky for me. But this stuff will change your mind. Use these keto breadcrumbs in place of normal breadcrumbs, and you can make anything taste like "the real thing." We love them for my Chicken Nuggets (page 174), fried pickles, and any and all casseroles as a topping. Don't be afraid to play around with this recipe, either. You can use any flavor of pork rinds and any seasonings you like. So versatile!

INGREDIENTS

1 (8-ounce) bag pork rinds

4 ounces Parmesan cheese, grated (about 1 cup)

1 tablespoon garlic powder

Special Equipment:
Food processor

DIRECTIONS

Place all the ingredients in a food processor and pulse until the mixture has the consistency of breadcrumbs. Store in the refrigerator for up to 1 month.

Nutritional information (per serving)

Calories: 53	Total Carbs: 1g
Fat: 3g	Fiber: 0g
Protein: 5g	Net Carbs: 1g

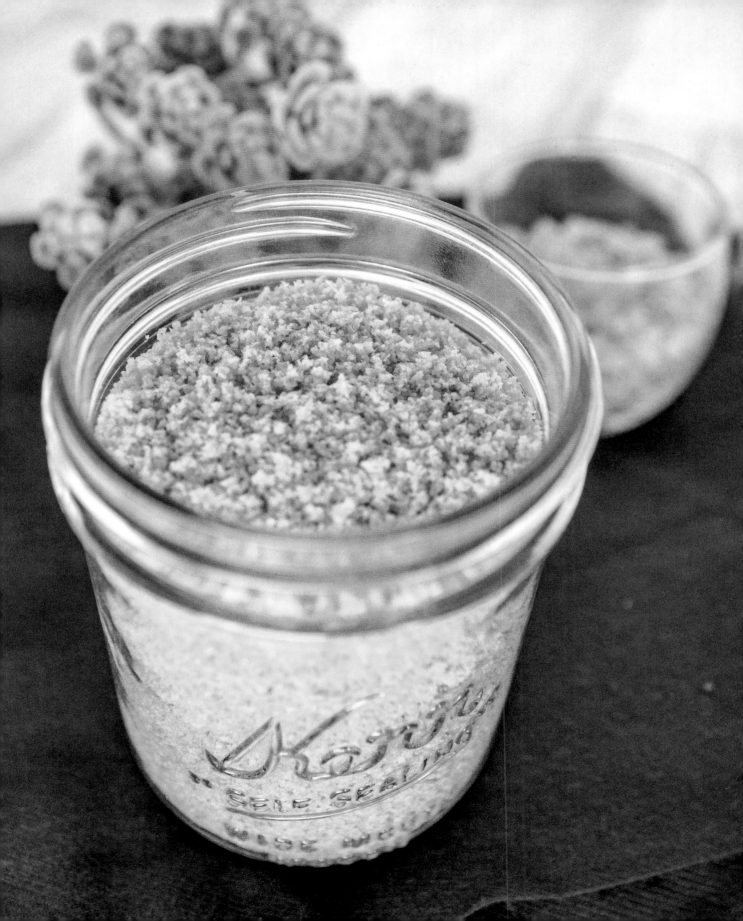

ONION SOUP MIX

MAKES ¼ cup   PREP TIME: 5 minutes   COOK TIME: —

I'm a big fan of making my own spice and seasoning blends. It's the best way to avoid hidden gluten and sugar. This onion soup mix is so tasty and perfect for my French Onion Soup (page 100). One batch is equal to one store-bought onion soup packet.

INGREDIENTS

3 tablespoons dried onion flakes

1 teaspoon garlic powder

1 teaspoon onion powder

1 teaspoon dried parsley

½ teaspoon celery salt

½ teaspoon turmeric powder

½ teaspoon salt

¼ teaspoon ground black pepper

DIRECTIONS

Put all the ingredients in a small bowl or jar with a lid and stir (or shake) to combine. Store in the pantry for up to 6 months.

Nutritional information (per batch)

Calories: 46	Total Carbs: 11g
Fat: 0g	Fiber: 1g
Protein: 1g	Net Carbs: 10g

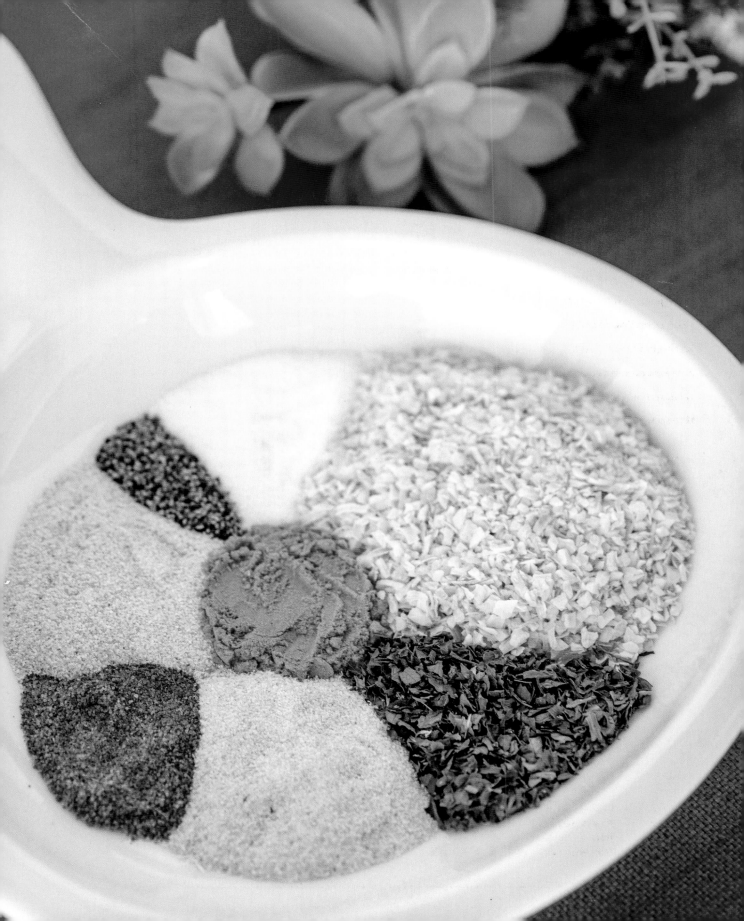

TACO SEASONING

NET CARBS
5g

MAKES 3 tablespoons   **PREP TIME: 5 minutes**   **COOK TIME:** —

Making your own taco seasoning is the best way to ensure that there's nothing sneaky going into your taco meat. Most store-bought taco seasonings contain sugar or gluten, so we prefer to make it at home! One batch of this seasoning mix is perfect for 1 pound of meat.

INGREDIENTS

1 tablespoon chili powder

1 teaspoon ground cumin

1 teaspoon garlic powder

1 teaspoon paprika

½ teaspoon onion powder

½ teaspoon dried oregano leaves

½ teaspoon salt

¼ teaspoon ground black pepper

¼ teaspoon red pepper flakes

DIRECTIONS

Place all the ingredients in a small bowl or jar with a lid and stir (or shake) to combine. Store in the pantry for up to 6 months.

Nutritional information (per batch)

Calories: 55	Total Carbs: 10g
Fat: 2g	Fiber: 5g
Protein: 3g	Net Carbs: 5g

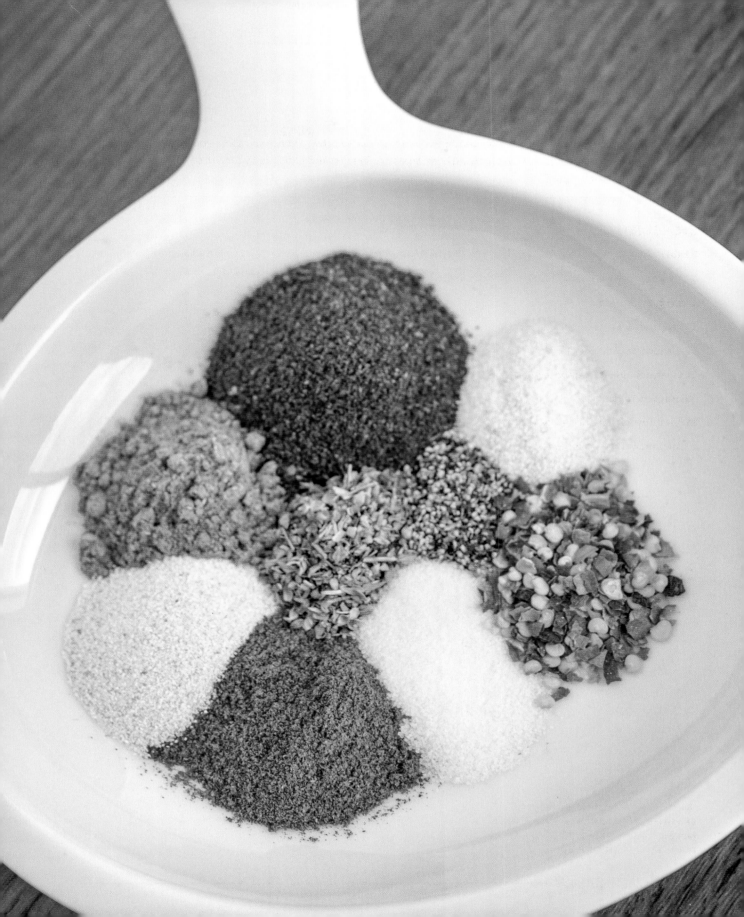

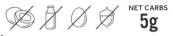

RANCH SEASONING MIX

MAKES ½ cup (2 tablespoons per serving)   **PREP TIME:** 5 minutes   **COOK TIME:** —

Homemade seasoning mixes are seriously so easy to make, and there's a good chance you already have these herbs and spices on hand. Two tablespoons of this mix is equal to one store-bought packet of ranch seasoning. Mix it with ⅓ cup mayonnaise, ¼ cup sour cream, and ¼ cup heavy whipping cream for the perfect gluten-free, sugar-free ranch dressing!

INGREDIENTS

2½ tablespoons dried parsley

1 tablespoon dried onion flakes

2½ teaspoons garlic powder

2½ teaspoons onion powder

1½ teaspoons salt

1 teaspoon dried chives

1 teaspoon ground black pepper

DIRECTIONS

Put all the ingredients in a small bowl or jar with a lid and stir (or shake) to combine. Store in the pantry for up to 6 months.

Nutritional information (per serving)

Calories: 28	Total Carbs: 6g
Fat: 0.1g	Fiber: 1g
Protein: 1g	Net Carbs: 5g

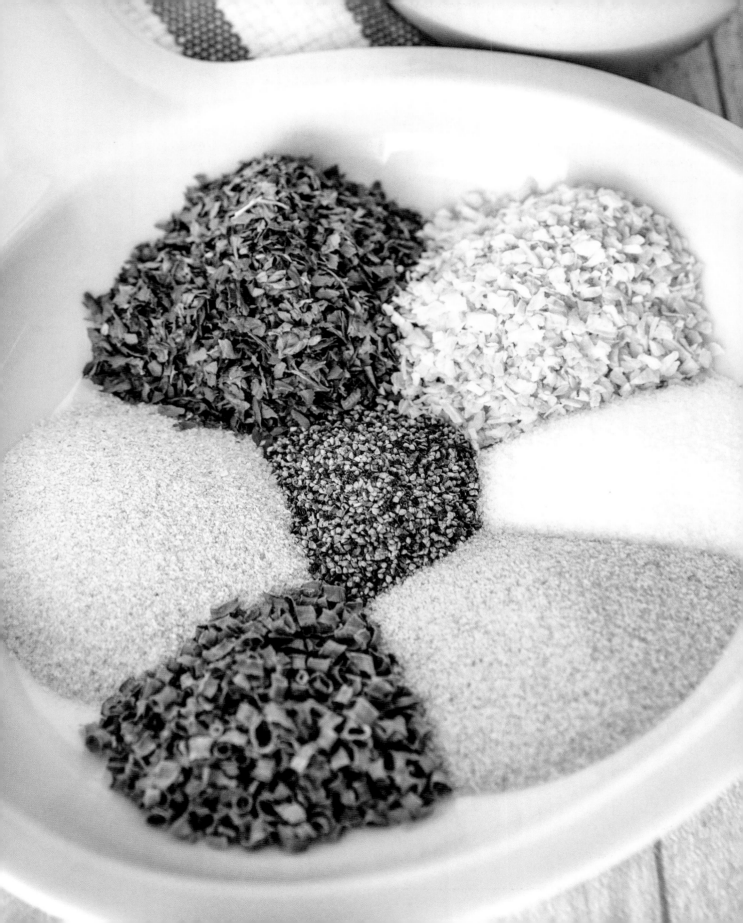

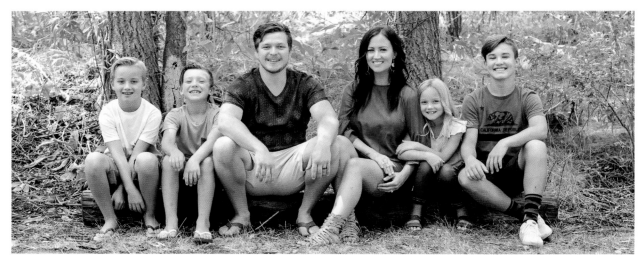

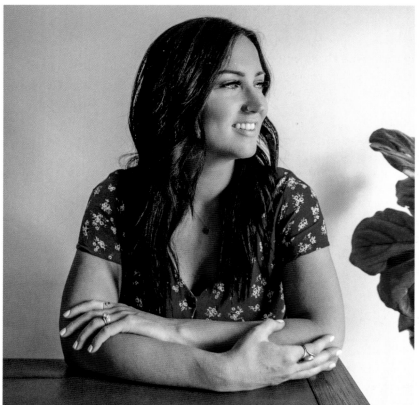

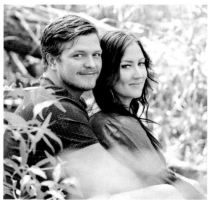

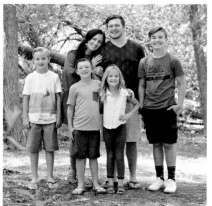

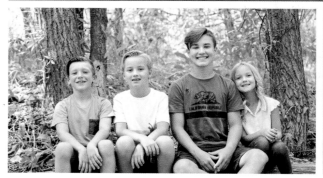

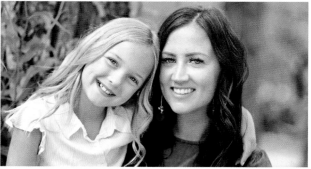

ACKNOWLEDGMENTS

To my husband, Cameron. I could not have written this book without you and your support! Thank you for carrying me through my hard days and always lifting me to higher head spaces. Your electric vibes are my saving grace. Thank you for always pushing me to new levels and seeing things in me that I can't see in myself. You always know what I need, and you are quick to make sure I get it. I could not ask for a better partner. I totally scored in the husband department. You are my life, my heart, my soul. I love you.

To my oldest son, Gavin, my favorite fellow foodie. It is a privilege to be your mom. You have raised me more than I've raised you. Thank you for stepping up as the man of the house during the years that we didn't have one. Your zest for life, good food, and good movies speak to my soul. Plus, you're like, really, really good-looking, so there's that.

To my second son, Roman, my goofball, my quirky weirdo, my carefree little man. You are my happy place. Thank you for your cuddles and constant compliments on the meals I prepare. Deep down I know you're just being nice, but I adore you for always trying to build me up. Your creative brain will take you incredibly far in life. Let it.

To my daughter, Mila. You are beautiful and kind and everything good in this world. Thank you for your morning smiles, your happy spirit, and your beaming soul. You are my best friend and favorite shopping buddy. You will grow up to move mountains, and I cannot wait to see it. The grass is always greener under you. I love you more than pickles and Diet Coke.

To my youngest son, Cylis, my most compassionate, empathetic little man. You are sweet and spicy combined. I always knew I had another son out there, and my family was made whole when you came along. Thank you for our Friday lunch dates, your honest opinions about my cooking, and your genuine excitement for all things keto. You challenge me to be better. I am lucky to have you call me "Mom."

To my mom and dad. Thank you for always being my greatest supporters and for raising me to love myself. I love you.

To my best friend, Kellie Jones. Thank you for always being a listening ear and a voice of reason in my life. I cherish your friendship more than you'll ever know.

To my @ketomadesimple Instagram followers, who have stood by my side since the beginning. You motivate me every day. Thank you.

To the Victory Belt team. Thank you for taking a chance on me. I am still in awe at how you turned my messy recipes into works of art. You have made my dreams a reality, and I will forever be thankful for you all.

ALLERGEN INDEX

RECIPE INDEX

GOOD MORNING

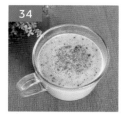
Bulletproof Coffee

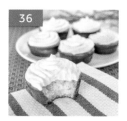
Banana Muffins

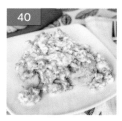
Cylis's Chia Pudding

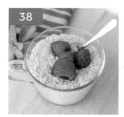
Country Sausage Gravy

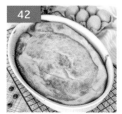
Dutch Baby

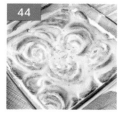
Orange Rolls

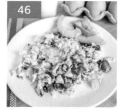
BAE (Bacon and Eggs)

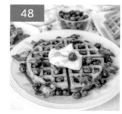
Flourless Waffles

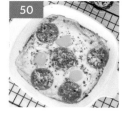
Mila's Pizza Eggs

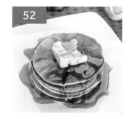
Banana Cream Cheese Pan-Crepes

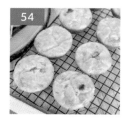
Bacon and Mozzarella Frittata Muffins

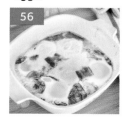
Buttery Baked Eggs

MUNCHIES

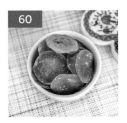
60
Pepperoni Chips

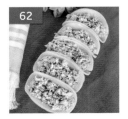
62
Tuna Avocado Tacos

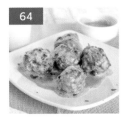
64
Swedish Meatballs

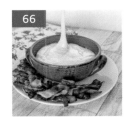
66
Smoked Gouda Fondue

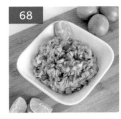
68
Gavin's Guac

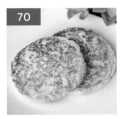
70
Best 90-Second Bread Ever

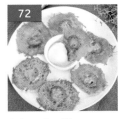
72
Jalapeño Cheese Crisps

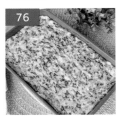
74
Bacon Cheese Dip

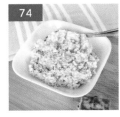
76
Spinach Artichoke Dip

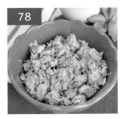
78
Tuna Avocado Salad

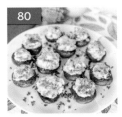
80
Sausage-Stuffed Mushrooms

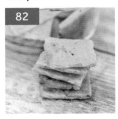
82
Cheese Crackers

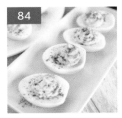
84
The Best Damn Deviled Eggs

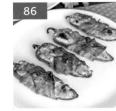
86
BBQ Jalapeño Poppers

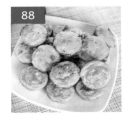
88
Oven-Baked Cheesy Tuna Bites

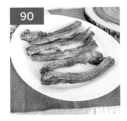
90
Pork Belly Strips

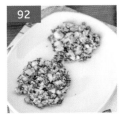
92
Spanakopita Bites

SOUPS & SALADS

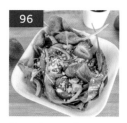
96
Strawberry Spinach Salad

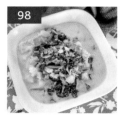
98
Zuppa Toscana

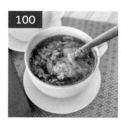
100
French Onion Soup

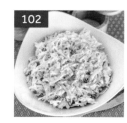
102
Classic Coleslaw

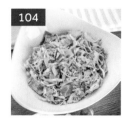
104
Reuben in a Bowl

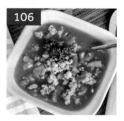
106
Buffalo Wing Chili

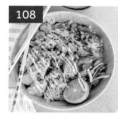
108
Salmon Bowls

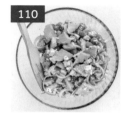
110
Tomato Cucumber Salad

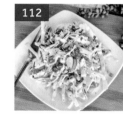
112
Chicken Cabbage Salad

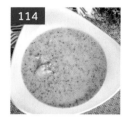
114
Broccoli Cheese Soup

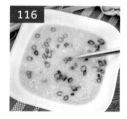
116
Egg Drop Soup

ON THE SIDE

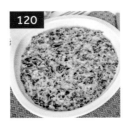
120

Creamed Spinach

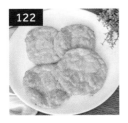
122

Cheddar Cheese Buns

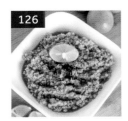
124

Roasted Eggplant

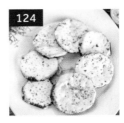
126

Spanish Cauli-Rice

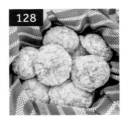
128

Sour Cream and Cheddar Biscuits

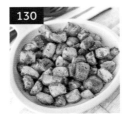
130

Faux-tatoes

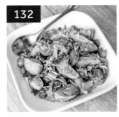
132

Bacon Parmesan Brussels Sprouts

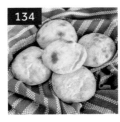
134

Dinner Rolls

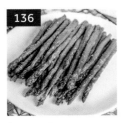
136

Simple Asparagus

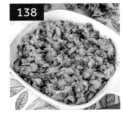
138

Pork Rind Stuffing

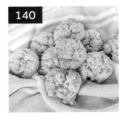
140

Damn Good Biscuits

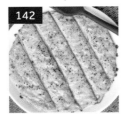
142

Cheesy Garlic Flatbread

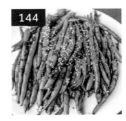
144

Garlicky Green Beans

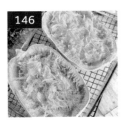
146

Simple Spaghetti Squash

MAIN DISHES

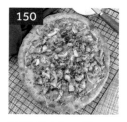

150

BBQ Chicken Pizza

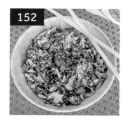

152

Egg Roll in a Bowl

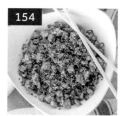

154

Ham Fried Rice

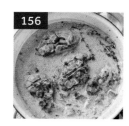

156

One-Pot
Mustard Chicken

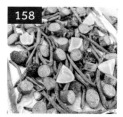

158

Sheet Pan Kielbasa
and Veggies

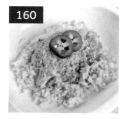

160

Jalapeño Popper
Chicken Bake

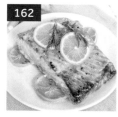

162

Maple-Glazed
Salmon

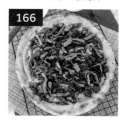

164

Beef Empanadas

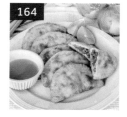

166

Caramelized Onion
Tart

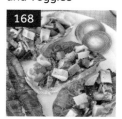

168

BLTA Wraps

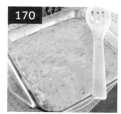

170

Cheesy Taco Bake

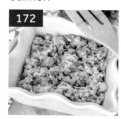

172

Green Chili Sausage
Casserole

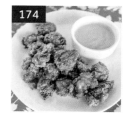

174

Chicken Nuggets

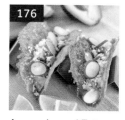

176

Avocado and Feta
Tacos

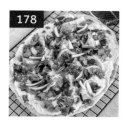

178

Bacon Chicken
Alfredo Pizza

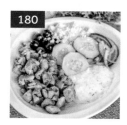

180

Greek Chicken

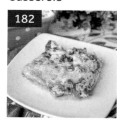

182

Zucchini Lasagna

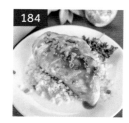

184

Maple-Glazed Dijon
Chicken

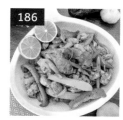

186

One-Pan Chicken
Fajitas

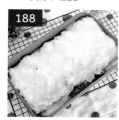

188

Green Chili Chicken
Enchiladas

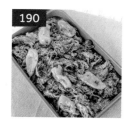

190

Mississippi
Pot Roast

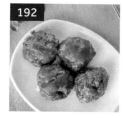

192

Mini Meatloaves

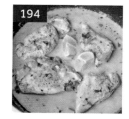

194

One-Pan Coconut
Lime Chicken

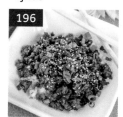

196

Korean BBQ Beef

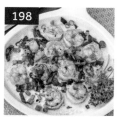

198

Shrimp and Grits

SWEET TOOTH

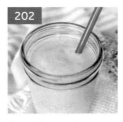
202
Strawberry Coconut Smoothie

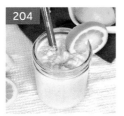
204
Lemon Julius

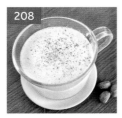
206
Butterbeer

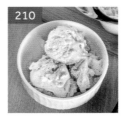
208
Eggnog

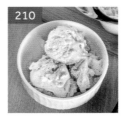
210
Cinnamon Ice Cream

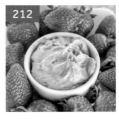
212
Caramel Dip

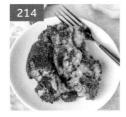
214
Ooey Gooey Monkey Bread

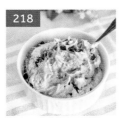
216
Pumpkin Fry Bread

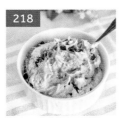
218
Loaded Fat Bomb

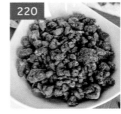
220
Puppy Chow

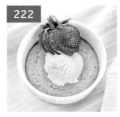
222
Vanilla Shortbread Cake for Two

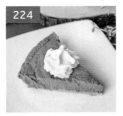
224
Pumpkin Pie

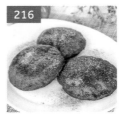
226
Old-Fashioned Chocolate Donuts

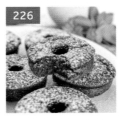
228
Peanut Butter Balls

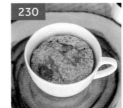
230
Snickerdoodle Mug Cake

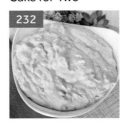
232
Cameron's Pink Stuff

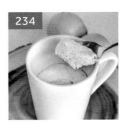
234
Lemon Mug Cake

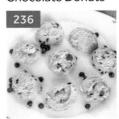
236
Chocolate Chip Peanut Butter Fat Bombs

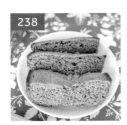
238
Cinnamon Spice Bread

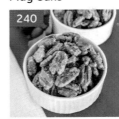
240
Candied Pecans

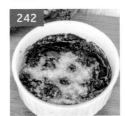
242
Blueberry Cobbler

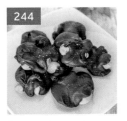
244
Salted Chocolate Macadamia Nut Clusters

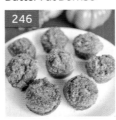
246
Pumpkin Pie Donut Muffins

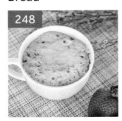
248
Strawberry Banana Mug Cake

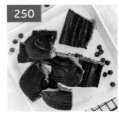
250
Roman's Chocolate-Covered Peanut Butter Bars

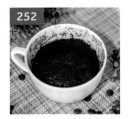
252

Flourless Chocolate
Mug Cake

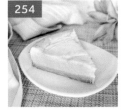
254

Cheesecake

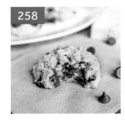
256

Crème Brûlée

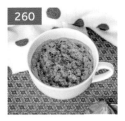
258

Chocolate Chip
Cookies

260

Egg-Free Peanut
Butter Mug Cake

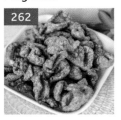
262

Cinnamon Crisps

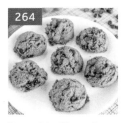
264

Pumpkin Chocolate
Chip Cookies

GET SAUCY

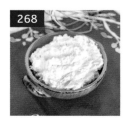
268

Next-Level
Whipped Cream

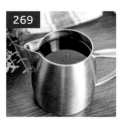
269

Maple Syrup

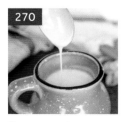
270

Sweetened
Condensed Milk

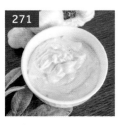
271

Aioli

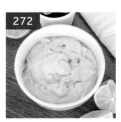
272

Chipotle Mayo

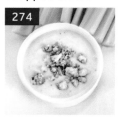
274

Blue Cheese
Dressing

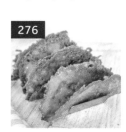
276

Cheese Shells

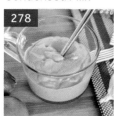
278

Avocado Cilantro
Lime Dressing

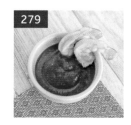
279

Cocktail Sauce

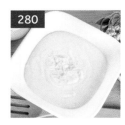
280

Easiest Alfredo
Sauce Ever

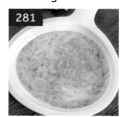
281

Sweet Cream Sauce

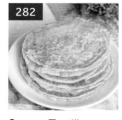
282

Savory Tortillas

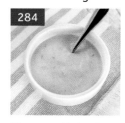
284

Thousand Island
Dressing

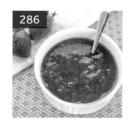
286

Jam on the Fly

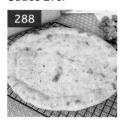
288

Fathead Pizza Crust

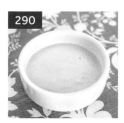
290

Copycat Chick-fil-A
Sauce

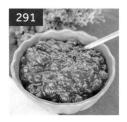
291

Thanksgiving
Cranberry Sauce

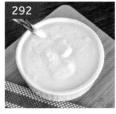
292

Creamy
Horseradish Sauce

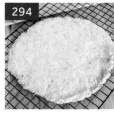
294

Chicken Pizza Crust

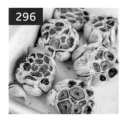
296

Roasted Garlic

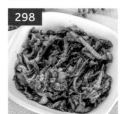
298

Caramelized Onions

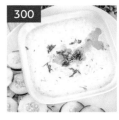
300

Tzatziki Sauce

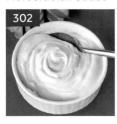
302

Cream Cheese
Frosting

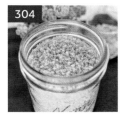
304

Savory
Breadcrumbs

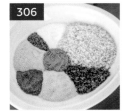
306

Onion Soup Mix

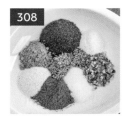
308

Taco Seasoning

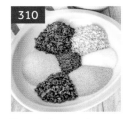
310

Ranch Seasoning
Mix

GENERAL INDEX

vanilla extract *(continued)*
    Sweet Cream Sauce, 281
    Sweetened Condensed Milk, 270
    Vanilla Shortbread Cake for Two,
      222–223
Vanilla Shortbread Cake for Two recipe,
    222–223
vegetables. *See also specific vegetables*
    about, 13
    bulk chopping, 25
vodka, 20

W

waffle iron, 30
way of eating (WOE), 12
weight loss stalls, 26
whipped cream
    Lemon Mug Cake, 234–235
    Pumpkin Pie, 224–225
    Vanilla Shortbread Cake for Two,
      222–223
whipped topping
    Cameron's Pink Stuff, 232–233
whiskey, 20
white wine, 20
wines, 20
WOE (way of eating), 12
Worcestershire sauce
    The Best Damn Deviled Eggs, 84–85
    Cocktail Sauce, 279
    Mini Meatloaves, 192–193
    Swedish Meatballs, 64–65

X

xanthan gum
    Blueberry Cobbler, 242–243
    Broccoli Cheese Soup, 114–115
    Cheddar Cheese Buns, 122–123
    Cheesy Garlic Flatbread, 142–143
    Country Sausage Gravy, 40–41
    Damn Good Biscuits, 140–141
    Egg Drop Soup, 116–117
    Faux-Tatoes, 130–131
    Garlicky Green Beans, 144–145
    Maple Syrup, 269
    One-Pan Coconut Lime Chicken,
      194–195
    Pumpkin Chocolate Chip Cookies,
      264–265
    Smoked Gouda Fondue, 66–67

Z

zinc, 27
Zucchini Lasagna recipe, 182–183
Zuppa Toscana recipe, 98–99